Cephalopod Cognition

Cephalopods are generally regarded as the most intelligent group among the invertebrates. Despite their popularity, relatively little is known about the range and function of their cognitive abilities. This book fills that gap, accentuating the varied and fascinating aspects of cognition across the group.

Starting with the brain, learning and memory, Part I looks at early learning, memory acquisition and cognitive development in modern cephalopods. An analysis of the Chambered *Nautilus*, a living fossil, is included, providing insight into the evolution of behavioural complexity. Part II surveys environmental responses, especially within the active and learning-dependent coleoids. The ever-intriguing camouflage abilities of octopuses and cuttlefish are highlighted, alongside bioluminescence, navigation and other aspects of visual and cognitive competence.

Covering the range of cognitive function, this text underscores the importance of the cephalopods within the field of comparative cognition generally. It will be highly valuable for researchers, graduates and senior undergraduate students.

Anne-Sophie Darmaillacq is a researcher in the Group Memory and Behavioural Plasticity Unit at Caen University in France. She studies embryonic cognition and early learning systems in the cuttlefish *Sepia officinalis* and lectures in ethology at graduate and undergraduate levels.

Ludovic Dickel is Professor of Behavioural Biology at Caen University, managing the Group Memory and Behavioural Plasticity Unit. His research interests are focused on brain development and cognition in cuttlefish as well as collaborative work on embryonic neuroethology in oviparous species.

Jennifer Mather is Professor in the Department of Psychology at the University of Lethbridge in Alberta, Canada. She is active in researching many aspects of cephalopod cognition and behaviour, especially in octopuses, including ground-breaking work in personality, play and consciousness.

Cephalopod Cognition

Edited by

ANNE-SOPHIE DARMAILLACQ

University of Caen Basse-Normandie, France

LUDOVIC DICKEL

University of Caen Basse-Normandie, France

JENNIFER MATHER

University of Lethbridge, Alberta, Canada

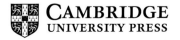

CAMBRIDGE
UNIVERSITY PRESS

University Printing House, Cambridge CB2 8BS, United Kingdom

One Liberty Plaza, 20th Floor, New York, NY 10006, USA

477 Williamstown Road, Port Melbourne, VIC 3207, Australia

314-321, 3rd Floor, Plot 3, Splendor Forum, Jasola District Centre, New Delhi - 110025, India

79 Anson Road, #06-04/06, Singapore 079906

Cambridge University Press is part of the University of Cambridge.

It furthers the University's mission by disseminating knowledge in the pursuit of
education, learning and research at the highest international levels of excellence.

www.cambridge.org
Information on this title: www.cambridge.org/9781108464697

First published 2014
First paperback edition 2018

A catalogue record for this publication is available from the British Library

Library of Congress Cataloging in Publication data
Cephalopod cognition / edited by Anne-Sophie Darmaillacq, University of Caen
Basse-Normandie, France, Ludovic Dickel, University of Caen Basse-Normandie,
France, Jennifer Mather, University of Lethbridge, Alberta, Canada.
  pages   cm
Includes bibliographical references and index.
ISBN 978-1-107-01556-2 (hardback)
1. Cephalopoda – Behavior.   2. Invertebrates – Behavior.   3. Cognition in animals.
I. Darmaillacq, Anne-Sophie, 1977–   II. Dickel, Ludovic.   III. Mather, Jennifer A.
QL785.C34   2014
594′.5 – dc23   2014009749

ISBN 978-1-107-01556-2 Hardback
ISBN 978-1-108-46469-7 Paperback

To the next generation

ASD and LD: To Nitzan and Pia

JM: To Charlotte and Nicky

Contents

Contributors

Roland C. Anderson
Former Biologist, Seattle Aquarium, Seattle, WA, USA

Jennifer A. Basil
Associate Professor, LIBE Laboratory, Department of Biology, Brooklyn College, CUNY, Brooklyn, New York, NY, USA

Cécile Bellanger
Assistant Professor, Groupe Mémoire et Plasticité comportementale, EA4259, Université de Caen Basse-Normandie, Caen, France

Jean G. Boal
Professor, Department of Biology, Millersville University, Millersville, PA, USA

Gordon M. Burghardt
Professor, Departments of Psychology and Ecology and Evolutionary Biology, University of Tennessee, Knoxville, TN, USA

Robyn Crook
Research Fellow, Department of Integrative Biology and Pharmacology, University of Texas Health Science Center, Houston, TX, USA

Anne-Sophie Darmaillacq
Assistant Professor, Groupe Mémoire et Plasticité comportementale, EA4259, Université de Caen Basse-Normandie, Caen, France

Ludovic Dickel
Professor, Groupe Mémoire et Plasticité comportementale, EA4259, Université de Caen Basse-Normandie, Caen, France

Frank W. Grasso
Associate Professor, Biomimetic and Cognitive Robotics Laboratory, Department of Psychology, Brooklyn College, CUNY, Brooklyn, New York, NY, USA

Tamar Gutnick
Doctoral Fellow, Department of Neurobiology, Institute of Life Science, Hebrew University, Jerusalem, Israel

Binyamin Hochner
Professor, Department of Neurobiology, Silberman Institute of Life Sciences and the Interdisciplinary Center for Neural Computation, Hebrew University, Jerusalem, Israel

Sönke Johnsen
Professor, Biology Department, Duke University, Durham, NC, USA

Noam Josef
Doctoral Fellow, Department of Life Sciences, Ben-Gurion University of the Negev, Eilat Campus, Eilat, Israel

Christelle Jozet-Alves
Assistant Professor, Groupe Mémoire et Plasticité comportementale, EA4259, Université de Caen Basse-Normandie, Caen, France

Michael J. Kuba
Research Fellow, Department of Neurobiology, Institute of Life Science, Hebrew University, Jerusalem, Israel

Tatiana S. Leite
Professor, Departamento de Oceanografia e Limnologia, Federale Universite do Rio Grande do Norte, Via Costeira s/n Mae Luiza, Natal, Brazil

Jennifer A. Mather
Professor, Department of Psychology, University of Lethbridge, Lethbridge, AB, Canada

Ronald O'Dor
Professor of Biology, Dalhousie University, Halifax, NS, Canada

Daniel Osorio
Professor, School of Life Sciences, University of Sussex, Sussex, UK

Nadav Shashar
Professor, Department of Life Sciences, Ben-Gurion University of the Negev, Eilat Campus, Eilat, Israel

Tal Shomrat
Postdoctoral Fellow, Department of Neurobiology, Silberman Institute of Life Sciences, Hebrew University, Jerusalem, Israel

James B. Wood
Mounts Botanical Garden, West Palm Beach, FL, USA

Sarah Zylinski
Lecturer, School of Biology, University of Leeds, Leeds, UK

Preface

In July of 2012, at the Francis Crick Memorial Conference on Consciousness in Human and Non-Human Animals, a group of researchers signed The Cambridge Declaration on Consciousness. What was important about this declaration was that it firmly stated that consciousness can emerge in animals that evolved along different evolutionary tracks, including cephalopod mollusks. This recognized what researchers in cephalopod behaviour, starting with the ground-breaking work of J. Z. Young and Martin Wells over 50 years ago, have been maintaining, that these animals are 'learning specialists' and capable of 'complex cognition'. The chapters of this book will help define and discuss this cephalopod cognition, giving insight not just into how their brain and behaviour work, but also a comparative view that can be contrasted to research in 'traditional' vertebrates.

Cognition has been difficult to define and has been described more or less broadly over the years (Shettleworth, 2010). In general terms, Neisser (1967) defined it as 'all the processes by which the sensory input is transformed, reduced, elaborated, stored, recovered and used' (and see chapter 6, this volume, by Mather et al.). Deukas (1998) defined it similarly as 'the neuronal processes concerned with the acquisition and manipulation of information by animals'. Richardson's (2010) definition that cognitive systems 'disambiguate confusing, incomplete and rapidly changing data, while generating equally unique, yet adaptive responses' reminds us that this information processing is not static and works across time. Shettleworth (2010) starts with a definition that is similar to these, but points out that many believe it to be too broad. She notes that cognition might need to be declarative (knowing that) rather than procedural (knowing how). Similarly, cognition might need to act on mental representations. First-order operation (operating directly on perceptual input) would not be cognitive, whereas second-order ones (acting on first order ones) would be. She reminds her readers that without experimental analysis, it is impossible to tell what kinds of processes are reflected in a behaviour, a point nicely analyzed by Webb (2012) for insects. She also notes that different kinds of animals might accomplish functionally similar behaviour in different ways, an important point for the comparison of cephalopod cognition with that or animals from other phyla (see the chapter 7, this volume, by Jozet-Alves et al.). All of these ideas are incorporated in different ways in the chapters of this book.

Although comparative cognition was probably not even defined when Martin J. Wells was doing research in the 1950s and 1960s, his work definitely fits into that category and was also the basis for much of the work we are doing on cephalopod cognition now.

His initial orientation was physiology, but Wells moved the study of octopus learning from visual to tactile, and located a second area in the brain concerned with learning. He conducted many of the lesion studies that laid the groundwork for our understanding of the brain's control of behaviour (see chapter 4, this volume, by Hochner & Shomrat). But his investigation of the function of the optic gland was a pioneering step in the understanding of invertebrate neuroendocrinology. He was always interested in cardiovascular physiology and his work was the foundation for later study in this area, particularly by Ronald O'Dor. Later in his career he became intrigued with the lifestyle and adaptation of nautiloids, and while he may have underestimated their ability (see chapter 2, this volume, by Basil & Crook), he laid the foundation for further research in this area too. And we still find his book, written in 1978, a useful source of information (Wells, 1978).

Part I: cognition, brain and evolution

Cephalopods are often described as amazing brainy creatures; this is probably why they are the first invertebrates considered as 'sensitive' beings and, hence, the use of them is now regulated by a European directive. This is fully explored in the first part of this book. Given the absence of parental care to the eggs and juveniles, Darmaillacq et al. (chapter 1) highlight how the cuttlefish is a suitable model to address developmental questions. They review the remarkable memory and other cognitive skills from embryonic stages. From a comparative point of view, Basil and Crook (chapter 2) illustrate learning in the ancient cephalopod *Nautilus pompilius*. This chapter addresses how *Nautilus* can be used for a better understanding of evolution of cognition and neural complexity in its more derived relatives, the coleoid cephalopods (octopuses, cuttlefish and squid). In contrast, Kuba et al. (chapter 3) underline the interest in the 'sophisticated' octopus as a model to study object play, a high-order behavioural emergence in the animal kingdom. Hochner and Shomrat (chapter 4) underline the spectacular functional and structural similarities of memory systems between octopus and mammals, despite very different brain organization. Lastly, chapter 5 by Grasso gives an authoritative account of current understanding of the octopus nervous system and a clearly personal view of the functional architecture. The hierarchical system proposed in this chapter could be applied in robotics and cybernetics, and the ideas are challenging and may be controversial.

Part II: cognition and the environment

Of course cognitive abilities evolved through and are used in the natural environment. But it is not always easy to study them or even to theorize how they are used in the marine environment. Given that cephalopods are mostly not social animals, their cognitive ability is not, as it is in the 'higher' vertebrates, used to solve social problems and understand the actions of conspecifics. Instead, Mather et al. (chapter 6) argue that foraging in the face of predator pressure is the foundation for the development of intelligence and perhaps consciousness, particularly of octopuses. All cephalopods are mobile, and Jozet-Alves et al. (chapter 7) point out the sensory processing and cognitive competence involved in both long-distance and local movement, including laboratory investigation of the latter activities. And one of the most fascinating aspects of the cephalopods' lives is their skin display system. Josef and Shashar (chapter 8) discuss the basic aspects of benthic cephalopods' camouflage and Zylinski and Osorio (chapter 9) review the recent in-depth research on how cuttlefish use visual information about the background to produce the precise matching that they perform so well. Finally, Zylinski and Johnsen (chapter 10) challenge us to look more widely at the many species across the class. They point out that the deep-sea cephalopods, though little known, have abilities in visual cognition and body pattern production quite different from the well-known near-shore species. This range of adaptations leaves us much more to investigate about cephalopod cognition as it is adapted to a wide variety of habitats.

References

Deukas, R. (ed.) (1998). *Cognitive Ecology*. Chicago, IL: University of Chicago Press.

Neisser, U. (1967). *Cognitive Psychology*. New York, NY: Appleton-Century-Crofts.

Richardson, K. (2010). *The Evolution of Intelligent Systems*. London: Palgrave Macmillan.

Shettleworth, S. J. (ed.) (2010). *Cognition, Evolution and Behaviour*. New York, NY: Oxford University Press.

Webb, B. (2012). Cognition in insects. *Philosophical Transactions of the Royal Society of London B*, **367**: 2715–2722.

Wells, M. J. (1978). *Octopus – Physiology and Behaviour*. Chichester, Sussex: John Wiley and Sons, Inc.

Acknowledgements

This book emerges from the symposia about cognition in cephalopods co-organized by A.-S. Darmaillacq, L. Dickel (University of Caen, France), N. Shashar (University of Ben Gurion, Israel) and Y. Ikeda (University of Ryukyus, Japan) at the 31st International Ethological Conference held in Rennes (France) in 2009, entitled 'Studying cephalopods' brain and behaviours: when molluscs allow a better understanding of the mechanisms and evolution of cognition: Part I and Part II'. We are very grateful to the scientific committee of the International Ethological Conference for having accepted these symposia. The editors would like to thank all of the contributors for their hard work and enthusiasm while producing this volume. They also thank all the reviewers whose comments have made valuable contributions to each of the chapters. We would like to thank Martin Griffith of Cambridge University Press for his support, enthusiasm and encouragements, and Megan Waddington for her patience. It is encouraging to see a range of contributors from both young researchers to more established experts in cephalopod cognition.

Financial support for the research of A.-S. Darmaillacq and L. Dickel on cognition in cuttlefish was supported by the French ministry of research, the regional council of Basse-Normandie and the University of Caen Basse-Normandie. We thank the Société Française pour l'Etude du Comportement Animal for promoting behavioural research.

Tribute to Martin J. Wells

Martin Wells, who died aged 80 in 2009, was not only a distinguished biologist with a passion for invertebrates, but also a colourful and stimulating personality who enthused generations of students with the sheer excitement and beauty of studying animals, especially cephalopods – squids and octopuses. He began his research into cephalopod learning when he and his wife, Joyce, abandoned their PhD programs at Cambridge to move to the Stazione Zoologica in Naples, Italy, as the Director in 1953. Acting on a suggestion from J. Z. Young, who had discovered a way of training octopuses to make visual discriminations, they began studying tactile learning in octopus. They soon showed that these animals could discriminate between objects on the basis of touch, using the suckers on their arms, and that octopus suckers contain chemoreceptors so they can learn to 'taste' what they touch. This 'tasting by touching' is extremely sensitive, enabling octopuses to distinguish between snails and stones as their arms explore their surroundings at night or in murky waters.

Collaborations with J. Z. Young continued into the 1970s, building up a map of octopus brain function based on surgically 'removing bits', seeing what functions changed and then documenting exactly what was removed microscopically. This eventually resulted in octopus brains becoming the best-known non-vertebrate biological data processor ever studied. Ultimately, cephalopods' brains were so different that they were referred to as 'the only alien intelligence that humans have encountered'. A bit later Martin tried to work backward towards the origins of this intelligence by studying ancient *Nautilus* brains, but they turned out to be not very smart, so he began referring to them as 'racing snails'.

Martin also discovered that in the cephalopod brain there is an analogue of the vertebrate pituitary gland: the optic gland, closely associated with sexual maturation. Martin and Joyce's 1959 paper in the *Journal of Experimental Biology* on this topic became a classic in the literature of invertebrate endocrinology. Martin's interest in the 1970s turned to various aspects of cephalopod cardiovascular and respiratory physiology. Collaborating with colleagues from around the world, he published a series of challenging papers attempting to relate physiology to the life of the whole animal in its environment. His more recent studies on nautiluses yielded fascinating data about the physiology of an animal that regularly moves from the surface to depths of more than 700 m, and also taught us much about the reasons for the eventual failure, from an evolutionary perspective, of the shelled cephalopods (the ammonites and belemnites) that once dominated the ancient seas.

On the basis of his work in Naples, Martin was elected to a prize fellowship at Trinity College, Cambridge, in 1956, and in 1959 he was appointed a university demonstrator in the Cambridge zoology department. He soon became one of five founder fellows of Churchill College, and a tutor and director of studies in biology. In 1966 Martin was awarded a Cambridge ScD and the silver medal of the Zoological Society of London in 1968. He was made a university reader in 1976. With Joyce, he travelled extensively in search of cephalopods, and colleagues with whom to study them. Among many destinations that he visited (often as a visiting professor) were Duke University in North Carolina, Hawaii, Ghana, Dalhousie in Canada, Papua New Guinea, Australia, Texas and Uganda.

Martin approached marine biology as a 'way of life'. He used his position in Cambridge to create a global cadre of marine biologists of the cephalopod persuasion. Post-doctoral fellows and graduate students from around the world were welcomed to his laboratory, his college, his house, his marine stations and his boats. They were expected to make wine and, occasionally, garden in the Bury, his home. Perhaps only half of the world's cephalopod biologists enjoyed Martin and Joyce's hospitality over the years, but this community will never forget their influence. Several generations now hark back to it. Martin's approach was not just a scientific but also an intellectual exercise that expanded the minds of those lucky enough to be involved. He was a writer of popular science books, essays and rigorous papers, a novelist, painter and a yachtsman, talents he came by honestly as the grandson of H. G. Wells. Living with the entire Wells family shaped minds.

Martin's philosophy was always, 'Why tackle easy questions when the hard ones are so much more interesting?' I think the hardest question he ever asked was, 'Why do cephalopods need to be so smart when they die so young?' The phrase 'live fast, die young' has become a popular descriptor of the cephalopod lifestyle, but perhaps the phrase should be expanded to 'live fast and smart, to leave your offspring fewer enemies'. Martin died on the first day of Darwin's bicentenary, so a Darwinian answer seems appropriate.

Ronald O'Dor

Part I

Cognition, brain and evolution

1 Cuttlefish preschool or how to learn in the peri-hatching period

Anne-Sophie Darmaillacq, Christelle Jozet-Alves, Cécile Bellanger and Ludovic Dickel

1.1   Introduction

One of the greatest challenges faced by many precocial young after hatching is that of finding food without being eaten. This challenge is particularly important in species where offspring receive no parental care. In these species, newly hatched young have at least two possible options in response to the problem of prey and predators: 'come prepared' (e.g. unlearned behaviour), which is safe but rigid, or 'learn as you go' (e.g. trial-and-error learning), which is risky if they do not learn quickly enough, but more flexible for adapting to a changing environment.

For a better understanding of how a newborn animal deals with environmental challenges, we need to study what is perceived and learned before hatching. Our understanding of prenatal cognitive activity is comparatively recent, compared for example with philosophical trends of the seventeenth century. A cognitive system can be defined as one which is able to perceive and extract information from its environment, and then use that information for the purpose of making appropriate decisions and developing suitable behaviour (Shettleworth, 2010; Vauclair, 1996). There is no longer any doubt about the embryo as a cognitive system, since it is now well established that fetal sensory experience has a crucial role in behavioural and cognitive development (Krasnegor, Blass, Hofer & Smotherman, 1987).

Although there are 700 cephalopod species, the common cuttlefish *Sepia officinalis* has been the focal subject of intensive developmental studies in neuroethology. Cuttlefish, like many other cephalopod species, start life under strong selective pressure from their environment; neither eggs nor juveniles benefit from parental care (Boletzky, 1987), and so young individuals must find their own means of feeding themselves and avoiding predators. Female *S. officinalis* lay hundreds of eggs in shallow water on various rigid supports: algae stems, tubeworms, ropes, nets, etc. (Boletzky, 1983). Eggs laid in clusters, popularly known as '*les raisins de mer*' (sea grapes), are abandoned after the death of the mother. The egg capsule consists of a chorion and spirally coiled black envelopes, which protect the embryos against microbial attack and predation (Boletzky, 2003). Throughout embryonic development, the capsule is enlarged as osmotic pressure increases due to water entering the perivitelline space, becoming more translucent shortly before the embryos hatch. Once the animals have hatched, egg envelopes decay after some weeks of degradation (Billings, Sullivan & Vine, 2000). Unlike many other cephalopods, there is no larval or paralarval stage in cuttlefish development; the hatchlings are very similar to adults in their general form, which facilitates comparative development studies. They possess the same benthic life style as adults; they can also swim in the water column, achieve elaborate forms of crypsis by colour pattern and posture changes, and use the same prey-catching strategies as adults, by striking out with their tentacles or by jumping on prey. They seem to possess a behavioural repertoire comparable with that of adults, although some adjustments in both predatory and defensive behaviour occur during development (for review, see Dickel et al., 2006). The brain of early juveniles has the same structure as that of adults, and all the brain lobes are present from hatching. Neurogenesis is intense during development (e.g. in octopus, the adult brain possesses a thousand times more neurones than that of the hatchling) and some brain structures develop faster than others during post-embryonic maturation (for a review, see Nixon & Young, 2003). From an experimental point of view, these characteristics make the cuttlefish a unique animal model in developmental neuroethology; firstly, because the absence of parental care allows a precise control of the experiential history of embryo and juvenile; and, secondly, because the absence of a paralarval stage in young cuttlefish allows longitudinal and comparative studies of brain and behaviour from hatching to adulthood.

This chapter is a review of the most recent studies addressing the influence of early experience in *S. officinalis*, from embryonic stages, to post-hatching behaviour and cognition. It will first describe the development of the sensory systems and the central nervous system in the embryo. It will then focus on the factors affecting the development of prey preference and the efficiency of primary defences in newly hatched cuttlefish and juveniles. It will also address the ontogeny of lateralization in cuttlefish, which may afford juveniles greater behavioural efficiency by enabling them to look out for escape routes while hunting. Finally, we will try to describe the scenario of the beginning of the life of a cuttlefish.

1.2   Development of the sensory systems

The study of cognition is concerned with how animals process information, beginning with how information is acquired by the senses (Shettleworth, 2010). As all of an animal's experience is founded on its ability to sense changes in its environment, measurement of the embryo's sensory capabilities allows us to define the limits of its potential for modifying its behaviour through experience (Smotherman & Robinson, 1992). The onset of sensory system function follows an invariant sequence in birds and mammals – i.e. tactile, vestibular, chemical, auditory and visual (Gottlieb, 1971; Lickliter, 1993). This process remains to be investigated in invertebrates. The sense organs of adult cuttlefish have been well described (Hanlon & Messenger, 1996), but we do not know at what point they begin to function during embryonic development. The stages of embryonic development in the cuttlefish have been precisely described by Lemaire (1970), from

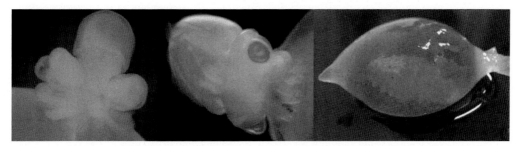

Figure 1.1 *Sepia officinalis* embryonic stages according to Lemaire (1970) from left to right: (A) stage 23, (B) stage 25 and (C) stage 30 (copyright L. Bonnaud and A.-S. Darmaillacq). See plate section for colour version.

segmentation to organogenesis. Organogenesis ranges from stage 18 to stage 30 (i.e. hatching). From stage 23 (about 4 weeks before hatching, incubation temperature 18°C, embryo size about 1 mm; Figure 1.1, left), rhythmic mantle contractions are visible through the outer covering of the egg (Romagny, Darmaillacq, Guibé, Bellanger & Dickel, 2012); stage 25 (about 3 weeks before hatching, incubation temperature 18°C, embryo size about 2 mm; Figure 1.1, middle) is easily identifiable by the reddish colouration of the retina and stage 30 (a few days before hatching, incubation temperature 18°C, embryo size from 7 to 9 mm; Figure 1.1, right), corresponds to the hatching stage where embryos resemble juveniles (Lemaire, 1970).

Variations in the frequency of mantle contractions in adult cuttlefish have been demonstrated to be a good indicator of stimulus detection (odour: Boal & Golden, 1999; visual stimuli: King & Adamo, 2006). Romagny, Darmaillacq, Guibé, Bellanger & Dickel (2012) used this behavioural characteristic to investigate whether tactile, chemical and visual sensory systems are functional in cuttlefish embryos. From stage 23, these authors observed an increase of the rate of mantle contractions immediately after a gentle prick on the ventral mantle of the embryo with a blunt needle through the membrane of the egg. At the same developmental stage, a predator odour introduced to the immediate environment of the egg induces the same behavioural response. Response to visual stimuli (sudden light) did not occur earlier than stage 25. This study shows for the first time that in cuttlefish sensory systems do not all become functional at the same stage of embryonic development. As in vertebrates (Lickliter, 1993), visual system maturation in the cuttlefish embryo occurs later than that of the tactile and chemical systems. This similarity between cuttlefish and vertebrates could merely be a coincidence but it could also suggest a unique evolutionary origin or, more likely, a similar convergent evolution. The latter hypothesis is reinforced by the other known evolutionary convergences between the sensory systems of cephalopods and vertebrates (e.g. eyes, statocysts, lateral line; Budelmann, 1994; Nixon & Young, 2003; Packard, 1972). Similar environmental pressures could have led to the same developmentally conserved sequence in vertebrates and in invertebrates. Further investigation on behavioural embryology in invertebrates could provide important insights into whether this phenomenon is conserved throughout different taxa.

One expression of structural and functional developments in the sensory systems of embryos is the ability to learn. Three types of learning have been documented, mainly in vertebrates, as originating from prenatal sensory stimulation by chemosensory and auditory stimuli: these are habituation, associative learning and exposure learning. Associative and exposure learning can only be assessed after hatching even if the process of acquisition occurs before hatching (see section 1.3.5) whereas habituation can be directly tested with embryos. Habituation, understood to be a simple form of learning, is defined as a decreasing response to an often-repeated stimulus. This has been demonstrated in mammal fetuses (Granier-Deferre & Busnel, 1983; van Heteren, Boekkooi, Jongsma & Nijhuis, 2001; Schaal, 1988; Smotherman & Robinson, 1992). In *S. officinalis* embryos, habituation to a light stimulus presented every 30 minutes occurs at stage 30 but not at stage 25 (Romagny, Darmaillacq, Guibé, Bellanger & Dickel, 2012). This learning is disrupted with a dishabituatory stimulus (a prick). Habituation is a central process which allows the subject to filter irrelevant information and focus on biologically meaningful stimuli. Before the egg capsule dilates and becomes transparent, the embryo develops in a visually buffered dark environment, in which light is attenuated by the capsule before reaching the developing embryo. This may explain why the visual habituation processes are not mature at stage 25. In the experiments described above, the outer dark layer of the eggs was removed. It, therefore, seems likely that habituation to tactile or chemical stimuli can occur before stage 30. There is a rich and varied array of stimuli in the prenatal environment and so it seems likely that the embryos would make 'sense' of these opportunities for learning about their future world. Firstly, a decrease of the response to repeated non-relevant stimuli may serve the embryo to avoid loss of energy. Secondly, its capabilities to memorize visual information from the environment perceived in the egg may potentially optimize behavioural adaptation of hatchlings to environmental pressure met at the hatching sites (available shelters, predators and prey).

1.3   Early learning about prey

1.3.1   Prey preference and early experience

Cuttlefish are active predators, feeding on different types of prey including fish and crustaceans (Guerra, 2006). They search for prey and find it mainly by visual means (Messenger, 1968), although one cannot exclude the possibility that other sensory means may be involved, and prey movement is of real significance. The question is: how do newly hatched cuttlefish recognize safe prey in the absence of parental assistance and/or observational learning? Wells (1962) presented newly hatched cuttlefish having no prior post-embryonic experience of food with a series of models, either rotating or moving up and down, to newly hatched cuttlefish without prior post-embryonic experience with food. He showed that they preferred elongate shapes moving along their longer axis (mysid-like prey) to rounded shapes (crab-like prey) that they almost never attacked.

Unfortunately Wells (1962) did not actually record the environmental conditions in which the eggs developed, conditions that might have influenced prey choice. When naïve 1-day-old cuttlefish are given a choice between shrimp, crabs and fish, again they prefer shrimp to the other two types of prey (Darmaillacq, Chichery, Poirier & Dickel, 2004). This finding not only confirms that cuttlefish have an innate preference for shrimp-like prey. It also suggests that prey recognition is based on identification processes of a higher order than the simple selection of elongate prey moving along their long axis, since hatchling cuttlefish prefer shrimp to fish which nevertheless share the same basic characteristics. This preference for shrimp continues throughout the first month of life but then seems to extend to other prey types even when cuttlefish are only fed shrimp. It is known that early experience exerts a particularly potent influence on subsequent food selection. For example, turtles retain a preference for the first food they experience in their life (Burghardt, 1967; Burghardt & Hess, 1966). This phenomenon, known as the primacy effect, has also been shown in other precocial species such as the lynx spider (reviewed in Stasiak, 2002 and see also Punzo, 2002). In cuttlefish, Darmaillacq, Chichery, Poirier & Dickel (2004) showed that juveniles that ate crab as their first meal 3 days after hatching subsequently preferred crabs to shrimp. The ability to learn the positive consequences of food ingestion may be adaptive to a young animal needing to select safe prey alone. However, it may be a risky option for the young to be genetically programmed to seek out a single type of prey, especially in the case of a changing environment.

1.3.2   Associative learning

Cuttlefish actively prey upon shrimp, capturing them by shooting out their two tentacles for a strike. This behaviour, visually driven, has been extensively used in the studies of learning and memory capabilities in cuttlefish since the 1940s. Shrimp are presented behind glass (or inside a glass tube; Figure 1.2); the cuttlefish then attacks the prey but does not obtain it (Agin, Chichery & Chichery, 2001; Agin, Chichery, Maubert & Chichery, 2003; Bellanger, Dauphin, Chichery & Chichery, 2003; Dickel, Boal & Budelmann, 2000; Dickel, Chichery & Chichery, 1997, 1998, 2001; Messenger, 1971; Sanders & Young, 1940; Wells, 1962).

Under these conditions, *S. officinalis* learns not to attack the shrimp and, hence, to inhibit the predatory motor pattern: the number of capture attempts (tentacle strikes) decreases with stimulus presentations. This learning has been recognized as a form of associative learning (Agin, Dickel, Chichery & Chichery, 1998; Agin et al., 2006; Messenger, 1973). Following a massed procedure (a single continuous 20-min training phase), with various retention times (between 2 min and 2 days), Messenger (1971) reported differential performance of memory recall in adult cuttlefish. He considered this retention curve to be a product of two memory stores: a labile short-term memory (STM) lasting for a period of some minutes, and a long-term memory (LTM) lasting at least 2 days, and probably more. The retention curves obtained in 30- and 90-day-old cuttlefish bear a close resemblance to those recorded in adults, suggesting that LTM is

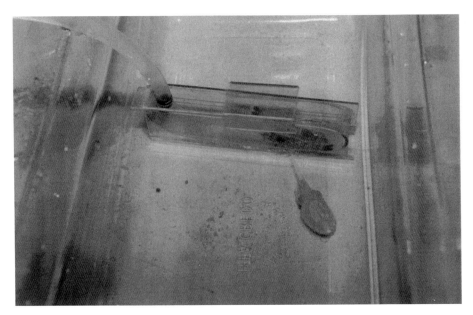

Figure 1.2 One-week-old cuttlefish striking at shrimp enclosed in a glass apparatus. The prey movement is kept constant by a continuous water flow (copyright L. Dickel).

fully operational from one month of age (Agin et al., 2006). STM appears earlier, as early as 8 days of age (Dickel, Chichery & Chichery, 1998), but 1-week-old cuttlefish have poor 60-minute retention performance. This improves progressively between 15 and 60 days of age (Dickel, Chichery & Chichery, 1998). These results suggest that there is a time lag between the establishment of short- and long-term memory systems during post-embryonic development and that LTM matures later than STM. Moreover, there is an improvement in the acquisition of learning ability during the first 2 months of life, as well as an increase of 24-hour retention performance between 30 and 90 days of age (Dickel, Boal & Budelmann, 2000; Dickel, Chichery & Chichery, 2001). As first suggested by Wirz (1954), this poor LTM performance in 8-day-old cuttlefish has been related to the immaturity of the brain's vertical complex (see below, section 6). This is particularly true of the vertical lobe, which, although the smallest lobe of the vertical complex at hatching, nearly doubles in size during the first month of post-embryonic development (Dickel, Chichery & Chichery, 1997, 2001).

However, this seems in contradiction with the findings of Darmaillacq, Chichery, Poirier & Dickel (2004) where cuttlefish fed on crab at 3 days of age, subsequently showed a preference for crab rather than their naturally preferred prey 4 days later. One can imagine that it is much more adaptive for a growing individual to learn quickly that available food is a positive alternative when their naturally preferred food is not accessible. Another possibility, not mutually exclusive with the first, is that such learning depends on different mechanisms and involves different brain structures than those involved in the retention of an associative task. This point will be discussed later in this chapter.

1.3.3   Food imprinting

Cuttlefish hatch with internal nutritive reserves. Even if active predation can begin before the inner yolk is entirely used up (Boletzky, 1987; Dickel, Chichery & Chichery, 1997), these reserves allow young cuttlefish to go without food for a few days. This period is probably critical in the life of young cuttlefish, since hatchlings can collect information about their environment (potential food, predation risk, shelters) before they start foraging. In cuttlefish from the English Channel, the prey-pursuit behaviour does not begin before the end of the first week after hatching (Dickel, Chichery & Chichery, 1997). From these data, it has been shown that the preference for crabs could be induced simply after visual familiarization with them during a sensitive period within the first hours of life after hatching (Darmaillacq, Chichery & Dickel, 2006; Darmaillacq, Chichery, Shashar & Dickel, 2006).

Interestingly, the efficiency of this familiarization depends on the length of the exposure as well as the density of prey exposed, i.e. the flow of information perceived during the sensitive period. Finally, it appears that the primacy of the early familiarization outweighs the untrained preference for shrimp (Darmaillacq, Chichery, Shashar & Dickel, 2006). This learning of the visual characteristics of a potential prey meets all the criteria of imprinting (Sluckin, 2007): no reinforcement, sensitive period, persistence (Darmaillacq, Chichery, Shashar & Dickel, 2006) and generalization (Guibé, Poirel, Houdé & Dickel, 2012; see next section). Food imprinting could account for the prey preference observed in 1-week-old cuttlefish, an effective compromise between the flexible but precarious strategy of trial and error, and the rigid, genetically driven response of non-learning. Such early learning capabilities would allow juveniles to take advantage of a changing environment and to deal with a world where shrimp (i.e. their "innate" food preference) was unavailable. To our knowledge, there is no available literature about fluctuation in prey availability on the English Channel coasts. Unlike filial or sexual imprinting, food imprinting might seem ineffective and even disadvantageous in the long term (Healy, 2006), in particular for long-lived individuals in a changeable environment. However, it could be helpful for juveniles to find available prey attractive in the weeks following hatching before they begin to forage.

It also appears that, if we compare these results with those obtained from the prawn-in-the-tube protocol, the two different types of learning may depend on the presence of different neural substrates.

1.3.4   Prey generalization

The preference for different types of prey observed in cuttlefish suggests that they are capable of interspecies discrimination (crab *vs* shrimp). Both crab and shrimp belong to the Class Crustacea, but they differ greatly in characteristic movement and morphology. A recent study has shown that naïve hatchlings preferred black crabs to white ones (Guibé, Poirel, Houdé & Dickel, 2012); this result is consistent with those obtained in the adult octopus, which spontaneously prefers to attack dark over white artificial objects (Fiorito & Scotto, 1992; Messenger & Sanders, 1972). However, if newly hatched cuttlefish have been exposed to white crabs, their spontaneous preference changes to white crabs. This demonstrates that cuttlefish have the ability to discriminate between two crabs from the same species but with different cephalothorax luminance. Moreover, if they are familiarized with white crabs at hatching, they subsequently prefer black crabs to shrimps. This means that they can generalize the learning of the characteristics of a prey to which they have been familiarized to a novel prey that shares some morphological features (Guibé, Poirel, Houdé & Dickel, 2012), and suggests a capacity for prey-generalization and possibly categorization in hatchling cuttlefish. This cognitive process, which consists in grouping distinguishable objects or events on the basis of a common feature or set of features and consequently to respond in a similar way to new stimuli, is a cognitive economy. Perceptual categorization has been extensively studied in pigeon, monkeys and honeybees using operant conditioning (Wasserman & Zentall, 2006), but still poorly investigated in marine molluscs.

It should be mentioned here that late juvenile cuttlefish (dorsal mantle length, DML, from 100 to 140 mm) from the wild systematically catch crabs (cephalothorax length, CL, from 40 to 60 mm) by the jumping strategy, although they capture shrimp by striking with their tentacles (Chichery, 1992). Results show that fewer than 60% of crab captured by inexperienced 5-day-old cuttlefish are caught by the jumping strategy (Dickel, 1997). These observations show that, even though crab identification is possible at hatching, there seems to be a correlation between the decision-making processes for catching prey and the experience and/or later brain maturation of juvenile cuttlefish. The frequency with which the jumping strategy is adopted in crab predation increases progressively during post-embryonic development to reach more than 80% after a month of life (Dickel, 1997). A possible hypothesis is that the later maturation of the vertical lobe system is a factor in these processes (see below).

1.3.5   Embryonic learning of visual features of potential prey

In *S. officinalis*, the egg envelopes are stained black with the ink of the female. As the embryo grows and the osmotic pressure of the perivitelline fluid increases (Boletzky, 1983), the elastic envelopes are dilated and some parts peel off so that the envelopes become more transparent. By the end of embryonic development the tactile, chemical and visual systems are all functional (see above, section 1.2), so that it is very likely that the embryo approaching the end of its development can perceive stimuli coming from its environment and, in particular, potential prey. Darmaillacq, Chichery, Shashar & Dickel (2006) showed that the sensitive window for food imprinting was open at hatching; given the characteristics of the egg capsules and the embryo's cognitive competencies, this sensitive period is likely to begin before hatching. Based on this assumption, Darmaillacq, Lesimple & Dickel (2008) exposed cuttlefish embryos to crabs for at least a week before hatching (Figure 1.3). They were able to show that these cuttlefish subsequently preferred crab to shrimp, unlike a control group of cuttlefish that had not seen crab during the sensitive period before hatching. Hence, embryos are able to learn the general shape of a potential prey in the late stages of their development. This preference was observed whether the outer layer of the egg envelope had been removed or not.

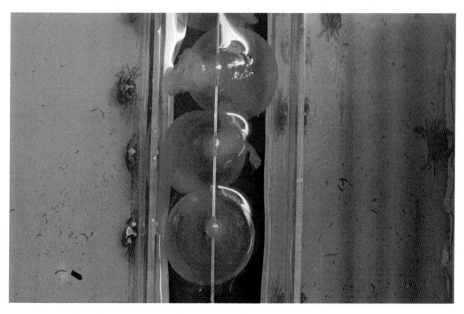

Figure 1.3 Embryonic exposure to crabs. Note the absence of pigmentation of the egg capsule usually stained in black in *Sepia officinalis* (copyright A.-S. Darmaillacq). For details about the apparatus see Darmaillacq, Lesimple and Dickel (2008).

Cephalopod ink is generally supposed to function in defence as a visual stimulus, either as a smoke screen or as a distraction for predators (Hanlon & Messenger, 1996). It has been hypothesized that it could function in the chemical realm as well (Derby, 2007) and be repellent to predators (e.g. moray eel: Hanlon & Messenger, 1996; green turtle: Caldwell, 2005). The ink contained in the egg envelope may also have the same function, providing, in addition to the visual screen, a repulsive smell to ward off predators. Other evidence that supports this idea is that female *Sepia pharaonis*, which lay transparent eggs, hide them in crevices, corals or under any potential shelter, whereas *S. officinalis* lay eggs in open fields without any additional protection. In *Sepia esculenta*, the eggs have a sticky clear exterior that accumulates sand and other material for cryptic colouration (Hanlon & Messenger, 1996). The results obtained by Darmaillacq, Lesimple & Dickel (2008) suggest that the envelopes, although black in appearance, do not prevent embryos from seeing outside during the last days of embryonic development, while continuing to protect them from predation. Guibé and collaborators recently confirmed that visual information can be used during the very last week, and specified that a 4-hour exposure to crabs either in the morning or in the afternoon was enough (L. Dickel & M. Guibé, unpublished data). From these results, one can argue that the sensitive period probably starts shortly before hatching.

Shrimp differ from crabs in morphology, way of moving and luminance. But to what extent does the embryo perceive the details of prey presented outside the egg? A partial answer to this question has recently been found. When offered a choice between white and black crabs, cuttlefish visually familiarized *in ovo* to white crabs preferred them, unlike the control cuttlefish that preferred black crabs; they also prefer black crabs to shrimp, unlike the control cuttlefish that prefer shrimp (Guibé, Poirel, Houdé & Dickel, 2012). This confirms that juvenile cuttlefish have the ability to categorize and generalize prey, but, interestingly, it also shows that embryos are capable of perception of one particular feature of prey, its luminance.

If vision is the predominant sense in cuttlefish, chemical perception is also important in the recognition of prey items, predators and conspecifics (Boal & Golden, 1999; Boal & Marsh, 1998; Hanlon & Messenger, 1996). In embryos, the chemical system is functional before the visual one (Romagny, Darmaillacq, Guibé, Bellanger & Dickel, 2012). To evaluate the effect of a chemical exposure on visual preference after hatching, embryos were exposed to odours from shrimp (*Crangon crangon*; preferred prey), crabs (*Carcinus maenas*; unpreferred prey), molluscs (*Mytilus edulis*; non-prey) or a seawater control (Guibé, Boal & Dickel, 2010). They were then tested for a visual preference between crabs and shrimp. Cuttlefish that had previously smelt shrimp had a visual preference for crabs, whereas cuttlefish that had previously smelt crabs preferred shrimp and cuttlefish that had previously smelt bivalves had no preference. To explain these puzzling results, the authors pointed out a cross-modal effect between the chemical and visual systems. Moreover, they hypothesized that an overstimulation of the chemical system during the embryonic development could have disturbed the onset of the visual system and, hence, the visual perception in juveniles (Honeycutt & Lickliter, 2003).

1.4   Lateralization

Cerebral lateralization is a universal and evolutionarily ancient trait in vertebrates (Vallortigara & Rogers, 2005). It is often revealed behaviourally by motor (e.g. handedness) and perceptual (e.g. preferential eye use) asymmetries. It now appears that in invertebrates, too, cerebral lateralization is probably widespread (Frasnelli, Vallortigara & Rogers, 2012). This suggests that lateralization of the nervous system may be a common feature of complex brains, even with completely different evolutionary histories. Very recent research has also begun to suggest evidence of lateralization in the cuttlefish brain. Several studies have investigated whether behavioural asymmetries are already present at hatching, whether the development of lateralization is dependent on both genes and environment, as in vertebrates, and the neural correlates of visual lateralization (see below, section 1.6).

1.4.1   Ontogenesis of lateralization

Visual lateralization

Adult cuttlefish show an untrained side-turning preference (preference for turning right or left) in a T-maze (Alves, Chichery, Boal & Dickel, 2007). Side-turning preference may be the result of an eye use preference (i.e. visual lateralization) in cuttlefish, as has been shown in octopus (Byrne, Kuba & Griebel, 2002; Byrne, Kuba & Meisel, 2004).

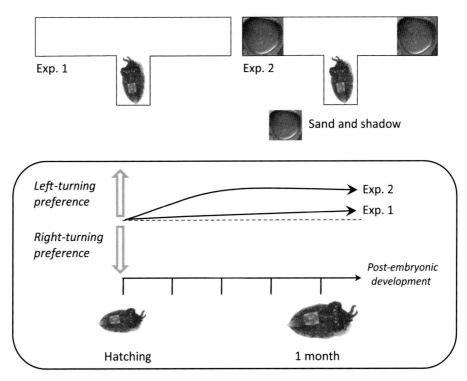

Figure 1.4 Postembryonic development of side-turning preference in *Sepia officinalis*. Exp. 1: Cuttlefish are tested in an empty apparatus; Exp. 2: Cuttlefish are tested with a shelter (i.e. sand and shadow) on both sides of the apparatus (Jozet-Alves et al., 2012).

The cuttlefish visual system consists of two eyes sitting laterally on the head (Nixon & Young, 2003) and asymmetry of eye use seems to be ubiquitous among vertebrates with laterally placed eyes (Vallortigara & Bisazza, 2002).

Jozet-Alves et al. (2012b) investigated the age at which the right- or left-turning preference appeared by testing cuttlefish in a T-shaped apparatus between 3 and 60 days post-hatching. To find out whether side-turning preferences were the result of an eye use preference, cuttlefish were tested either inside a plain T-shaped apparatus or in one with an attractive shelter on each arm of the T-maze (Figure 1.4). In the first case, juveniles did not show any side-turning preference. However, when shelters were available in both arms of the T-shaped apparatus, the authors observed a progressive development from 3 to 60 days post-hatching of a bias to turn leftwards, even though when going out of the start box, cuttlefish simultaneously saw both shelters, one on each side. In the natural environment, an eye-use preference may be very adaptive for cuttlefish to decide rapidly which shelter to choose.

The emergence of visual lateralization in juvenile cuttlefish coincides with other ontogenetic events such as the progressive diversification of their diet (Darmaillacq, Chichery, Poirier & Dickel, 2004), increasing efficiency in matching the background (Hanlon & Messenger, 1988) and dispersal (Dickel et al., 2006). One potential advantage of visual lateralization is the ability to process two types of information simultaneously. It is possible that the lateralization affords the cuttlefish greater behavioural efficiency at the time of dispersal, by enabling them to look out for escape routes while hunting.

Lateralization of food imprinting

In invertebrates, there is growing evidence for perceptual and motor lateralization, but few examples of lateralization of learning are available. Researchers have demonstrated asymmetrical performance favouring the right antenna when bees have to learn to respond to particular odours to obtain a food reward (in honeybees: Letzkus et al., 2006; in bumble bees: Anfora et al., 2011). More recently, Letzkus, Boeddeker, Wood, Zhang & Srinivasan (2008) also found that honeybees learn a colour cue better with their right eye to obtain a food reward.

C. Jozet-Alves and A.-S. Darmaillacq (unpublished data) investigated lateralization of food imprinting (see above) in cuttlefish. They familiarized cuttlefish with crab with the right eye, the left eye or both eyes. This study revealed that the efficiency of the familiarization depends on the eye exposed to crab: only cuttlefish exposed to crab with their right eye were significantly more likely than control cuttlefish to choose crab. This study indicates: (i) that some types of behavioural lateralization are already established in hatchlings; and (ii) that the right-eye pathway is sufficient for food imprinting. The right eye may play a predominant role in learning the characteristics of a potential prey. It is then possible that the right visual field is more generally specialized for foraging and feeding behaviour, as in many species of vertebrates (such as chicks and fish; Rogers, 2007) and in honeybees (Letzkus, Boeddeker, Wood, Zhang & Srinivasan, 2008).

1.4.2   Influence of early experience on visual lateralization

In vertebrates, some well-known examples of lateralization indicate that the ontogeny of lateralization depends on the interaction of genes and experience. For example, in fish, the degree of lateralization varies between populations of the same species that have been exposed to different ecological pressures (e.g. predation pressure: Brown, Western & Braithwaite, 2007). In invertebrates, no study has yet explored the influence of early experience on the development of lateralization. The cuttlefish appears to offer an ideal opportunity for addressing questions pertaining to the ontogenesis of lateralization in invertebrates as their incubation and rearing conditions are easy to control.

Recently, Jozet-Alves and Hébert (2013) investigated a modulation of lateralization by chemical signals of predation in cuttlefish. Cuttlefish embryos differed according to the type of olfactory stimulation [predator odour (sea bass), non-predator odour (sea urchins), no odour (plain sea water)] to which they were exposed before hatching. Whereas hatchlings that had not been exposed to predator odour during embryonic development (control and non-predator groups) showed no side-turning bias in a T-shaped apparatus, as found previously by Jozet-Alves et al. (2012b; see above), hatchlings that had been exposed to predator odour (predator group) preferentially turned to the left in the T-maze. The exposure to predator odour could possibly be an acute predictor of a high predation risk in the environment. Differences in strength of lateralization might provide fitness benefits to cuttlefish that hatch in high-predation areas, enabling them to hunt and watch predators simultaneously. Indeed, it has been shown that strongly lateralized individuals possess cognitive advantages over their less-lateralized counterparts both in vertebrates (e.g. Magat & Brown, 2009, Rogers, Zucca & Vallortigara, 2004) and invertebrates (drosophila: Pascual, Huang, Nevue & Préat, 2004). Cerebral lateralization may enhance brain efficiency in cognitive tasks that demand the simultaneous but different use of both hemispheres.

1.4.3   Discussion on lateralization

In vertebrates, the right visual field is usually associated with the response to an identified target such as a prey item, while the left visual field is specialized for the control of rapid responses (e.g. response to a predator). This common pattern of visual lateralization has led some researchers to argue in favour of a homology of cerebral lateralization, at least in vertebrates (Rogers, 2007). The different studies on lateralization in cuttlefish described above seem to indicate a dominance of the left visual field (i.e. left-turning preference in a T-shaped apparatus to reach a shelter) in a defensive context, and a dominance of the right visual field in learning the characteristics of a potential prey. Moreover, as in vertebrates, visual lateralization in cuttlefish is markedly influenced by early experience; genetic influences on lateralization are not paramount even in invertebrates. The similarities observed between vertebrates and cuttlefish could merely be a coincidence or be indicative of a common origin of visual lateralization in vertebrates and invertebrates. This last hypothesis implies that lateralization evolved once in the common ancestor. Regardless of whether the various types of lateralization are homologous or not, allocating some functions to one half of the brain, and other functions to the other half appears a common solution to enhance brain's capacity. This solution appears to be more widely adopted in the animal kingdom than an increase in brain size. Evidence of lateralization now available from invertebrates, and more specifically from cephalopods, will offer an instructive comparison for a better understanding of lateralization in vertebrates.

1.5   Phenotypic plasticity and defensive behaviour

Predation is a constant threat faced by prey animals, especially young individuals, and Brown and Chivers (2006) have suggested that there may be strong selection pressure for the early detection and avoidance of potential predators. Another option is to avoid being detected, a strategy that includes primary defensive behaviour. In the cuttlefish, primary defence is generally called crypsis (see chapter 9, this volume, by Zylinski & Osorio) and comprises camouflage and sand digging (Hanlon & Messenger, 1996). Cuttlefish hatchlings spontaneously show the Disruptive pattern (see chapter 9, this volume, by Zylinski & Osorio) whatever the substrate they settle on (Uniform grey or

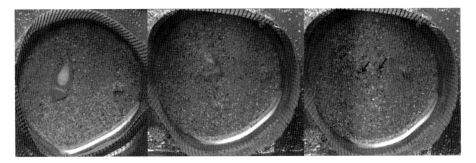

Figure 1.5 Sand-digging behaviour in 15-day-old cuttlefish. From left to right: cuttlefish not buried, partially buried (50%) and completely buried (the arrows indicate the eyes) (copyright C. Di Poi).

a chequerboard). Then, throughout the first 2 months of post-embryonic development, the cuttlefish's ability to blend into a Uniform background improves, resulting in closer general background resemblance and a much reduced display of the Disruptive pattern; this is especially true of cuttlefish reared in enriched conditions (i.e. tanks provided with sand, shelters, rocks, conspecific, etc.: Poirier, Chichery & Dickel, 2005). This suggests that sensory and cognitive enrichment affects the maturation of defensive strategies. The same result was obtained for sand digging behaviour, where cuttlefish reared on sand had shorter latencies to dig and were much better covered with sand than those reared without sand (Poirier, Chichery & Dickel, 2004; Figure 1.5). Although this behaviour is at least partially experience-dependent, what really stands out is that camouflage behaviours in hatchlings are immature and hence inefficient.

We have already pointed out that embryos were able to perceive external information concerning potential prey from inside the egg. However, a question remains: if embryos can see potential prey, can they also see the risk of predation to which they will be exposed after hatching? A very recent study showed cuttlefish that, as embryos, had been exposed to sea bass, *Dicentrarchus labrax*, and crabs, *Carcinus maenas* (which can be considered as potential predators), displayed a more effective camouflage on a Uniform substrate or on sand (A.-S. Darmaillacq & L. Dickel, unpublished data). This suggests that sensory-motor maturation could have begun during the last stages of embryonic development. The type of stimulus to which cuttlefish respond (movement, shape, size, etc.) is still not clear, and more experiments are needed. Nevertheless, in cuttlefish, camouflage is used to prevent being detected by not only predators but also by prey. As a consequence, it could be very advantageous for young cuttlefish to be well camouflaged, so that they are effective in catching prey present in the vicinity of the eggs. Such behavioural plasticity makes sense for a small and highly vulnerable organism. When predation risk is high, it is likely that there is more movement around the eggs and, hence, better camouflage at hatching will be highly adaptive, whereas this is not necessary in an area of low predation risk. This suggests a cost of camouflage. Body colouration may also serve functions other than defence (communication, hunting strategy, etc.) that do not require the expression of an efficient camouflage.

1.6   The brain and its neurotransmitters

1.6.1   Brain patterning

The cephalopod brain originates from four pairs of molluscan ganglia, known as the pedal, palliovisceral, cerebral and optic ganglia. Baratte and Bonnaud (2009) described ganglionic proneural cells forming dendrites at stage 16 of embryogenesis, which demonstrate early neural differentiation. These ganglia converge at stage 21 to become a central circumoesophageal brain, lying between the eyes. Thus, the central nervous system comprises supra- and sub-oesophageal masses connected by peri-oesophageal lobes. On each side of the peri-oesophageal lobes are the large optic lobes, connected to the supra-oesophageal mass by short optic tracts. The cephalopod brain has been described in great detail (for a review, see Nixon & Young, 2003). A review of brain development requires a preliminary summary of its anatomy and the main functions of the lobes in adult cuttlefish. The central mass lobes all have the same pattern: a central neuropil (area of nerve fibres) and a surrounding cortex (cell bodies). The optic lobes comprise an outer cortex and a central medulla. They are involved in higher-order visual processing, in the control of motor programmes (Chichery & Chanelet, 1976) as well as in memory (in connection with the vertical system, see below). In the hilum of the optic lobes, the peduncle lobes are small structures lying horizontally and dorsally to the optic tracts. The peduncle lobes are higher motor centres that may play a role in the fine control of locomotion, body colour and pupil dilatation (Chichery & Chanelet, 1978). The vertical system corresponds to the dorsal part of the supra-oesophageal mass and contains various structures such as the vertical, sub-vertical and superior frontal lobes, involved in learning and memory (Sanders & Young, 1940), and the inferior frontal lobe involved in sensory-motor integration (Young, 1979). The ventral part (basal lobes) of the supra-oesophageal mass comprises some higher centres implicated in the control of motor programmes. The sub-oesophageal mass (brachial, pedal and palliovisceral lobes) and the peri-oesophageal mass (magnocellular lobes) contain the premotor and motor neurones responsible for swimming, escape behaviour, ink ejection and arm and tentacle movements (Nixon & Young, 2003).

1.6.2   Brain maturation

The central nervous system in cephalopods grows throughout life, but some lobes develop in size or in function earlier than others (Nixon & Mangold, 1998; Figure 1.6). This brain maturation has been investigated in juvenile cuttlefish from hatching until the age of 3 months through three sets of studies: (i) measurement of the relative growth of the different lobes (volume of a lobe/total brain volume) (Dickel, Chichery & Chichery, 1997); (ii) quantification of cell proliferation in the brain of juvenile cuttlefish (5-bromo-2′-deoxyuridine incorporation) (Poirier, 2004); (iii) Determination of the presence of heavy neurofilaments (pNF-H, 220 kD) in the optic lobes of late embryos (Darmaillacq, 2005) and in the brain of early juveniles (Dickel, 1997). These highly phosphorylated neurofilaments in the cytoskeleton are considered as strong markers of a stabilized neural

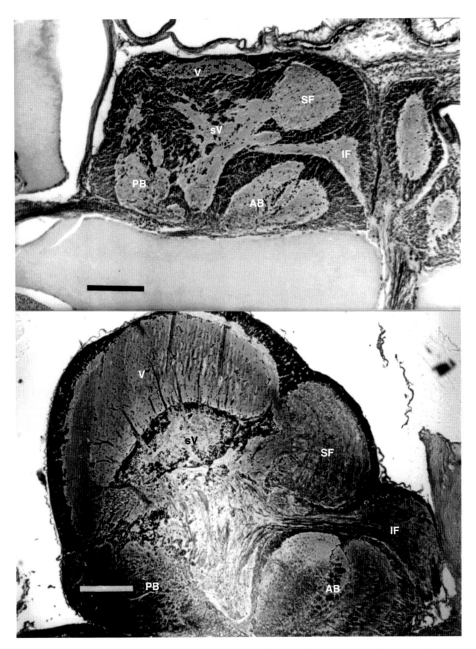

Figure 1.6 Supra-oesophageal mass of the brain: cuttlefish hatchling (top) and 3-month-old cuttlefish (bottom) (sagittal sections). Note the dramatic increase of the vertical lobe (V) size. Abbreviations: AB, anterior basal lobe; IF, inferior frontal lobe; PB, posterior basal lobe; SF, superior frontal lobe; sV, subvertical lobe; V, vertical lobe. Upper scale bar = 200 μm; lower scale bar = 400 μm (copyright L. Dickel).

network in both the vertebrate and the invertebrate nervous system (Darmaillacq, 2005; Dickel, 1997; Grant, Tseng, Gould, Gainer & Pant, 1995; Riederer, 1992).

Optic lobes

Each optic lobe receives input from the retina and their cortex corresponds to the deeper layers of the vertebrate retina (second and third-order neurones; Nixon & Young, 2003). The behavioural response of embryos to a visual stimulus (see section 1.2) and their ability to learn visual features of potential prey (see section 1.3.5) indicate that the visual system, including the optic lobes, is functional before hatching. The presence of pNF-H in the plexiform layer of the cortex at embryonic stage 29 suggests that first-order visual inputs (plexiform layer) are already mature (Darmaillacq, 2005). At hatching, the optic lobes are similar in relative size and tissue organization to those of adults. Their connexions with the arms are already mature at hatching. This early maturation could be linked to the early visuo-motor abilities of hatchlings. As described in section 1.3.4, newly hatched cuttlefish are able to perform prey-generalization and categorization (Guibé, Poirel, Houdé & Dickel, 2012). Investigations of neural circuits involved in prey identification are still very preliminary, but the optic lobes seem likely to be the neural substrates of these early processes of visual integration. Apart from their involvement in the integration of visual information, the optic lobes have been supposed to be the site of the visual memory store in octopus (Sanders 1975; Young, 1965). No study has been undertaken so far in cuttlefish, but here, again, they seem likely candidates for neural substrates of food imprinting based on visual familiarization (see section 1.3.3). These structures are more developed in newly hatched cuttlefish than the vertical lobe system (see above). In addition to their early neural and functional maturation, the optic lobes also undergo further post-embryonic maturation. Even though the rate of cell divisions in these lobes decreases from hatching to age 2 months, this decrease is less marked than in other brain structures (Poirier, 2004). The increase in size of the optic lobes is mainly due to the development of neurites; indeed, plexiform layers of the deep retina thicken during the first days of post-hatching development. pNF-H immunostaining in the cortex and neuropil is of low intensity at birth and the neurites show a gradual post-embryonic stabilization during the first 6 days (Dickel, 1997). This post-embryonic maturation means that the development of the optic lobe can still be affected by the environment of the juvenile. Accumulating evidence in vertebrates shows that sensory experience modulates brain development during a critical period, especially before the maturation of the brain wiring (Bengoetxea et al., 2012).

Motor centres

Several lobes of the supra-, sub- and peri-oesophageal mass control the various actions of the cuttlefish. Those lobes are gathered into lower, intermediate and higher motor centres. The lower and intermediate motor centres (sub-oesophageal, chromatophore and magnocellular lobes) contain the motor neurones, whereas the higher motor centres (peduncle lobes and basal lobes of the supra-oesophageal mass) are responsible for the combined movements of different effectors. At hatching, juveniles display prey capture and cryptic behaviours. Brain studies have shown that the lobes involved in such behaviours (e.g. basal, chromatophore and sub-oesophageal lobes) are well developed, as are their connections. Moreover, the sub-oesophageal lobes show some mature neurones at embryonic stage 29. The higher motor centres are mature soon after hatching since a high staining of pNF-H has been observed in their neuropil (basal part of the supra-oesophageal mass and peduncle lobes). Cell proliferation decreases gradually (peduncle, chromatophore and basal lobes) until the age of 2 months. This can be linked to the improvement of predation and camouflage strategies observed during the first 2 months (see Section 1.5).

The vertical lobe system (memory system)

The vertical system contains associative structures receiving signals from different sensory systems and is known to be involved in learning and memory (Agin et al., 2006; Graindorge et al., 2006). If the optic lobes have been suggested as a location for information storage, Young (1965) hypothesized that this stored information is not available for use in the absence of the vertical lobe system. This seems to be particularly true in the case of associative learning. Short- and long-term synaptic plasticity has recently been shown in the vertical lobe of adult cuttlefish (Shomrat et al., 2011). Apart from the inferior frontal lobe, which shows some mature neurons from embryonic stage 29, the vertical system is quite immature at hatching. The associative nervous structures (vertical and superior frontal lobes) are the most poorly developed regions of the brain in hatchlings. Their volume increases during the first months of life, and the post-embryonic growth of the vertical lobe is dramatic when compared to that of other supra-oesophageal lobes (7% of the total brain volume in hatchlings against 12% in 12-month-old animals; Figure 1.6). As first suggested by Wirz (1954), poor long-term memory performance of an associative learning task in 8-day-old cuttlefish has been related to the immaturity of the vertical complex. Moreover, the growth of the superior frontal and vertical lobes appears to be significantly linked with the improvement of long-term retention performances (Dickel, Chichery & Chichery, 2001, see section 1.3.2). This increase in volume may be due to neuritic growth and cell proliferation, especially during the first months of life. In vertebrates, an increase in neurogenesis underlies brain growth in early postnatal development (during the first week of life in rats); afterwards neurogenesis decreases to reach a relatively stable state in adulthood (Bandeira, Lent & Herculano-Houzel, 2009; Jabès, Lavenex, Amaral & Lavenex, 2010). Even if the neuropil of the frontal superior lobe and its connexions to the vertical lobe show some pNF-H stained fibres at hatching, the fibres in this lobe keep on stabilizing, at least in the week after hatching (intensification of the pNF-H staining). In the sub-vertical lobe, cell proliferation increases during the 2 weeks after hatching, the rate then decreasing until 2 months of age, as in the other lobes of the vertical system. The tracts connecting the vertical lobe to the sub-vertical lobe – sites of long-term potentiation (Shomrat et al., 2011) – are lacking at hatching (Dickel, Chichery & Chichery, 1997). These nervous tracts grow between day 1 and day 9 and appear really stable at the age of 1 month (Dickel, Chichery & Chichery, 1997). From a functional standpoint, their appearance is concomitant with the maturation of short-term retention of some visual information during the first days of life (see section 1.3.2). In addition to this involvement in memory processes, one can also hypothesize that the late maturation of the vertical lobe system could be related to decision-making processes for catching prey (see section 3.4).

Brain maturation is strongly influenced by environment. The maturation of the vertical–subvertical lobe tracts depends on the water temperature (Dickel, Chichery & Chichery, 1997), and when juveniles are reared in enriched conditions (in large tanks, with conspecifics, sand, shelters, seaweed), the vertical system develops faster, especially during the first month of life (Dickel, Chichery & Chichery, 2001). Poirier (2004) showed that enrichment did not modify the intensity of cell proliferation in the vertical system, so it might optimize neurite growth. The development of the optic lobes is also environment-sensitive. When cuttlefish are reared in the dark, there is a significant decrease in cell proliferation in the optic lobe neuropils at 15 days compared to cuttlefish reared in a natural light–dark cycle, whatever the other rearing conditions (Poirier, 2004). On the contrary, at 30 days of age enriched rearing conditions induce an increase in cell proliferation in the deep retina and in the neuropil of optic lobes. These results highlight the importance of sensory stimulation on brain maturation.

1.6.3   Brain correlates of visual lateralization

Little is known about how the ontogenesis of behavioural asymmetry is related to the development of cerebral asymmetry. Jozet-Alves, Romagny, Bellanger & Dickel (2012a) have investigated whether anatomical or neurochemical asymmetries are present in the cuttlefish brain at 30 days post-hatching, and whether these asymmetries correlate with side-turning preferences. The authors found individual variation in the size of the optic lobe and the degree of vertical lobe asymmetry. Some cuttlefish possessed relatively symmetrical optic and vertical lobes, and others possessed a larger right optic lobe and right half of the vertical lobe. A striking correlation emerged from the behavioural results: the larger the right optic lobe and the right part of the vertical lobe, the stronger the bias to turn leftwards. The absence of correlation between other brain asymmetry measurements and behavioural lateralization indicates that these correlations are exclusive to these structures and not part of a more general brain asymmetry. It remains to be determined how the optic/vertical lobes interact with other neural systems to produce lateralization of behaviour.

1.6.4   Neurotransmitters in the developing brain

Neurotransmitters have diverse roles in the developing nervous system from embryonic developmental functions in morphogenesis to synapse formation (Buznikov, Shmukler & Lauder, 1996). The few neurotransmitters studied in the developing brain of *S. officinalis* will be reviewed here.

Acetylcholine
The central cholinergic system is involved in cognitive processes, as extensively reported in vertebrates (Everitt & Robbins, 1997) and, to a lesser extent, in invertebrates (e.g. insects: Fresquet, Fournier & Gauthier, 1998; molluscs: Mpitsos, Murray, Creech &

Barker, 1988). Acetylcholine has been studied in the cuttlefish central nervous system (Bellanger, Dauphin, Belzunce & Chichery, 1998; Messenger, 1996) including during memory formation (Bellanger, Dauphin, Chichery & Chichery, 2003). Unlike the muscarinic type, nicotinic-like receptors are widely present in the brain of adult cuttlefish. We have not yet investigated the development of these nicotinic-like receptors during post-embryonic life but preliminary results show that, except in the optic and superior frontal lobes, density and distribution of the nicotinic-like receptors in the different brain structures are relatively unchanged from 3 months to 15 months of age (Bellanger, Halm, Dauphin & Chichery, 2005).

Serotonin

In addition to its physiological role as a neuromodulator (e.g. in mood regulation, memory, food motivation, etc.), serotonin also modulates cellular migration and cytoarchitecture throughout development (Daubert & Condron, 2010). The distribution of serotonin immunoreactive cells in the brain of newly hatched cuttlefish is quite similar to that described in the adult's brain (unpublished data; Boyer, Maubert, Charnay & Chichery, 2007). Monoamines were quantified in the whole head of juveniles (by high performance liquid chromatography). Circulating monoamines may have been included in our measurements but are likely to be in negligible amounts (little remaining haemolymph). The median serotonin content was 0.43 ± 0.07 ng/mg tissue at hatching and seems to have remained quite stable during the first week of life, but it was subject to considerable inter-individual variations (0.35 ± 0.34 ng/mg tissue at day 7; unpublished data). The spatio-temporal distribution of serotonin was investigated in the visual system during embryogenesis by immunohistochemistry (Romagny, 2010). Serotonin is not present in the embryos before stage 26. Few immunoreactive fibres were observed in the retina and optic lobes (cortex and neuropil) from stages 27. Then the number of serotonin immunoreactive fibres increased gradually until hatching. A strong light stimulus significantly increased serotonin staining in the visual system in newly hatched cuttlefish. This argues for the implication of serotonin in the functioning of this sensory system in embryos. Nevertheless, we cannot yet determine whether the increase in serotonin content results from activation of the visual pathways or to a general reaction of the young to a stressor.

Catecholamines

In the brain, catecholamines are known to be involved in major functions in vertebrates including motor control, cognition, emotion, positive reinforcement and visceral regulation (Iversen & Iversen, 2007). They contribute to the development of neuronal pathways and synapse formation (Dobson, Dmetrichuk & Spencer, 2006). Catecholamines occur in the embryonic ganglia of cuttlefish at stage 16 in some proneural cells exhibiting neurites (Baratte & Bonnaud, 2009). Baratte and Bonnaud (2009) suggested an early differentiation of catecholamine-containing neurones in the future brain and in the primary retina. Catecholamines may also play a modulatory role, such as axonal guidance, during gangliogenesis. Dopamine and particularly noradrenaline are more concentrated in the head of newly hatched cuttlefish than serotonin (0.78 ± 0.42 ng dopamine/mg tissue and 19.51 ± 496.27 ng noradrenaline/mg tissue).

Oxytocin

Brain oxytocin plays an important role in behavioural regulation in mammals and may influence the development of the central nervous system during the postnatal period (Carter, 2003). The spatio-temporal distribution of a peptide has been investigated in the central nervous system during the postnatal development of *S. officinalis* (Bardou et al., 2010). The central oxytocin-like system is well developed at birth and continues to mature throughout the postnatal weeks until it reaches clear maturity in 2-month-old animals. After hatching very few changes occur in the relative abundance of fibres containing oxytocin-like elements; the maturation of this neuropeptidic system is mainly seen in the spatial distribution of cell bodies. Most of the central lobes show a mature oxytocin-like pattern in 15-day-old animals. Surprisingly, the central vertical lobe and the medulla of the optic lobes have the earliest maturation. Indeed, no change in the relative abundance of oxytocin-like cell bodies was observed between hatching and age 3 months. The sub-oesophageal lobes continue maturation until the age of 2 months.

Our knowledge of the processes of brain development in cuttlefish is incomplete. Nevertheless, we can see that the structures involved in motor programme and sensory integration mature earlier than the associative lobes. This heterogeneity can certainly be linked to the behavioural abilities of hatchlings and the post-embryonic optimization of learning capacities.

1.7   Conclusion

The starting point of this chapter was to find out whether, as in vertebrates, prenatal experience could shape postnatal behaviour in a sophisticated invertebrate and if so, whether cuttlefish embryos could be considered to have complex cognitive systems. In fact, the studies reviewed here show that cuttlefish, which are known to have good learning and memory capabilities as adults, seem already to be very good learners as embryos. In the absence of parental care, young cuttlefish have to find edible prey and protect themselves from predators. The studies showed that embryos can collect visual information concerning prey and predators and use it after hatching. This validates the existence of continuities in learning from prenatal to postnatal life even in invertebrates. For this, embryos need efficient sense organs, the onset of whose functioning follows the same sequence as in vertebrates, and which are functional even before they have completed their maturation. They also need a sophisticated nervous system that will integrate and process all the information collected by the sensory system, which is indeed the case. Cuttlefish are at the same time potential prey and predators, so that they need to have both efficient anti-predator and predatory behaviour; this requires cognitive abilities such as prey/predator categorization and generalization. In the cuttlefish which, like the other coleoids, 'live fast and die young', such cognitive abilities seem to be established very early, even at the embryonic stage. Female cuttlefish lay relatively large eggs with abundant yolk reserves. As a consequence embryos have resources for neural development in the egg compared with other molluscs, which seem to have a more random approach (more offspring and some will survive by luck – see chapter 2, this volume, by Basil & Crook). Embryos could then benefit from a large brain and adapt to a wide range of environments.

At this point it might be useful to describe the early stages of the life of a cuttlefish, as it is now understood. The cuttlefish embryo develops inside an opaque egg, sheltered from predators. As the embryo grows, the envelope of the egg stretches and becomes thinner and more transparent. This allows the embryo to become familiar with its future biotic and abiotic environment through its chemical and visual senses as each perceptual system becomes functional. At hatching, the cuttlefish is able to dig into the sand and to camouflage itself, although it will probably prefer to find a shelter (Guibé & Dickel, 2011), until its more classical defensive behaviour becomes more efficient. Meanwhile, since from inside the egg it has had a 'preview' of prey type, it is prepared to feed in the immediate environment on what is available immediately after hatching, switching to its innately preferred (elongate-shaped) prey if this becomes available.

Cuttlefish are usually described as animals that receive no parental care. However, it is still not known whether a kind of indirect parental care exists, in that the mother could in laying her eggs choose a place where suitable prey will be available, or she may, as birds are known to do, deposit chemical information (steroid hormones, prey odours, etc.) in the yolk (Henriksen, Rettenbacher & Groothuis, 2011).

In conclusion, cuttlefish are both the most important cephalopod fishery resource in Europe, and also an important component in the marine ecosystem. At the present time, cuttlefish in Europe face a major problem. Each year, billions of eggs are laid on fishermen's traps, which are an ideal available surface for females, but they are destroyed during harvest when the traps are cleaned. To counterbalance this, future programmes for the reintroduction of eggs/hatchlings will soon be necessary. In depth ethological knowledge, as described in this chapter, will be necessary to ensure that conditions on the spawning ground do not interfere with embryos and hatchling viability. Survival of young animals in the wild depends largely on their behavioural plasticity and their embryonic experience. For this reason, as a major contribution to the programme's success, attention will have to be given to the quality of the released individuals, in particular ensuring the development of strategies to include the encouragement of the best possible performance and robustness from the eggs or hatchlings concerned.

Acknowledgements

We are very grateful to Frédéric Guyon who takes care of the cuttlefish at the Marine Station (CREC, Luc sur Mer, France) and to Jean-Paul Lehodey who helps us design and build the experimental apparatus. We also thank all the voluntary students (from undergraduate to graduate levels) who participated in some of the experiments. Lastly, we are particularly grateful to Prs Raymond and Marie-Paule Chichery who worked for decades to develop cephalopod research in Normandy.

References

Agin, V., Chichery, R. and Chichery, M.-P. (2001). Effects of learning on cytochrome oxidase activity in cuttlefish brain. *Neuroreport*, **12**: 1–4.

Agin, V., Chichery, R., Chichery, M-P., Dickel, L., Darmaillacq, A.-S. and Bellanger, C. (2006). Behavioural plasticity and neural correlates in adult cuttlefish. *Vie et Milieu*, **56**: 81–87.

Agin, V., Chichery, R., Maubert, E. and Chichery, M.-P. (2003). Time-dependent effects of cyclo-heximide on long-term memory in the cuttlefish. *Pharmacology Biochemistry and Behavior*, **75**: 141–146.

Agin, V., Dickel, L., Chichery, R. and Chichery, M.-P. (1998). Evidence for a specific short-term memory in the cuttlefish, *Sepia*. *Behavioural Processes*, **43**: 329–334.

Alves, C., Chichery, R., Boal, J. G. and Dickel L. (2007). Orientation in the cuttlefish *Sepia officinalis*: response versus place learning. *Animal Cognition*, **10**: 29–36.

Anfora, G., Rigosi, E., Frasnelli, E., Ruga, V., Trona, F. and Vallortigara, G. (2011). Lateralization in the invertebrate brain: left-right asymmetry of olfaction in bumble bee, *Bombus terrestris*. *Public Library of Science One*, **6**: e18903.

Bandeira, F., Lent, R. and Herculano-Houzel, S. (2009). Changing numbers of neuronal and non-neuronal cells underlie postnatal brain growth in the rat. *Proceedings of the National Academy of Sciences of the United States of America*, **106**: 14108–14113.

Baratte, S. and Bonnaud, L. (2009). Evidence of early nervous differentiation and early cate-cholaminergic sensory system during *Sepia officinalis* embryogenesis. *Journal of Comparative Neurology*, **517**(4): 539–549.

Bardou, I., Maubert, E., Leprince, J., Chichery, R., Dallérac, G., Vaudry, H. and Agin, V. (2010). Ontogeny of oxytocin-like immunoreactivity in the cuttlefish, *Sepia officinalis*, central nervous system. *Developmental Neuroscience*, **32**(1): 19–32.

Bellanger, C., Dauphin, F., Belzunce, L. and Chichery, R. (1998). Parallel regional quantification of choline acetyltransferase and cholinesterase activity in the central nervous system of an invertebrate (*Sepia officinalis*). *Brain Research. Brain Research Protocols*, **3**: 68–75.

Bellanger, C., Dauphin, F., Chichery, M.-P. and Chichery, R. (2003). Changes in cholinergic enzyme activities in the cuttlefish brain during memory formation. *Physiology and Behavior*, **79**: 749–756.

Bellanger, C., Halm, M.-P., Dauphin, F. and Chichery, R. (2005). *In vitro* evidence and age-related changes for nicotinic but not muscarinic acetylcholine receptors in the central nervous system of *Sepia officinalis*. *Neuroscience Letters*, **387**(3): 162–167.

Bengoetxea, H., Ortuzar, N., Bulnes, S., Rico-Barrio, I., Lafuente, J. V. and Argandoña, E. G. (2012). Enriched and deprived sensory experience induces structural changes and rewires connectivity during the postnatal development of the brain. *Neural Plasticity*, **2012**: 1–10.

Billings, V. C., Sullivan, M. and Vine, H. (2000). Sighting of *Thysanoteuthis rhombus* egg mass in Indonesian waters and observations of embryonic development. *Journal of the Marine Biological Association of the United Kingdom*, **80**: 1139–1140.

Boal, J. G. and Golden, D. K. (1999). Distance chemoreception in the common cuttlefish, *Sepia officinalis* (Mollusca cephalopoda). *Journal of Experimental Marine Biology and Ecology*, **235**: 307–317.

Boal, J. G. and Marsh, S. E. (1998). Social recognition using chemical cues in cuttlefish (*Sepia officinalis* Linnaeus, 1758). *Journal of Experimental Marine Biology and Ecology*, **230**: 183–192.

Boletzky, S. v. (1983). *Sepia officinalis*. In *Cephalopod Life Cycles, Species Accounts*, Boyle P. R. (ed.), vol. 1. New York: Academic Press.

Boletzky, S. v. (1987). Juvenile behaviour. In *Cephalopod Life Cycles, Comparative Reviews*, Boyle P. R. (ed.), vol. 2. New York: Academic Press.

Boletzky, S. v. (2003). Biology of early stages in cephalopod molluscs. *Advances in Marine Biology*, **44**: 143–203.

Boyer, C., Maubert, E., Charnay, Y. and Chichery, R. (2007). Distribution of neurokinin A-like and serotonin immunoreactivities within the vertical lobe complex in *Sepia officinalis*. *Brain Research*, **1133**(1): 53–66.

Brown, C., Western, J. A. C. and Braithwaite, V. A. (2007). The influence of early experience on, and inheritance of, cerebral lateralization. *Animal Behaviour*, **74**: 231–238.

Brown, G. E. and Chivers, D. P. (2006). Learning about danger: chemical alarm cues and the assessment of predation risk by fishes. In *Fish Cognition and Behavior*, Brown, C., Laland, K. and Krause, J. (eds.). Oxford (UK): Wiley-Blackwell.

Budelmann, B. U. (1994). Cephalopod sense organs, nerves and the brain: adaptations for high performance and life style. *Marine and Freshwater Behaviour and Physiology*, **25**: 13–33.

Burghardt, G. M. (1967). The primacy effect of the first feeding experience in the snapping turtle. *Psychonomic Science*, **7**: 383–384.

Burghardt, G. M. and Hess, E. H. (1966). Food imprinting in the snapping turtle, *Chelydra serpentina*. *Science*, **151**: 108–109.

Buznikov, G. A., Shmukler, Y. B. and Lauder, J. M. (1996). From oocyte to neuron: do neurotransmitters function in the same way throughout development? *Cellular and Molecular Neurobiology*, **16**: 533–559.

Byrne, R. A., Kuba, M. and Griebel, U. (2002). Lateral asymmetry of eye use in *Octopus vulgaris*. *Animal Behaviour*, **64**: 461–468.

Byrne, R. A., Kuba, M. J. and Meisel, D. V. (2004). Lateralized eye use in *Octopus vulgaris* shows antisymmetrical distribution. *Animal Behaviour*, **68**: 1107–1114.

Caldwell, R. L. (2005). An observation of inking behavior protecting adult *Octopus bocki* from predation by green turtle (*Chelonia mydas*) hatchlings. *Pacific Science*, **59**: 69–72.

Carter, C. S. (2003). Developmental consequences of oxytocin. *Physiology and Behavior*, **79**(3): 383–397.

Chichery, M.-P. (1992). Approche neuroéthologique du comportement prédateur de la seiche *Sepia officinalis*. Doctorat d'Etat de l'Université de Caen Basse-Normandie.

Chichery, R. and Chanelet, J. (1976). Motor and behavioural responses obtained by stimulation with chronic electrodes of the optic lobe of *Sepia officinalis*. *Brain Research*, **105**: 525–532.

Chichery, R. and Chanelet, J. (1978). Motor responses obtained by stimulation of the peduncle lobe of *Sepia officinalis* in chronic experiments. *Brain Research*, **150**: 188–193.

Darmaillacq, A.-S. (2005). Plasticité des préférences alimentaires chez la seiche Sepia officinalis: approches ontogénétique et neuro-ethologique. Unpublished thesis (PhD), Université de Paris-Nord.

Darmaillacq, A.-S., Chichery, R. and Dickel, L. (2006). Food imprinting, new evidence from the cuttlefish *Sepia officinalis*. *Biology Letters*, **2**: 345–347.

Darmaillacq, A.-S., Chichery, R., Poirier, R. and Dickel, L. (2004). Effect of early feeding experience on subsequent prey preference by cuttlefish, *Sepia officinalis*. *Developmental Psychobiology*, **45**: 239–244.

Darmaillacq, A.-S., Chichery, R., Shashar, N. and Dickel, L. (2006). Early familiarization over-rides innate prey preference in newly-hatched *Sepia officinalis* cuttlefish. *Animal Behaviour*, **71**(3): 511–514.

Darmaillacq, A.-S., Lesimple, C. and Dickel, L. (2008). Embryonic visual learning in the cuttlefish, *Sepia officinalis*. *Animal Behaviour*, **76**: 131–134.

Daubert, E. A. and Condron, B. G. (2010). Serotonin: a regulator of neuronal morphology and circuitry. *Trends in Neuroscience*, **33**(9): 424–434.

Derby, C. D. (2007). Escape by inking and secreting: marine molluscs avoid predators through a rich array of chemicals and mechanisms. *The Biological Bulletin*, **213**: 274–289.

Dickel, L. (1997). Comportement prédateur et mémoire chez la seiche (*Sepia officinalis*), approches développementale et neuro-éthologique. Unpublished thesis (PhD), Université de Caen Basse-Normandie.

Dickel, L, Boal, J. G. and Budelmann, B. U. (2000). The effect of early experience on learning and memory in cuttlefish. *Developmental Psychobiology*, **36**(2): 101–110.

Dickel, L., Chichery, M.-P. and Chichery, R. (1997). Postembryonic maturation of the vertical lobe complex and early development of predatory behavior in the cuttlefish (*Sepia officinalis*). *Neurobiology of Learning and Memory*, **67**(2): 150–160.

Dickel, L., Chichery, M.-P. and Chichery, R. (1998). Time differences in the emergence of short- and long-term memory during post-embryonic development in the cuttlefish, *Sepia*. *Behavioural Processes*, **44**: 81–86.

Dickel, L., Chichery, M.-P. and Chichery, R. (2001). Increase of learning abilities and matura-tion of the vertical lobe complex during postembryonic development in the cuttlefish, *Sepia*. *Developmental Psychobiology*, **39**(2): 92–98.

Dickel, L., Darmaillacq, A.-S., Poirier, R., Agin, V., Bellanger, C. and Chichery, R. (2006). Behavioural and neural maturation in the cuttlefish *Sepia officinalis*. *Vie et Milieu*, **56**: 89–95.

Dobson, K. S., Dmetrichuk, J. M. and Spencer, G. E. (2006). Different receptors mediate the electrophysiological and growth cone responses of an identified neuron to applied dopamine. *Neuroscience*, **141**(4): 1801–1810.

Everitt, B. J. and Robbins, T. W. (1997). Central cholinergic systems and cognition. *Annual Review of Psychology*, **48**: 649–684.

Fiorito, G. and Scotto, P. (1992). Observational learning in *Octopus vulgaris*. *Science*, **256**: 545–247.

Frasnelli, E., Vallortigara, G. and Rogers, L. J. (2012). Left–right asymmetries of behaviour and nervous system in invertebrates. *Neuroscience and Biobehavioral Reviews*, **36**: 1273–1291.

Fresquet, N., Fournier, D. and Gauthier, M. (1998). A new attempt to assess the effect of learn-ing processes on the cholinergic system: studies on fruitflies and honeybees. *Comparative Biochemistry and Physiology B*, **119**(2): 349–353.

Gottlieb, G. (ed.) (1971). *Ontogenesis of Sensory Function in Birds and Mammals*. New York: Academic Press.

Graindorge, N., Alves, C., Darmaillacq, A.-S., Chichery, R., Dickel, L. and Bellanger, C. (2006). Effects of dorsal and ventral vertical lobe electrolytic lesions on the spatial learning and locomotor activity in *Sepia*. *Behavioral Neuroscience*, **120**: 1151–1158.

Granier-Deferre, C. and Busnel, M. C. (1983). Stimulations acoustiques au cours du développement du système auditif et adaptation au bruit chez la souris. *International Journal of Audiology*, **22**: 280–310.

Grant, P., Tseng, D., Gould, R. M., Gainer, H. and Pant, H. C. (1995). Expression of neurofilament proteins during development of the nervous system in the squid *Loligo pealei*. *Journal of Comparative Neurology*, **356**(2): 311–326.

Guerra, A. (2006). Ecology of *Sepia officinalis*. *Vie et Milieu*, **56**: 97–107.

Guibé, M., Boal, J. G. and Dickel, L. (2010). Early exposure to odors changes later visual prey preferences in cuttlefish. *Developmental Psychobiology*, **52**: 833–837.

Guibé, M. and Dickel, L. (2011). Embryonic visual experience influences posthatching shelter preference in cuttlefish. *Vie Milieu*, **61**(4): 243–246.

Guibé, M., Poirel, N., Houdé, O. and Dickel, L. (2012). Food imprinting and visual generalization in embryos and newly hatched cuttlefish (*Sepia officinalis*). *Animal Behaviour*, **84**: 213–217.

Hanlon, R. T. and Messenger, J. B. (1988). Adaptive coloration in young cuttlefish (*Sepia officinalis* L.): the morphology and development of body patterns and their relation to behaviour. *Philosophical Transactions of the Royal Society of London. Series B*, **320**: 437–487.

Hanlon, R. T. and Messenger, J. B. (eds.) (1996). *Cephalopod Behaviour*. Cambridge (UK): Cambridge University Press.

Healy, S. D. (2006). Imprinting: seeing food and eating it. *Current Biology*, **13**: R501.

Henriksen, R., Rettenbacher, S. and Groothuis, T. G. G. (2011). Prenatal stress in birds: pathways, effects, function and perspectives. *Neuroscience and Biobehavioral Reviews*, **35**: 1484–1501.

van Heteren, C. F., Boekkooi, P. F., Jongsma, H. W. and Nijhuis, J. G. (2001). Fetal habituation to vibroacoustic stimulation in relation to fetal states and fetal heart rate parameters. *Early Human Development*, **61**: 135–145.

Honeycutt, H. and Lickliter, R. (2003). The influence of prenatal tactile and vestibular stimulation on auditory and visual responsiveness in bobwhite quail: a matter of timing. *Developmental Psychobiology*, **43**(2): 71–81.

Iversen, S. D. and Iversen, L. L. (2007). Dopamine: 50 years in perspective. *Trends in Neuroscience*, **30**(5): 188–193.

Jabès, A., Lavenex, P. B., Amaral, D. G. and Lavenex, P. (2010). Quantitative analysis of postnatal neurogenesis and neuron number in the macaque monkey dentate gyrus. *European Journal of Neuroscience*, **31**: 273–285.

Jozet-Alves, C. and Hébert, M. (2012). Embryonic exposure to predator odour modulates visual lateralization in cuttlefish. *Proceedings of the Royal Society. B: Biological Sciences*, **280**(1752): 20122575.

Jozet-Alves, C., Romagny, S., Bellanger, C. and Dickel, L. (2012). Cerebral correlates of visual lateralization in *Sepia*. *Behavioural Brain Research*, **234**: 20–25.

Jozet-Alves, C., Viblanc, V., Romagny, S., Dacher, M., Healy, S. D. and Dickel, L. (2012). Visual lateralization is task- and age-dependent in cuttlefish (*Sepia officinalis*). *Animal Behaviour*, **83**: 1313–1318.

King, A. J. and Adamo, S. A. (2006). The ventilatory, cardiac and behavioural responses of resting cuttlefish (*Sepia officinalis* L.) to sudden visual stimuli. *Journal of Experimental Biology*, **209**: 1101–1111.

Krasnegor, N. A., Blass, E. M., Hofer, M. A. and Smotherman, W. (eds.) (1987). *Perinatal Development: A Psychobiological Perspective*. New York: Academic Press.

Lemaire, J. (1970). Table de développement embryonnaire de *Sepia officinalis* L. (Mollusque céphalopode). *Bulletin de la Société Zoologique de France*, **95**: 773–782.

Letzkus, P., Boeddeker, N., Wood, J. T., Zhang, S. W. and Srinivasan, M. V. (2008). Lateralization of visual learning in the honeybee. *Biology Letters*, **4**: 16–19.

Letzkus, P., Ribi, W. A., Wood, J. T., Zhu, H., Zhang, S. W. and Srinivasan, M. V. (2006). Lateralization of olfaction in the honeybee *Apis mellifera*. *Current Biology*, **16**: 1471–1476.

Lickliter, R. (1993). Timing and the development of perinatal perceptual organization. In *Developmental Time and Timing*, Turkewitz G. and Devenny D. A. (eds.). Hillsdale, NJ: Erlbaum.

Magat, M. and Brown, C. (2009). Laterality enhances cognition in Australian parrots. *Proceedings of the Royal Society. B: Biological Sciences*, **276**: 4155–4162.

Messenger, J. B. (1968). The visual attack of the cuttlefish, *Sepia officinalis*. *Animal Behaviour*, **16**: 342–357.

Messenger, J. B. (1971). Two stage recovery of a response in *Sepia*. *Nature*, **232**: 202–203.

Messenger, J. B. (1973). Learning performance and brain structure: a study in development. *Brain Research*, **58**: 519–523.

Messenger, J. B. (1996). Neurotransmitters of cephalopods. *Invertebrate Neuroscience*, **2**(2): 95–114.

Messenger, J. B. and Sanders, G. D. (1972). Visual preference and two-cue discrimination learning in *Octopus*. *Animal Behaviour*, **20**: 580–585.

Mpitsos, G. J., Murray, T. F., Creech, H. C. and Barker, D. L. (1988). Muscarinic antagonist enhances one-trial food-aversion learning in the mollusc Pleurobranchaea. *Brain Research Bulletin*, **21**(2): 169–179.

Nixon, M. and Mangold, K. (1998). The early life of *Sepia officinalis*, and the contrast with that of *Octopus vulgaris* (Cephalopoda). *Journal of Zoology*, **245**(4): 407–421.

Nixon, M. and Young, J. Z. (eds.) (2003). *The Brains and Lives of Cephalopods*. New York: Oxford University Press.

Packard, A. (1972). Cephalopods and fish: the limits of convergence. *Biological Reviews*, **47**: 241–307.

Pascual, A., Huang, K.-L., Nevue, J. and Préat, T. (2004). Brain asymmetry and long-term memory. *Nature*, **427**: 605–606.

Poirier, R. (2004). Expérience précoce et ontogenèse des comportements défensifs chez la seiche (*Sepia officinalis*): approches comportementales et neurobiologiques. Unpublished thesis (PhD), Université de Caen Basse-Normandie.

Poirier, R., Chichery, R. and Dickel, L. (2004). Effect of rearing conditions on sand digging efficiency in juvenile cuttlefish. *Behavioural Processes*, **67**(2): 273–279.

Poirier, R., Chichery, R. and Dickel, L. (2005). Early experience and postembryonic maturation of body patterns in cuttlefish (*Sepia officinalis*). *Journal of Comparative Psychology*, **119**(2): 230–237.

Punzo, F. (2002). Food imprinting and subsequent prey preference in the lynx spider, *Oxyopes salticus*. *Behavioural Processes*, **58**: 177–181.

Riederer, B. M. (1992). Differential phosphorylation of some proteins of the neuronal cytoskeleton during brain development. *The Histochemical Journal*, **24**: 783–790.

Rogers, L. J. (2007). Lateralization in its many forms, and its evolution and development. In *The Evolution of Hemispheric Specialization in Primates, Special Topics in Primatology*, Hopkins, W. D. (ed.), vol. 5. Amsterdam: Elsevier.

Rogers, L. J., Zucca, P. and Vallortigara, G. (2004). Advantages of having a lateralized brain. *Proceedings of the Royal Society. B: Biological Sciences*, **271**(Suppl): S420–422.

Romagny, S. (2010). Ontogeny of the sensory systems and early learning in the cuttlefish, *Sepia officinalis*: behavioural and neurobiological approaches. Unpublished thesis (MSc), Université Paris 13.

Romagny, S., Darmaillacq, A.-S., Guibé, M., Bellanger, C. and Dickel, L. (2012). Feel, smell and see: emergence of perception and learning in an immature invertebrate, the cuttlefish embryo. *Journal of Experimental Biology*, **215**: 4125–4130.

Sanders, F. K. and Young, J. Z. (1940). Learning and other functions of the higher nervous centres of *Sepia*. *Journal of Neurophysiology*, **3**: 501–526.

Sanders, G. D. (1975). The cephalopods. In *Invertebrate Learning*, Corning, W. C., Dyal, J. A. and Willows, A. O. D. (eds.), vol 3. New York: Plenum Press.

Schaal, B. (1988). Olfaction in infants and children: developmental and functional perspectives. *Chemical Senses*, **13**: 145–190.

Shettleworth, S. J. (ed.) (2010). *Cognition, Evolution and Behaviour*. New York: Oxford University Press.

Shomrat, T., Graindorge, N., Bellanger, C., Fiorito, G., Loewenstein, Y. and Hochner, B. (2011). Alternative sites of synaptic plasticity in two homologous "Fan-out Fan-in" learning and memory networks. *Current Biology*, **21**: 1773–1782.

Sluckin, W. (ed.) (2007). *Imprinting and Early Learning*, 2nd edn. Piscataway, NJ: Aldine Transaction.

Smotherman, W. P. and Robinson, S. R. (1992). Prenatal experience with milk: fetal behavior and endogenous opioid systems. *Neuroscience and Biobehavioral Reviews*, **16**: 351–364.

Stasiak, M. (2002). The development of food preferences in cats: the new direction. *Nutritional Neuroscience*, **5**: 221–228.

Vallortigara, G. and Bisazza, A. (2002). How ancient is brain lateralization? In *Comparative Vertebrate Lateralization*, Andrew R. J. and Rogers L. J. (eds.). Cambridge: Cambridge University Press.

Vallortigara, G. and Rogers, L. J. (2005). Survival with an asymmetrical brain: advantages and disadvantages of cerebral lateralization. *Behavioral and Brain Sciences*, **28**: 575–633.

Vauclair, J. (1996). *La cognition animale. Que sais-je?* Paris: Presses Universitaires de France.

Wasserman, E. A. and Zentall, T. R. (eds.) (2006). *Comparative Cognition: Experimental Explorations of Animal Intelligence*. New York: Oxford University Press.

Wells, M. J. (1962). Early learning in *Sepia*. *Symposia of the Zoological Society of London*, **8**: 149–159.

Wirz, K. (1954). Etudes quantitatives sur le système nerveux des Céphalopodes. *Comptes rendus de l'Académie des sciences, Paris*, **238**: 1353–1355.

Young, J. Z. (1965). Influence of previous preferences on the memory of *Octopus vulgaris* after removal of the vertical lobe. *Journal of Experimental Biology*, **43**: 595–603.

Young, J. Z. (1979). The nervous system of *Loligo*. V: the vertical complex. *Philosophical Transactions of the Royal Society of London. Series B*, **285**: 311–354.

2 Evolution of behavioral and neural complexity: learning and memory in Chambered *Nautilus*

Jennifer Basil and Robyn Crook

We study learning in the ancient cephalopod *Nautilus pompilius* as a way of understanding how cognition and neural complexity may have evolved in its more derived relatives, the coleoid cephalopods (octopuses, cuttlefish and squid), whose brains are heavily invested in learning and memory. *Nautilus* retains a relatively primitive brain compared with the brains of coleoids, which are among the most complex of all the invertebrates. Coleoid brains contain several discrete lobes dedicated to learning and memory storage – the vertical and frontal lobe complexes. The nautilus central nervous system lacks known homologs or analogs of these regions, and instead the brain more likely approximates those of the ancestors of the two extant subclasses. Nautilus is, therefore, uniquely placed in this lineage for studies of the evolution and origin of cognition, including learning and memory. Our laboratory identifies and characterizes learning, memory formation, composition and retrieval in *Nautilus* through controlled classical-conditioning studies and behavioral assays with free-moving animals. In studies of classical conditioning where a light predicted the reward of food, nautiluses learned rapidly, expressing temporally separated short-term and long-term memory. Short-term memory in *Nautilus* was similar to that of coleoids, but long-term memory was of shorter duration. Spatial-memory studies in mazes reveal far more complex learning and memory than the "primitive brain" of nautiluses might predict. Providing increasingly complex cue arrays to be learned for spatial navigation to a goal, we tested nautiluses in cognitive tasks similar to those studied in coleoids. Our studies suggest that despite lacking the dedicated neural structures of its more derived relatives, nautiluses perform surprisingly well at cognitive tasks, and show flexibility in what they can learn and remember, even simultaneously. Perhaps the antecedent of the vertical or frontal lobe may be present in the *Nautilus* brain or there is an analogue in existing structures. Either of these possibilities may be identified through future electrophysiological and neuroanatomical experiments.

2.1 Introduction and comparative approaches

Cephalopod mollusks are a unique taxon for the comparative study of cognition because: (1) they exhibit complex behavior; (2) there is substantial variety in the natural histories

Cephalopod Cognition, eds A.-S. Darmaillacq, L. Dickel and J. Mather. Published by Cambridge University Press. © Cambridge 2014.

of the cephalopods that may contribute to behavioral differences; (3) their neuroanatomy shares many convergent features with vertebrate organization; (4) the brain of extant Chambered *Nautilus* retains primitive features of the cephalopod lineage, while the coleoid brain is highly derived and specialized; yet (5) we have discovered complex behaviors in nautiluses that overlap with those of their relatives, offering an exceptional opportunity for phylogenetic analysis of cognition not available in many other closely related lineages. To this end we characterize underlying factors shaping associative learning of ecologically relevant stimuli in nautiluses. Our aim is to reveal adaptive constraints contributing to cognition, large brains and fast and flexible processing by careful comparative study of a class that expresses both the ancestral and derived conditions in extant species.

Cephalopods are a diverse and successful group of mollusks. All living species belong to either the coleoidea (internal, reduced or absent shell: squids, octopuses, cuttlefishes, 600–800 species) or the nautiloidea (external, chambered shell: limited to two genera and perhaps five total species (Bonnaud, Ozouf-Costaz & Boucher-Rodoni, 2004; Saunders & Landman, 1987; Ward & Saunders, 1997)). A major contributing factor to the divergence of these two subclasses was a period of intense competition with vertebrates about 380 million years ago (MYA) (Aronson, 1991; Chamberlain, 1993; Grasso & Basil, 2009; Packard, 1972). The complex behavioral abilities of coleoids are thought to have developed from a "cognitive radiation" during this period, which minimized competition with fishes, as coleoids cannot outperform them (Chamberlain, 1993). Nautiloids also avoid fishes, but in a fundamentally different way. Coleoids opt for a "live fast/die young," r-selected, reproductive lifestyle characterized by rapid growth, fast metabolic rates, active hunting and voracious feeding. Nautiloids rely instead upon a "live slow/die old," k-selected lifestyle, where they dwell in cold, deep waters, avoiding predation and competition with most teleosts by scavenging in darkness rather than active hunting. Because they spend most of their time at depth, little is known of the cognitive behavior of the *Nautilus* and the theory that a "cognitive radiation" in coleoids served to minimize niche overlaps with day-hunting teleosts (Aronson, 1991; Chamberlain, 1990, 1993; Packard, 1972) developed largely in the absence of much information on the behavior of nautiluses. In the past few years, researchers have identified surprising cognitive abilities in *Nautilus*, casting these theories in a new light. Perhaps the cephalopod brain entering this period of intense competition millions of years ago was already large and capable of complex behaviors (Grasso & Basil, 2009) having previously coped with repeated periods of rapid diversification and competition following mass die offs.

2.2   Sensory ecology

An understanding of the internal world view of *Nautilus* (Figure 2.1) is essential to develop hypotheses about their cognitive abilities and to identify relevant ecological pressures shaping their behavior (Kamil, 1994; Tinbergen, 1963). *Nautilus* lives among

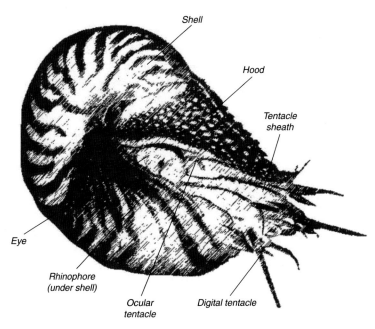

Shell

Hood

Tentacle
sheath

Eye

Rhinophore
(under shell)

Ocular
tentacle

Digital tentacle

Figure 2.1 Chambered *Nautilus*, with pertinent anatomical features labeled. External shell is chambered, with the animal residing in the front chamber only. Hood can close, protecting the animal inside the first chamber. Up to 90 distinct tentacles can be retracted into sheaths when at rest. Olfactory rhinophores lie below each eye, exposed to the exterior by a narrow pore.

the coral reefs of the Indo-Pacific, remaining in dimly lit waters at depths up to 300 m for most of its life. They undergo daily vertical migrations, traveling to shallower, warmer waters (75 m) to forage amidst coral reefs during night-time hours and make brief excursions throughout the day (Carlson, McKibben & De Gruy, 1984; Dunstan, Ward & Marschall, 2011; Ward, Carlson, Weekly & Brumbaugh, 1984). At depth nautiluses are likely to rely heavily upon chemical and tactile sensory modalities, especially since they are primarily nocturnal. The structure of the large but primitive pinhole eye of *Nautilus* also suggests vision may not be an essential sensory system for foraging (Messenger, 1991) as it is for other modern cephalopods (Hanlon & Messenger, 1996; Messenger, 1991; Muntz, 1986, 2010a; Muntz & Raj, 1984). Coleoid cephalopods have well-developed eyes with acute vision (Budelmann, 1995) and large optic lobes for processing visual input (Nixon & Young, 2003). While the eyes of *Nautilus* lack lenses, they are extremely large to capture as much light as possible in a dim environment and tuned to wavelengths (470 nm) commonly produced by bioluminescent organisms. Nautiluses are also positively phototactic (Muntz, 1986, 2010a, 2010b). Recent laboratory experiments (Crook & Basil, 2008a, 2013; Crook, Hanlon & Basil, 2009) reveal that nautiluses can use visual stimuli to learn simple associations and also to locate goals in complex spatial arrays (horizontal shallow-water mazes and vertical artificial reefs). Vision may play a greater role in their lives than previously thought, and it may be that food items such as decaying organisms provide both visual and olfactory cues to a scavenging nautilus in the wild. Nautiluses associating these kinds of stimuli to predict the presence or location of a food item based upon experience is likely important for their survival. Recalling good hiding locations in the coral reefs where they live would also be adaptive for an animal with few defenses other than an external shell (nautiluses lack ink, are relatively slow moving and do not have the capacity for active crypsis).

Nautiluses seem to be specialized for a "smelling and groping" lifestyle (Hanlon & Messenger, 1996; Saunders, 1985). A pair of olfactory organs (rhinophores), one located below each eye, is open to the exterior by a narrow pore (Figure 2.1; Barber & Wright, 1969; Ruth, Schmidtberg, Westermann & Schipp, 2002). Coleoids also bear rhinophores (Gilly & Lucero, 1992; Woodhams & Messenger, 1974) and have extensive tactile and chemical sensitivity in their suckers (Graziadei, 1964). The rhinophores of nautiluses are similar to the olfactory organs in *Octopus* and other cephalopods but are significantly larger, as are the olfactory lobes in the brain of *Nautilus* to which they project (Young, 1965a). The epithelium of their rhinophores possesses cells that are similar to chemoreceptors located in the sucker of *Octopus*, the olfactory structure of squids and the lip of *Sepia* (Emery, 1975; Gilly & Lucero, 1992; Graziadei, 1964; Lucero, Horrigan & Gilly, 1992; Ruth, Schmidtberg, Westermann & Schipp, 2002). The paired rhinophores are essential for orientation to food odor, especially at a distance (Basil et al., 2005; Basil, Hanlon, Sheikh & Atema, 2000), and nautiluses use odor to discriminate between males and females at short range (Basil, Lazemby, Nakanuku & Hanlon, 2002; Westermann & Beuerlein, 2005). Odor on a variety of spatial scales is, therefore, an important source of information to nautiluses in their complex coral-reef environment. Olfactory memory for predators and prey, along with possible mates, may be important to their survival in the wild.

Cephalopod arms and tentacles actively collect sensory information from their environment and nautiluses are no exception. Coleoid cephalopods have either 8 or 10 sucker-bearing appendages, while nautiluses possess a large array of up to 90 tentacles, lacking suckers and retracted into sheaths when the animals are at rest. These tentacles are covered in both mechanosensory (Kier, 1987) and chemosensory structures (Fukuda, 1980). Ruth, Schmidtberg, Westermann and Schipp (2002) described ciliated cells on the epithelium of the tentacles, suggesting they serve both a chemosensory and mechanosensory function at a variety of spatial scales. When the rhinophore is stimulated by odor, nautiluses extend their tentacles up to a shell length in a stereotyped posture and swim in the odor plume toward the source of the odor (Basil, Hanlon, Sheikh & Atema, 2000; Bidder, 1962), from up to 10 m away. Tentacle extension is in general a reliable and quantifiable measure of arousal in nautiluses (Basil et al., 2005; Basil, Hanlon, Sheikh & Atema, 2000; Bidder, 1962; Crook & Basil, 2008a; Ruth, Schmidtberg, Westermann & Schipp, 2002). We have demonstrated in a naturalistic odor-tracking paradigm, and by reversible rhinophore blockage, that *Nautilus*: (1) detects highly dilute odors at a distance of up to 10 m; (2) uses turbulent odor-plume information to locate the distant odor source; and (3) relies upon its paired rhinophores to track the odor accurately (Basil et al., 2005; Basil, Hanlon, Sheikh & Atema, 2000). Stimulation of the digital tentacles initiates near-field food-searching behavior (digging, etc; Basil et al., 2005). Clearly, complex odor and tactile stimuli are of great importance to these animals in their deep-sea, coral-reef habitat where little light penetrates.

Another possible source of environmental information in deep water is vibration and nautiluses detect and respond to underwater vibrations (Soucier & Basil, 2008). Nautiluses slowed their breathing in response to vibrations, especially when the source of the vibration was within 20 cm. When the amplitude and frequency of vibrations increased, nautiluses decreased their respirations further (Soucier & Basil, 2008). Potential receptors for environmental vibratory stimuli (e.g. snapping shrimp, etc.) include the mechanosensory receptors found on their tentacles and also at the base of their rhinophores (Ruth, Schmidtberg, Westermann & Schipp, 2002). Based on their responses to environmentally relevant stimuli, nautiluses can collect detailed information on many scales about a suite of environmental factors. Learning to associate these stimuli and remember their location would be advantageous in an animal with few defenses living in a complex, deep-sea environment.

2.3   Neural systems

Coleoid cephalopods have developed heavily modified brains that include dedicated learning and memory centers (Figure 2.2; vertical lobe and superior frontal lobe; Agin, Chichery, Maubert & Chichery, 2003; Boycott & Young, 1955; Dickel, Chichery & Chichery, 2001; Graindorge et al., 2006; Hochner, Shomrat & Fiorito, 2006; Young, 1960, 1988; Young & Boycott, 1971). In fact, coleoid brains have been proposed to converge with the vertebrate brain in organization (see Hochner, Shomrat & Fiorito, 2006 for review; Boyle, 1986; Kandel, 1976; Nixon & Young, 2003; Wells, 1978; Young, 1965b, 1991), with shorter connectives and synaptic morphology consistent with fast and flexible neural processing (Hochner, Shomrat & Fiorito, 2006). When the vertical lobe is ablated or lesioned in octopuses and cuttlefishes, learning and memory of certain stimuli are abolished (Boycott, 1961; Boycott & Young, 1955; Graindorge et al., 2006; Maldonado, 1965; Wells, 1978; Young, 1991). Observational learning, a complex cognitive behavior exhibited by coleoids (Fiorito & Scotto, 1992), also requires the vertical lobe (Fiorito & Chichery, 1995). Ecology impacts the organization of the coleoid brain. There is parametric variation in memory abilities and neural systems among coleoids depending upon their primary habitat. Many octopods have a well developed chemo-tactile memory system (subfrontal lobe) suited for their benthic habitat. This area of the brain is absent or poorly developed in pelagic octopods, which do not display complex chemo-tactile learning and memory, illustrating an ecological impact on brain and behavior (Young, 1964). On a cellular level, long-term memory formation in cuttlefish is dependent upon de novo protein synthesis at distinct time points after learning (Agin, Chichery, Maubert & Chichery, 2003) as in other animals (Davis & Squire, 1984; Stork & Welzl, 1999). Short-term memory in vertebrates and in invertebrates is mediated by transient changes in synaptic morphology (for a review of invertebrates and vertebrates, see Stork & Welzl, 1999). The neuroanatomy of dedicated learning

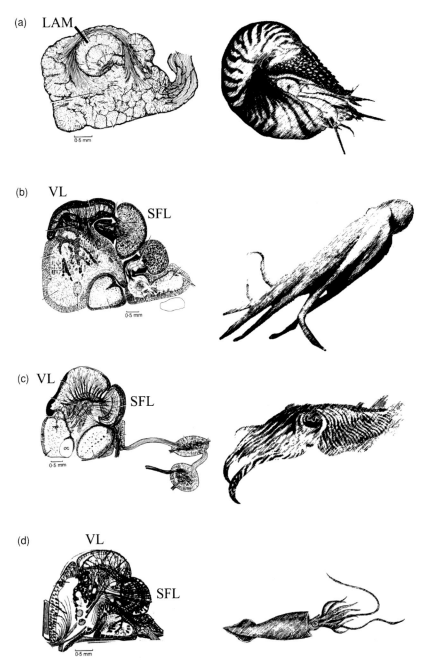

Figure 2.2 Comparison of cephalopod brains. (a) Nautiloids, (b) Octopods, (c) Cuttlefishes, (d) Squids. The vertical lobe complex (VL) plays a substantial role in learning and memory in coleoids, but is not found in nautiluses. The laminated area of the olfactory lobe (LAM) in nautiloids lies in a similar position to the vertical lobe complex in coleoids. SFL = subfrontal lobe complex. (Modified from Maddock & Young, 1987; figure reproduced from Grasso & Basil, 2009, with permission from S. Karger AG, Medical and Scientific Publishers, Basel.)

and memory structures of coleoids supports the hypothesis of anatomical convergence with vertebrates, especially since the cellular spiking properties and neuroanatomical arrangement conserve ancient molluskan features (for a review, see Hochner, Shomrat & Fiorito, 2006).

Nautiluses have a simple ring-shaped brain with little internal differentiation (Figure 2.2; Maddock & Young, 1987; Young, 1965a) and with only 13 lobes in contrast to the 38 found in squid and 40 in Octopus (Hochner, Shomrat & Fiorito, 2006; Young, 1965b; Young & Boycott, 1971), though the nautilid brain is considerably larger than the brains of other mollusks (Aplysia: Carew & Sahley, 1986; Kandel & Schwartz, 1982; Hermissenda: Alkon et al., 1990; Blackwell, 2006; Snails: Benjamin, 2000; Gelperin & Culligan, 1984). Recent embryological evidence (Sasaki, Shigeno & Tanabe, 2010; Shigeno et al., 2008; Shigeno, Takenori & Boletzky, 2010) suggests that nautilus retains features of the neural arrangement of the common cephalopod ancestor, which may help to illuminate how brain and cognitive complexity arose in the cephalopod lineage as a whole.

Of crucial importance is the apparent *absence* in nautilus of any defined structures analogous to the vertical or superior frontal lobe of coleoids (e.g. Boycott & Young, 1955; Young, 1965a). It is not surprising that the brain of *Nautilus* has a greatly expanded olfactory lobe, with their reliance on olfactory stimuli. One possible analog to coleoid learning-and-memory centers is the laminated area of the olfactory lobe (Figure 2.2, LAM) and surrounding cerebral nerve cord, located in a similar region in nautilus as the vertical lobe in coleoids (Young, 1965a). This laminated area receives input from the plexiform region (Figure 2.2), which integrates information from the visual and tactile systems of the animal (Young, 1965a). Based on its location and projections, the plexiform region is a likely comparator to the superior frontal lobes of coleoids. Perhaps the basic neural arrangement of nautiloids is conserved, although greatly expanded in coleoids, or nautiluses use another area of the brain entirely to support their learning (Grasso & Basil, 2009). There are currently no studies identifying regions in the nautilus brain essential for learning and memory as there are for coleoids.

2.4   Associative conditioning

Animals with simple neural organization, including mollusks, have proven invaluable to our understanding of learning and memory (for a review, see: Burrell & Sahley, 2001; Carew & Sahley, 1986; Milner, Squire & Kandel, 1998). A number of feeding and avoidance reflexes in the marine mollusk *Aplysia* can be classically conditioned and the neural, synaptic and cellular properties mediating learning have been well characterized (Baxter & Byrne, 2006; Brembs, Baxter & Byrne, 2004; Carew & Sahley, 1986; Kandel, 1976; Kandel & Schwartz, 1982). The marine mollusk *Hermissenda* can learn to associate a light with turbulence, which is adaptive for an organism that must brace itself against incoming wave action during storms (Blackwell, 2006; Crow, 2004; Crow & Alkon, 1978). Importantly, simple invertebrate learning systems share fundamental physiological and molecular features in common with variety of animal groups (e.g. Burrell & Sahley, 2001; Kandel & Tauc, 1965; *Hermissenda*: Blackwell, 2006; *Aplysia*: Walters, 1991; Walters, Alizadeh & Castro, 1991; *Lymnaea*: Benjamin, 2000; Snails: Gelperin & Culligan, 1984; Insects: Davis, 2005, including vertebrates, e.g. Fanselow & Poulos, 2005). Even in animals with simple neural systems, learning can occur rapidly and memory can persist for long periods of time. This is true of *Nautilus* (Crook & Basil, 2008a, 2008b, 2013; Crook, Hanlon & Basil, 2009; Grasso & Basil, 2009) and also coleoids. It is probably adaptive for animals to detect salient features in their environment and predict them, but there are also costs from a high investment in learning and memory (and supporting structures). Since nautilus retains pleisiomorphic neural features of the cephalopod lineage – a lineage known for its advanced learning capabilities – a thorough understanding of the capabilities of nautilus allows us to predict and test what adaptive role learning and memory has played in shaping cephalopod cognition.

Coleoids exhibit a range of cognitive behaviors (reviewed in Alves, Chichery, Boal & Dickel, 2007; Hanlon & Messenger, 1996; Mather, 1995; Nixon & Young, 2003; Wells, 1978) including imprinting (Darmaillacq, Chichery & Dickel, 2006; Darmaillacq, Chichery, Shashar & Dickel, 2006), associative learning (Agin, Chichery, Dickel & Chichery, 2006; Agin, Dickel, Chichery & Chichery, 1998; Agin, Poirier, Chichery, Dickel & Chichery, 2006; Darmaillacq, Dickel, Chichery, Agin & Chichery, 2004), discriminative learning (Boal, 1996; Cole & Adamo, 2005; Hvorecny et al., 2007; Sutherland, 1963), observational learning (Fiorito & Scotto, 1992; Suboski, Muir & Hall, 1993) and short- and long-term memory (Agin, Poirier, Chichery, Dickel & Chichery, 2006; Sanders, 1970). Behavioral changes as a result of learning are long lasting in relation to coleoids' typically brief lifespan (Agin, Dickel, Chichery & Chichery, 1998; Alves, Chichery, Boal & Dickel, 2007; Boal, 1991; Boal, Dunham, Williams & Hanlon, 2000; Darmaillacq, Dickel, Chichery, Agin & Chichery, 2004; Hanlon & Messenger, 1996; Messenger, 1973). Coleoid cephalopods can be operantly conditioned to avoid attacking a prawn contained within a hard Plexiglas tube (Agin, Chichery, Dickel & Chichery, 2006; Cartron, Darmaillacq & Dickel, 2013) and with this paradigm researchers have discovered that cuttlefish possess temporally separated short and long-term memory stores (Agin, Dickel, Chichery & Chichery, 1998; Agin, Poirier, Chichery, Dickel & Chichery, 2006; Messenger, 1973). For comparison, we have used associative-conditioning techniques to probe the memory profile of Chambered *Nautilus*.

In classical associative conditioning, an initially neutral conditioned stimulus (CS, e.g. bell) becomes associated with an unconditioned stimulus (US, e.g. food) and subsequently elicits a response on its own (the conditioned response, CR, e.g. salivation) previously only initiated by the US (Pavlov, 1927). Models of classical conditioning (e.g. Pavlov, 1927; Rescorla & Wagner, 1972) posit that: (1) learning can be thought of in terms of a change in association strength between the CS and the US; and that (2) variation in stimulus salience and CS/US timing or pairing can contribute to changes in the strength of the association. A hallmark of classical conditioning is that the CS must precede the US in a reliable way. The period between them should not be too great or the associative strength will lessen. This is true across a variety of animal phyla (e.g. Bees: Bitterman, Menzel, Fietz & Schäfer, 1983; Menzel, Leboulle & Eisenhardt, 2006; Mollusks: Blackwell, 2006; Vertebrates: Rescorla & Wagner, 1972). According

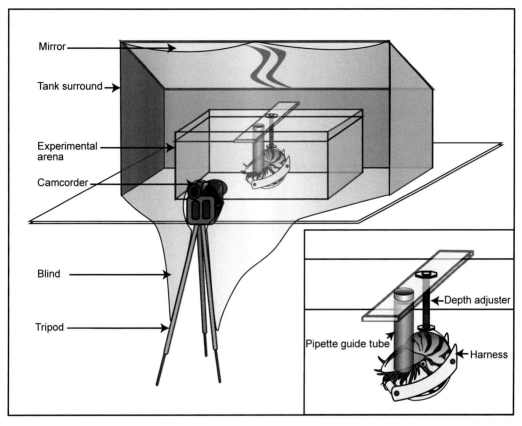

Figure 2.3 Classical conditioning aquarium. A small light is flashed onto the back of the tank (conditioned stimulus) to create a dispersed 470 nm illumination of the tank for 1 s and to avoid direct contact with the eye of the animal. The harness holding the shell (inset) aids in controlled delivery of the odor reward (unconditioned stimulus) via the guide tube, 1 s later. Tentacles are free to respond to either of the stimuli and behavior is captured on video by a camera 0.5 m from the harness. (Reproduced from Crook and Basil (2008a), with permission from Company of Biologists, Ltd.)

to models like those of Rescorla and Wagner (1972), after the association is learned associative strength will decline if the CS is occasionally not followed by the US in a predictable way, or at all. When there is no US present as expected, a discrepancy arises. This results in both unlearning of the association and a learning of the absence of the US. The CS subsequently loses associative strength on each trial where this is the case until it has none at all and the animal no longer responds (extinction).

For our studies, we used a pairing of light (CS) to signal a food-odor reward (US) in an experimental aquarium where the nautilus was held in place in a harness by its shell, allowing it tentacles to freely extend (CR) (Figure 2.3, conditioning apparatus; Crook & Basil, 2008a). In forward-paired conditioning, or CS+ trials, 2 ml of fish-head stimulus (US) was taken into a pipette, which was inserted into a guide tube attached to the harness for release onto the rhinophores. A blue light (470 nm, CS) was flashed for 500 ms against a predetermined spot on the back of the experimental tank. With a

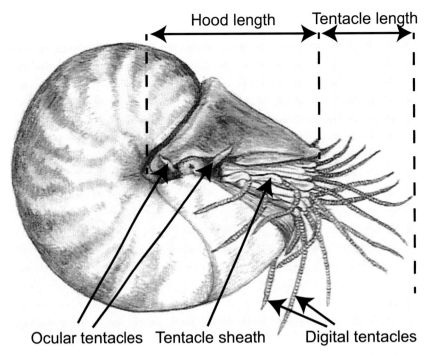

Figure 2.4 Tentacle extension response (TER), calculated from tentacle length/hood proportion. TER is used as a conditioned response in associative conditioning as a measure of learning the association between a light pulse (conditioned stimulus) and an odor reward (unconditioned stimulus). Tentacles are retracted when at rest and can extend up to a full body length from their sheaths when the animals are aroused. (Reproduced from Crook and Basil (2008a), with permission from Company of Biologists, Ltd.)

delay of 1 s, the odor reward was released from the pipette (Figure 2.3, inset). We ranked stereotyped tentacle extension over the following 10 min, as the CR during acquisition and then at various delays after training, to probe the nature of short-term (ST) and long-term (LT) memory (tentacle extension response [TER], Figure 2.4; modified from bee proboscis extension response [PER]; Bitterman, Menzel, Fietz & Schäfer, 1983; Chandra, Hosler & Smith, 2000; Menzel, Leboulle & Eisenhardt, 2006; Smith, 1997; Smith & Cobey, 1994).

Memory testing began after the last trial of training to map the time course of short-term and long-term memory. We tested the following memory-retention intervals: 3 min, 30 min, 1 h, 6 h, 12 h and 24 h post training (counterbalanced to control for any experiential effects). For each retention interval, separate animals were tested with a single unrewarded presentation of the light (CS) and their tentacle extension responses measured for 3 min. Excitatory conditioning is thought to be pairing dependent, with the CS predicting the US in a reliable way. To determine that excitatory conditioning had occurred, we also assessed learning and memory with an explicitly unpaired group, where the US was presented at random intervals relative to the CS (CS−). After training, retention was tested in this group at the same intervals as above.

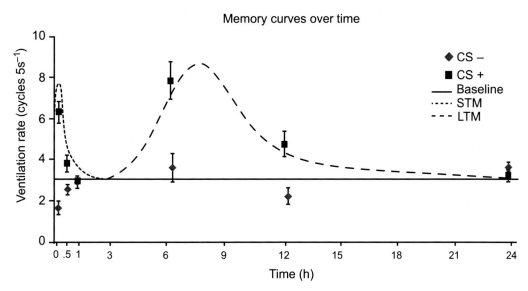

Figure 2.5 Biphasic memory profile during associative conditioning. Y axis: Proportion of trials with a tentacle extension response; X axis: Time after initial training. In excitatory forward-paired (CS+) , trials (black), there is a peak of memory at 1 h after training that drops and then rises again at about 6 h, declining until 24 h. No such learning curve is detected in explicitly unpaired (CS–) , trials (grey). Bars indicate SEM.

　　Our studies revealed that nautiluses exhibit a biphasic learning curve with identifiable short-term and long-term memory peaks (Figure 2.5, Crook & Basil, 2008a) as found in cuttlefishes (Agin, Poirier, Chichery, Dickel & Chichery, 2006; Messenger, 1973). Duration of short-term memory in nautiluses is comparable to other cephalopods (up to 1 h; Agin, Poirier, Chichery, Dickel & Chichery, 2006) but long-term memory is much shorter, at least under these conditions (~12 h in *Nautilus* versus up to a week in *Octopus*, (Young, 1961; Figure 2.5). In contrast, in explicitly unpaired controls, where the delivery of odor was not reliably signaled by the flash of light, there was no increase in tentacle extension during training or retention testing. More tentacle extension (CR) in response to the light (CS) during training in the excitatory-conditioning group demonstrates that excitatory learning occurs only when there is a predictable temporal relationship between the light (CS) and the odor (US).

　　Nautiluses exhibit almost no memory for the task 6 h after initial training, hypothetically because that is when short-term memory is being consolidated into long-term memory. We do not know the exact time-course or mechanism of consolidation between 1 and 6 h. We currently determine if the memory stores are separate, as may be the case in cuttlefish, or if there is some form of functional intermediate-term memory (McGaugh, 2000) as in the snail *Lymnaea* (Lukowiak, Adatia, Krygier & Syed, 2000; Sangha, Scheibenstock, McComb & Lukowiak, 2003). Long-term memory formation in cuttlefishes is dependent upon translational processes at critical time points after learning (Agin, Chichery, Maubert & Chichery, 2003; Pedreira & Maldonado, 2003), but the timing of long-term memory formation (and perhaps intermediate-term memory) in nautiluses is unknown and we continue to probe their memory processing in a variety of tasks. Identifying the location and processes guiding learning and memory in nautiluses (e.g. cuttlefishes, Agin, Chichery & Chichery, 2001) will allow us to understand how behavioral complexity emerges from the variety of neuroanatomical solutions found in this lineage.

2.5   Spatial navigation

For questions of adaptation and cognition, an analysis of the spatial abilities of cephalopods is illustrative because: (1) a direct link can be made to spatial problems they solve in the wild; (2) given the variability in natural environments, some form of flexibility is required of any animal navigating; and (3) similar tasks have been tested in both the coleoids and nautiloids, so direct comparisons can be made within this lineage. Coleoid cephalopods are adept at solving spatial problems (e.g. Wells, 1964) – not surprising, given the complexity of their natural environment and pressures they experience in the wild (predator avoidance, food localization, returning to known locations and dens, and finding conspecifics (for a review, see Alves, Boal & Dickel, 2008; Hanlon & Messenger, 1996; see also chapter 7, this volume, by Jozet-Alves et al.). Learning the complex layout of an environment requires: (1) exploration of the space (Gallistel, 1990; O'Keefe & Nadel, 1978) – with animals often exhibiting (2) habituation to the space over time once the layout has been learned (e.g. voles: Shillito, 1963; hamsters: Poucet, Chapuis, Durup & Thinus-Blanc, 1986; blind cave fish: Teyke, 1985, 1988, 1989; crayfish: Basil & Sandeman, 2000). If a familiar environment is altered in some way, (3) the level of exploratory behavior increases (dishabituation), presumably because the previously gathered environmental information must be updated (fish: Welker & Welker, 1958; hamsters: Poucet, Chapuis, Durup & Thinus-Blanc, 1986; blind cave fish: Teyke, 1985, 1988, 1989; crayfish: Basil & Sandeman, 2000). Octopuses in a complex environment habituate to the space over time, supporting the notion that they were actively exploring and learning (Boal, Dunham, Williams & Hanlon, 2000; Karson, Boal & Hanlon, 2003). After having been removed for a period from the space, they were still able to locate a preferred den, illustrating their memory for the environment. Nautiluses, too, explore and become habituated to a vertical, three-dimensional artificial reef over time (Crook, Hanlon & Basil, 2009), spending more time in contact with the reef as they became familiar with it. When the spatial configuration of the reef was changed, nautiluses altered their swimming behavior and proximity to the reef, indicating that during exploration they had learned something about the original configuration of the reef and had detected it had changed.

The ability to competently navigate on different spatial scales requires an animal detect and perhaps learn the relevant topography of its environment. They can simply remember a series of turns to return to a goal (Gallistel, 1990), which are called response strategies, including route memory, or, when overall distance and net direction has been determined and remembered from the movements made on the outgoing journey, known as dead reckoning or path integration. Alternatively, they can use single visual cues as "beacons" (Gallistel, 1990, beacon homing), coding the location of a goal in space with a landmark nearby (e.g. *Octopus*, Mather, 1991). A more complex alternative is arranging more than one beacon in a "chain" to be followed to a goal (coleoids: Alves, Boal & Dickel, 2008; Alves, Chichery, Boal & Dickel, 2007; arthropods: Collett, Dillmann, Giger & Wehner, 1992; Gallistel, 1990). Animals may also use numerous landmarks distal to the goal to cue its location (piloting or place learning, Kamil & Jones, 1997), taking multiple bearings from these various landmarks to increase their accuracy (Kamil & Cheng, 2001). Karson, Boal and Hanlon (2003) and Alves, Chichery, Boal and Dickel (2007) demonstrated that cuttlefishes can use route information to find a goal location (a dark spot with a sandy bottom). Depending upon the kinds of cues available and/or reliable (either outside or inside a maze or spatial array), cuttlefishes can also switch flexibly between tactics to find a familiar spatial goal, using cues within the maze or outside the maze to varying degrees. Given their complex natural environment and the importance of quickly locating home, food and safety, it is perhaps not surprising octopuses and cuttlefish would have well-developed, complex spatial abilities, probably based upon constellations of visual cues in their environment.

The spatial abilities of *Nautilus* are particularly interesting because of their unique daily vertical migration in the wild, as they swim up and down coral-reef slopes during night-time hours to forage (Carlson, McKibben & De Gruy, 1984; Dunstan, Alanis & Marshall, 2010; Ward, Carlson, Weekly & Brumbaugh, 1984). It may be that they can collect and use spatial information on a large scale during these vertical movements, relying upon smaller-scale spatial cues (visual, tactile, olfactory) as they hug the coral-reef face during foraging. In the laboratory, nautiluses are adept at solving spatial problems and are cognitively flexible in the solutions they use: relying upon a variety of landmark cues in various subsets to locate a learned escape hole in a shallow-water maze (Crook, 2008; Crook & Basil, 2013; Crook, Hanlon & Basil, 2009). Nautiluses can use visual cues as beacons or as a complex array of cues to locate the goal and demonstrate flexibility in cue use depending upon availability and reliability (Crook & Basil, 2013; Crook, Hanlon & Basil, 2009). They can also switch dynamically between beacon homing and route memory to find a goal in response to changes in the environment (Crook & Basil, 2013). Ecologically, nautiluses' accommodation of the spatial changes they encounter on their nightly vertical migrations along coral reefs would benefit from such a flexible system. The simpler neural architecture of nautiloids, relative to coleoids at least, seems to belie their true capabilities.

In our spatial experiments, when an escape hole in a horizontal, 1-m diameter, shallow-water maze (Figure 2.6) is cued only with a simple visual beacon (a white striped ring of bubble wrap) surrounding the hole, nautiluses learned the goal quickly and memory persisted for up to 3 weeks, rivaling the performance of octopuses (Crook, Hanlon & Basil, 2009; Figure 2.7). When the beacon was shifted from the goal, nautiluses first directed their search over the beacon, only finding the goal after extensive search of the maze. At least in this case, route-memory tactics did not compensate and allow the animals to find the goal quickly, with the learning and presence of the beacon taking priority over the alternate available tactic. In a later control series and with more experience, however, route memory was likely invoked when the beacon was removed entirely (Crook, Hanlon & Basil, 2009; Crook & Basil, 2013). In related experiments with a constellation of objects positioned in the maze in various subsets, nautiluses could

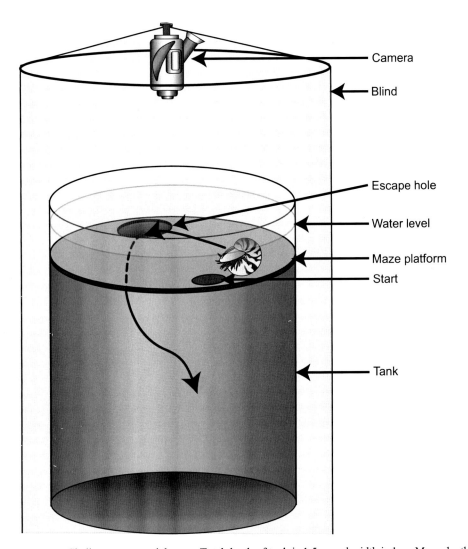

Figure 2.6 Shallow-water spatial maze. Total depth of tank is 1.5 m and width is 1 m. Maze depth is the shell diameter of the animal subject and width matches that of the tank. Goal location (exit to deeper water) located 80 cm from animal's start position and is 18 cm in diameter. Landmark, or beacon, is a 5 cm-wide concentric ring of white-striped bubble wrap surrounding the escape hole. (Reproduced from Crook, Hanlon & Basil, 2009, with permission from the American Psychological Association.)

use each subset flexibly, within the maze (both proximate to the goal and distant from the goal) and outside the maze, to navigate to the escape point. Prior learning of the beacon during training did not affect the ability of nautiluses to subsequently use local intra-maze cues alone in tests as long as they did not shift from the configuration in training (e.g. rats: Thein, Westbrook & Harris, 2008). Nautiluses also expressed a hierarchy for cues that shifted with cue reliability (Crook, 2008; Crook & Basil, 2013). The salience of a particular cue and the choice to include it in decision making was dependent on

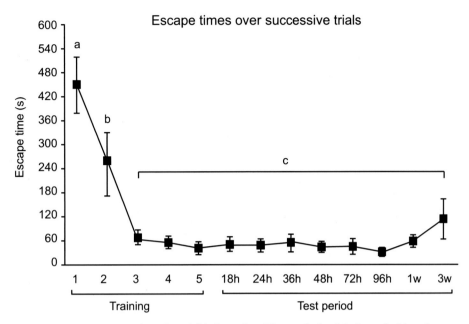

Figure 2.7 Long-term retention of spatial information. Time to find exit hole marked by a beacon in the spatial maze on successive 10-minute trials improves rapidly across 5 training trials and is retained for at least 3 weeks Points labeled with a different letter are significantly different ($P < 0.05$, two-tailed). (Reproduced from Crook, Hanlon & Basil, 2009, with permission from the American Psychological Association.)

the array of other cues that were present during learning and their reliability in testing. Similarly, Alves, Boal and Dickel (2008) showed that cuttlefish (*Sepia officinalis*) were capable of making spontaneous choices between response- and place-based strategies based on the type of cues available and the perception of their reliability. Nautiluses also detect and learn the layout of an artificial reef constructed from black and white cinder blocks introduced into their home tank. Over time, nautiluses increase their exploration of the artificial coral reef – coming into closer contact with the structure over a period of hours, touching the reef extensively with their tentacles and, finally, attaching to the reef with a few tentacles and remaining still. The nautiluses always detected when the vertical three-dimensional layout of the artificial coral reef was altered (Crook, Hanlon & Basil, 2009), swimming at a distance from the reef until, over a period of hours, they were familiarized with it and made contact. Animals did not behave this way when the visual pattern, the black and white components of the reef, simply swapped colors, with the three-dimensional layout remaining the same. In the dark waters where nautiluses live, this kind of tactile familiarization of local features could contribute to locating good hiding or foraging locations along the reef.

   In our initial studies examining beacon navigation, animals trained with a beacon (and potentially movement/route memory information as they navigated toward the beacon) did not seem to use their memory of the path to the beacon when the beacon was removed during testing (Crook, Hanlon & Basil, 2009). It seemed that route information was not available to the animals in the absence of visual cues signaling the goal. However, with subsequent training in more complex cue arrays, including a beacon, animals did find the escape point when the landmarks and beacon were removed during testing (Crook, 2008; Crook & Basil, 2013). We inferred that perhaps route/movement information is learned at the same time as visual cues and beacons, but at a slower rate requiring more experience. Beacon learning can be considered a form of associative learning, with the beacon signaling the reward of deep water. The path taken, too, results in the reward. Models of associative learning propose that the total expectation of a reward when learning is determined by the associative strengths of all the stimuli present during training (elemental models: Brandon & Wagner, 1998; Rescorla & Wagner, 1972; configurational models: Pearce, 1987, 1994) and not just the temporal relationship between the stimuli and reward. When an animal is learning more than one stimulus, for instance a beacon and the path to the beacon, the associative strengths of each of the components combine to equal a proportion of what is learned entirely (compound stimulus, Brandon & Wagner, 1998; Pearce, 1987, 1994; Rescorla & Wagner, 1972; Thein, Westbrook & Harris, 2008). If an animal is first trained to a compound stimulus and then tested with the component stimuli on their own, they should perform less well than with the stimuli in combination during testing (overshadowing, Rescorla & Wagner, 1972). In essence, the two sources of information being learned share a finite amount of memory space and each on its own only supports a portion of the information available during testing. An alternative would be that the two sources of information do not compete for memory space, but are stored and accessed separately, which has been demonstrated in vertebrates (e.g. rats: Cheng, Shettleworth, Huttenlocher & Rieser, 2007; Gibson & Shettleworth, 2005; Shettleworth & Sutton, 2005). If this is so, animals trained with a compound of beacon and route/movement information would perform less well in tests without a beacon than those trained only with dead reckoning and no beacon as a solution. Our experiments on the timing and nature of associations guide studies of the neural architecture and cellular properties underlying learning in nautiluses.

In coleoid cephalopods, the use of visual cues in various learning tasks is well documented (reviewed in Mather, 2008) and unsurprising given the complex structure of their eye and reliance on visual input in hunting, communication and defense. However, nautiluses have simple eyes that are probably not capable of forming distinct images (Muntz & Raj, 1984; Muntz, 2010b) and an optic lobe that is small compared with its relatives (Young, 1965a, 1988). We were, therefore, surprised that they used visual cues to orient and navigate in our maze studies and that they could dynamically switch among navigation tactics to find a goal. Thus, in spatial ability it appears that both the nautiloids and coleoids share a foundational set of abilities that may be conserved from their common ancestor, or may reflect that both lineages had to solve similar problems.

2.6   Evolution

The divergent modern lifestyles of nautiloids and coleoids are thought to have arisen during a period of intense competition with bony fishes before and during the

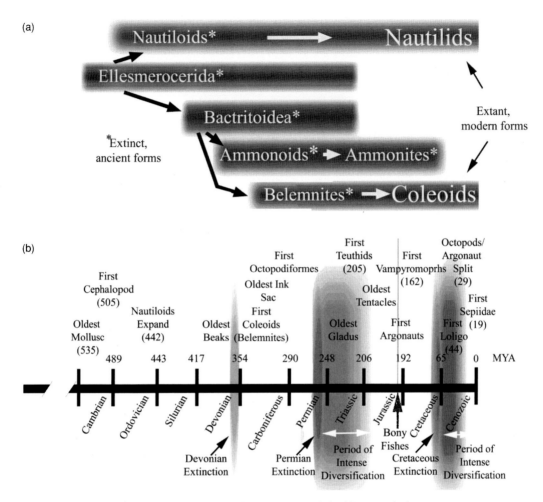

Figure 2.8 Timeline for cephalopod divergences and significant evolutionary event.
(a) Divergences; (b) timeline with significant events in cephalopod evolution above the line and
geological and speciation events below the line. MYA = millions of years ago. Note the
mass-extinction events and periods of rapid diversification thereafter. (Figure reproduced from
Grasso & Basil, 2009, with permission from S. Karger AG, Medical and Scientific Publishers,
Basel.)

Cretaceous, canalizing these two lineages into entirely different niches: "live fast, die
young" (coleoids) versus "live slow, die old" (nautilids) (Aronson, 1991; Chamberlain,
1990, 1993; Grasso & Basil, 2009; Landman & Cochran, 2010; Packard, 1972) The
cephalopod fossil record (Clarke & Trueman, 1988; Dzik, 1981; Strugnell, Jackson,
Drummond & Cooper, 2006; Strugnell, Norman, Jackson, Drummond & Cooper 2005;
Teichert, Clarke & Trueman, 1988) supports the idea that the ancestors of coleoids separated about 380 MYA, radiating into three orders and hundreds of species (Figure 2.8;
Bonnaud, Lu & Boucher-Rodoni, 2006; Carlini, Young & Vecchione, 2001; Teichert,
Clarke & Trueman, 1988; Teichert & Matsumoto, 2010; Young & Vecchione, 1996;

Young, Vecchione & Donovan, 1998). The coleoid expansion in direct competition with marine vertebrates is thought to be responsible for the evolution of their vertebrate-like eye, their speed and their complex behavior (Hochner, Shomrat & Fiorito, 2006; Nixon & Young, 2003; Packard, 1972). Coleoids are believed to have developed their fast-and-flexible cognitive abilities as a means to hide and escape from their fast, visual predators. Nautiloids likely remained in deep-water niches that avoided direct competition with vertebrates and adopted a slow-moving, scavenging lifestyle (Jurassic/Cretaceous; Chamberlain, 1993; Packard, 1972). Today, they are represented by only two genera, *Nautilus* and *Allonautilus* (Bonnaud, Ozouf-Costaz & Boucher-Rodoni, 2004; Saunders & Landman, 1987; Ward & Saunders, 1997). It has long been assumed that their slower lifestyle would not support much in the way of learning and memory. However, they are long lived and while they occupy a different niche from coleoids, their niche is quite complex, and they too must find food and avoid predation without the predatory (speed, poison) and defensive tools (active crypsis and ink release) of the coleoids. Learning and returning to reliable foraging and hiding places along the coral reef is likely adaptive to long-lived nautiluses. We argue based on the learning and memory capabilities of Chambered *Nautilus* and their ancestral state, that perhaps the brain that entered this period of competition was already large and capable of complex behaviors (Grasso & Basil, 2009) having coped with, and been refined, during periods of rapid diversification and competition following numerous mass extinctions (Figure 2.8).

2.7   Conclusions

The study of cognitive abilities in *Nautilus* is valuable because of their close phylogenetic relationship to the most neuroanatomically complex invertebrates, their unique ecological niche and their own brain organization, which despite lacking the known learning centers of coleoids, is more complex than those of other mollusks (for which much is known of their mechanisms of learning and memory). Their longevity, natural complex environment, unique foraging range and susceptibility to predation (for a review, see Crook & Basil, 2008b; Hanlon & Messenger, 1996) are likely to promote learning and memory in nautiluses. While the cephalopods are a perfect group for a comparative study of adaptive constraints promoting cognitive behavior and complex brains, a complete picture is not possible without a thorough understanding of the complex behavior of nautiluses – providing insight into historical and current evolutionary pressures shaping behavioral and brain complexity in all cephalopods and in other lineages with a heavy investment in brains.

Acknowledgements

We thank the members of the Laboratory for Invertebrate Behavior and Ecology (LIBE) for their invaluable intellectual input and for animal care. The Aquatic Research and

Environmental Assessment Center (AREAC) provided top-knotch facilities for our animals. Robert Dickie was instrumental in designing our recirculating systems. Thank you to the Biomimetic and Cognitive Robotics laboratory (BCR) for help with sea-water production and animal care. Doctors Binyamin Hochner and Roger Hanlon supported recent advances in the understanding of *Nautilus* brains. We appreciate our extensive discussions on this subject with Dr. Michael Kuba. The opportunity and time to write this chapter were generously supplied by a sabbatical (J. B., Brooklyn College) in the laboratory of Dr. Binyamin Hochner at the Hebrew University in Jerusalem.

References

Agin, V., Chichery, R. and Chichery, M.-P. (2001). Effects of learning on cytochrome oxidase activity in cuttlefish brain. *Neuroreport*, **12**: 1–4.

Agin, V., Chichery, R., Dickel, L. and Chichery, M.-P. (2006). The "prawn-in-the-tube" procedure in the cuttlefish: Habituation or passive avoidance learning? *Learning and Memory*, **13**: 97–101.

Agin, V., Chichery, R., Maubert, E. and Chichery, M.-P. (2003). Time-dependent effects of cycloheximide on long-term memory in the cuttlefish. *Pharmacology Biochemistry and Behavior*, **75**: 141–146.

Agin, V., Dickel, L., Chichery, R. and Chichery, M.-P. (1998). Evidence for a specific short-term memory in the cuttlefish, *Sepia*. *Behavioural Processes*, **43**: 329–334.

Agin, V., Poirier, R., Chichery, R., Dickel, L. and Chichery, M.-P. (2006). Developmental study of multiple memory stages in the cuttlefish, *Sepia officinalis*. *Neurobiology of Learning and Memory*, **86**: 264–269.

Alkon, D. L., Ikeno, H., Dworkin, J., McPhie, D. L., Olds, J. L., Lederhendler, I., Matzel, L., Schreurs, B. G., Kuzirian, A. and Collin, C. (1990). Contraction of neuronal branching volume: An anatomic correlate of Pavlovian conditioning. *Proceedings of the National Academy of Sciences*, **87**: 1611–1614.

Alves, C., Boal, J. G. and Dickel, L. (2008). Short-distance navigation in cephalopods: A review and synthesis. *Cognitive Processing*, **9**: 239–247.

Alves, C., Chichery, R., Boal, J. G. and Dickel, L. (2007). Orientation in the cuttlefish *Sepia officinalis*: Response versus place learning. *Animal Cognition*, **10**: 29–36.

Aronson, R. B. (1991). Ecology, paleobiology and evolutionary constraint in the octopus. *Bulletin of Marine Science*, **49**: 1–2.

Barber, V. C. and Wright, D. E. (1969). The fine structure of the sense organs of the cephalopod mollusc *Nautilus*. *Cell and Tissue Research*, **102**: 293–312.

Basil, J. A., Bahctinova, I., Kuroiwa, K., Lee, N., Mims, D., Preis, M. and Soucier, C. (2005). The function of the rhinophore and the tentacles of *Nautilus pompilius* L. (Cephalopoda, Nautiloidea) in orientation to odor. *Marine and Freshwater Behaviour and Physiology*, **38**: 209–221.

Basil, J. A., Hanlon, R. T., Sheikh, S. I. and Atema, J. (2000). Three-dimensional odor tracking by *Nautilus pompilius*. *Journal of Experimental Biology*, **203**: 1409–1414.

Basil, J. A., Lazenby, G. B., Nakanuku, L. and Hanlon, R. T. (2002). Female nautilus are attracted to male conspecific odor. *Bulletin of Marine Science*, **70**: 217–225.

Basil, J. A. and Sandeman, D. (2000). Crayfish (*Cherax destructor*) use tactile cues to detect and learn topographical changes in their environment. *Ethology*, **106**: 247–259.

Baxter, D. A. and Byrne, J. H. (2006). Feeding behavior of *Aplysia*: A model system for comparing cellular mechanisms of classical and operant conditioning. *Learning and Memory*, **13**: 669–80.

Benjamin, P. R. (2000). A systems approach to the cellular analysis of associative learning in the pond snail *Lymnaea*. *Learning and Memory*, **7**: 124–131.

Bidder, A. M. (1962). Use of the tentacles, swimming and buoyancy control in the pearly nautilus. *Nature*, **196**: 451–454.

Bitterman, M. E., Menzel, R., Fietz, A. and Schäfer, S. (1983). Classical conditioning of proboscis extension in honeybees (*Apis mellifera*). *Journal of Comparative Psychology*, **97**: 107–119.

Blackwell, K. T. (2006). Subcellular, cellular, and circuit mechanisms underlying classical conditioning in *Hermissenda crassicornis*. *Anatomical Record. Part B, New Anatomist*, **289**: 25–37.

Boal, J. G. (1991). Complex learning in *Octopus bimaculoides*. *American Malacological Bulletin*, **9**: 75–80.

Boal, J. G. (1996). A review of simultaneous visual discrimination as a method of training octopuses. *Biological Reviews*, **71**: 157–190.

Boal, J. G., Dunham, A. W., Williams, K. T. and Hanlon, R. T. (2000). Experimental evidence for spatial learning in octopuses (*Octopus bimaculoides*). *Journal of Comparative Psychology*, **114**: 246–252.

Bonnaud, L., Lu, C. C. and Boucher-Rodoni, R. (2006). Morphological character evolution and molecular trees in sepiids (Mollusca: Cephalopoda): Is the cuttlebone a robust phylogenetic marker? *Biological Journal of the Linnean Society*, **89**: 139–150.

Bonnaud, L., Ozouf-Costaz, C. and Boucher-Rodoni, R. (2004). A molecular and karyological approach to the taxonomy of *Nautilus*. *Comptes Rendus de Biologie*, **327**: 133–138.

Boycott, B. B. (1961). The functional organization of the brain of the cuttlefish *Sepia officinalis*. *Proceedings of the Royal Society. B: Biological Sciences*, **153**: 503–534.

Boycott, B. B. and Young, J. Z. (1955). A memory system in *Octopus vulgaris* Lamarck. *Proceedings of the Royal Society. B: Biological Sciences*, **143**: 449–480.

Boyle, P. R. (1986). Neural control of cephalopod behavior. *The Mollusca*, **9**: 1–97.

Brandon, S. E. and Wagner, A. R. (1998). Occasion setting: Influences of conditioned emotional responses and configured ural cues. In *Occasion setting: Associative learning and cognition in animals*. Schmajuk, N. A. and Holland, P. C. (Eds), pp. 343–382. Washington, DC, USA: American Psychological Association.

Brembs, B., Baxter, D. A. and Byrne, J. H. (2004). Extending *in vitro* conditioning in Aplysia to analyze operant and classical processes in the same preparation. *Learning and Memory*, **11**: 412–20.

Budelmann, B. U. (1995). Cephalopod sense organs, nerves and the brain: Adaptations for high performance and life style. *Marine and Freshwater Behaviour and Physiology*, **25**: 13–33.

Burrell, B. D. and Sahley, C. L. (2001). Learning in simple systems. *Current Opinion in Neurobiology*, **11**: 757–764.

Carew, T. J. and Sahley, C. L. (1986). Invertebrate learning and memory: From behavior to molecules. *Annual Review of Neuroscience*, **9**: 435–487.

Carlini, D. B., Young, R. E. and Vecchione, M. (2001). A molecular phylogeny of the Octopoda (Mollusca: Cephalopoda) evaluated in light of morphological evidence. *Molecular Phylogenetics and Evolution*, **21**: 388–397.

Carlson, B. A., McKibben, J. N. and De Gruy, M. V. (1984). Telemetric investigation of vertical migration of *Nautilus belauensis* in Palau. *Pacific Science*, **38**: 183–188.

Cartron, L., Darmaillacq, A. S. and Dickel, L. (2013). The "prawn-in-the-tube" procedure: What do cuttlefish learn and memorize? *Behavioural Brain Research*, **240**: 29–32.

Chamberlain, J. A. (1990). Jet propulsion of *Nautilus*: A surviving example of early paleozoic cephalopod locomotor design. *Canadian Journal of Zoology*, **68**: 806–814.

Chamberlain, J. A. (1993). Locomotion in ancient seas: Constraint and opportunity in cephalopod adaptive design. *Geobios*, **26**: 49–61.

Chandra, S. B. C., Hosler, J. S. and Smith, B. H. (2000). Heritable variation for latent inhibition and its correlation with reversal learning in honeybees (*Apis mellifera*). *Journal of Comparative Psychology*, **114**: 86–97.

Cheng, K., Shettleworth, S. J., Huttenlocher, J. and Rieser, J. J. (2007). Bayesian integration of spatial information. *Psychological Bulletin*, **133**: 625–637.

Clarke, M. R. and Trueman, E. R. (1988). Evolution of recent cephalopods. A brief review. *The Mollusca*, **12**: 11–79.

Cole, P. D. and Adamo, S. A. (2005). Cuttlefish (*Sepia officinalis*: Cephalopoda) hunting behavior and associative learning. *Animal Cognition*, **8**: 27–30.

Collett, T. S., Dillmann, E., Giger, A. and Wehner, R. (1992). Visual landmarks and route following in desert ants. *Journal of Comparative Physiology A*, **170**: 435–442.

Crook, R. J. (2008). *Behavioral correlates of learning and memory in Chambered Nautilus, Nautilus pompilius*. New York, NY, USA: City University of New York.

Crook, R. J. and Basil, J. A. (2008a). A biphasic memory curve in the chambered nautilus, *Nautilus pompilius* L. (Cephalopoda: Nautiloidea). *Journal of Experimental Biology*, **211**: 1992–1998.

Crook, R. J. and Basil, J. A. (2008b). A role for nautilus in studies of the evolution of brain and behavior. *Communicative and Integrative Biology*, **1**: 18–19.

Crook, R. J. and Basil, J. A. (2013). Flexible spatial orientation and navigational strategies in chambered *Nautilus*. *Ethology*, **119**: 77–85.

Crook, R. J., Hanlon, R. T. and Basil, J. A. (2009). Memory of visual and topographical features suggests spatial learning in nautilus (*Nautilus pompilius* L.). *Journal of Comparative Psychology*, **123**: 264–274.

Crow, T. (2004). Pavlovian conditioning of *Hermissenda:* Current cellular, molecular, and circuit perspectives. *Learning and Memory*, **11**: 229–238.

Crow, T. J. and Alkon, D. L. (1978). Retention of an associative behavioral change in *Hermissenda*. *Science*, **201**: 1239–1241.

Darmaillacq, A.-S., Chichery, R. and Dickel, L. (2006). Food imprinting, new evidence from the cuttlefish *Sepia officinalis*. *Biology Letters*, **2**: 345–347.

Darmaillacq, A.-S., Chichery, R., Shashar, N. and Dickel, L. (2006). Early familiarization overrides innate prey preference in newly hatched *Sepia officinalis* cuttlefish. *Animal Behaviour*, **71**: 511–514.

Darmaillacq, A. S., Dickel, L., Chichery, M.-P., Agin, V. and Chichery, R. (2004). Rapid taste aversion learning in adult cuttlefish, *Sepia officinalis*. *Animal Behaviour*, **68**: 1291–1298.

Davis, H. P. and Squire, L. R. (1984). Protein synthesis and memory: A review. *Psychological Bulletin*, **96**: 518–559.

Davis, R. L. (2005). Olfactory memory formation in *Drosophila*: From molecular to systems neuroscience. *Annual Review of Neuroscience*, **28**: 275–302.

Dickel, L., Chichery, M.-P. and Chichery, R. (2001). Increase of learning abilities and maturation of the vertical lobe complex during postembryonic development in the cuttlefish, *Sepia*. *Developmental Psychobiology*, **39**: 92–98.

Dunstan, A. J. , Alanis, O. and Marshall, J. (2010). *Nautilus pompilius* fishing and population decline in the Philippines: A comparison with an unexploited Australian *Nautilus* population. *Fisheries Research*, **106**: 239–247.

Dunstan, A. J., Ward, P. D. and Marshall, N. J. (2011). Vertical distribution and migration patterns of *Nautilus pompilius*. *Public Library of Science One*, **6**: e16311.

Dzik, J. (1981). Origin of the Cephalopoda. *Acta Palaeontologica Polonica*, **26**: 161–191.

Emery, D. G. (1975). The histology and fine structure of the olfactory organ of the squid *Lolliguncula brevis* blainville. *Tissue and Cell*, **7**: 357–367.

Fanselow, M. S. and Poulos, A. M. (2005). The neuroscience of mammalian associative learning. *Annual Review of Psychology*, **56**: 207–234.

Fiorito, G. and Chichery, R. (1995). Lesions of the vertical lobe impair visual discrimination learning by observation in *Octopus vulgaris*. *Neuroscience Letters*, **192**: 117–120.

Fiorito, G. and Scotto, P. (1992). Observational learning in *Octopus vulgaris*. *Science*, **256**: 545–547.

Fukuda, Y. (1980). *Observations by SEM, Nautilus macromphalus in captivity*. Tokyo, Japan: Tokai University Press.

Gallistel, C. R. (1990). *The organization of learning*. Cambridge, MA, USA: MIT Press.

Gelperin, A. and Culligan, N. (1984). In vitro expression of in vivo learning by an isolated molluscan CNS. *Brain Research*, **304**: 207–213.

Gibson, B. M. and Shettleworth, S. J. (2005). Place versus response learning revisited: Tests of blocking on the radial maze. *Behavioral Neuroscience*, **119**: 567–586.

Gilly, W. F. and Lucero, M. T. (1992). Behavioral responses to chemical stimulation of the olfactory organ in the squid *Loligo opalescens*. *Journal of Experimental Biology*, **162**: 209–229.

Graindorge, N., Alves, C., Darmaillacq, A.-S., Chichery, R., Dickel, L. and Bellanger, C. (2006). Effects of dorsal and ventral vertical lobe electrolytic lesions on spatial learning and locomotor activity in *Sepia officinalis*. *Behavioral Neuroscience*, **120**: 1151–1158.

Grasso, F. W. and Basil, J. A. (2009). The evolution of flexible behavioral repertoires in cephalopod molluscs. *Brain, Behavior and Evolution*, **74**: 231–245.

Graziadei, P. (1964). Receptors in the sucker of the cuttlefish. *Nature*, **203**: 384–386.

Hanlon, R. T. and Messenger, J. B. (1996). *Cephalopod behaviour*. Cambridge, MA, USA: Cambridge University Press.

Hochner, B., Shomrat, T. and Fiorito, G. (2006). The octopus: A model for a comparative analysis of the evolution of learning and memory mechanisms. *The Biological Bulletin*, **210**: 308–317.

Hvorecny, L. M., Grudowski, J. L., Blakeslee, C. J., Simmons, T. L., Roy, P. R., Brooks, J. A., Hanner, R. M., Beigel, M. E., Karson, M. A. and Nichols, R. H. (2007). Octopuses (*Octopus bimaculoides*) and cuttlefishes (*Sepia pharaonis*, *S. officinalis*) can conditionally discriminate. *Animal Cognition*, **10**: 449–459.

Kamil, A. C. (1994). A synthetic approach to the study of animal intelligence. *Behavioural Mechanisms in Evolutionary Ecology*, 11–45.

Kamil, A. C. and Cheng, K. (2001). Way-finding and landmarks: The multiple-bearings hypothesis. *Journal of Experimental Biology*, **204**: 103–113.

Kamil, A. C. and Jones, J. E. (1997). The seed-storing corvid Clark's nutcracker learns geometric relationships among landmarks. *Nature*, **390**: 276–279.

Kandel, E. R., 1976. *Cellular basis of behavior: An introduction to behavioral neurobiology*. New York, NY, USA: W. H. Freeman.

Kandel, E. R. and Schwartz, J. H. (1982). Molecular biology of learning: Modulation of transmitter release. *Science*, **218**: 433–443.

Kandel, E. R. and Tauc, L. (1965). Heterosynaptic facilitation in neurones of the abdominal ganglion of *Aplysia depilans*. *Journal of Physiology*, **181**: 1–27.

Karson, M. A., Boal, J. G. and Hanlon, R. T. (2003). Experimental evidence for spatial learning in cuttlefish (*Sepia officinalis*). *Journal of Comparative Psychology*, **117**: 149–155.

Kier, W. M. (1987). The functional morphology of the tentacle musculature of *Nautilus pompilius*. In *Nautilus: The biology and paleobiology of a living fossil*. Saunders, W. B. and Landman, N. (Eds), pp. 257–269. New York, NY, USA: Springer.

Landman, N. H. and Cochran, J. K. (2010). Growth and longevity of *Nautilus*. In *Nautilus: The biology and paleobiology of a living fossil*. Saunders, W. B. and Landman, N. (Eds), pp. 401–420. New York, NY, USA: Springer.

Lucero, M. T., Horrigan, F. T. and Gilly, W. M. F. (1992). Electrical responses to chemical stimulation of squid olfactory receptor cells. *Journal of Experimental Biology*, **162**: 231–249.

Lukowiak, K., Adatia, N., Krygier, D. and Syed, N. (2000). Operant conditioning in Lymnaea: Evidence for intermediate-and long-term memory. *Learning and Memory*, **7**: 140–150.

Maddock, L. and Young, J. Z. (1987). Quantitative differences among the brains of cephalopods. *Journal of Zoology*, **212**: 739–767.

Maldonado, H. (1965). The positive and negative learning process in *Octopus vulgaris* Lamarck. Influence of the vertical and median superior frontal lobes. *Journal of Comparative Physiology A*, **51**: 185–203.

Mather, J. A. (1991). Navigation by spatial memory and use of visual landmarks in octopuses. *Journal of Comparative Physiology A*, **168**: 491–497.

Mather, J. A. (1995). Cognition in cephalopods. *Advances in the Study of Behavior*, **24**: 317–353.

Mather, J. A. (2008). To boldly go where no mollusc has gone before: Personality, play, thinking, and consciousness in cephalopods. *American Malacological Bulletin*, **24**: 51–58.

McGaugh, J. L. (2000). Memory – a century of consolidation. *Science*, **287**: 248–251.

Menzel, R., Leboulle, G. and Eisenhardt, D. (2006). Small brains, bright minds. *Cell*, **124**: 237–239.

Messenger, J. B. (1973). Learning in the cuttlefish, *Sepia*. *Animal Behaviour*, **21**: 801–826.

Messenger, J. B. (1991). Photoreception and vision in molluscs. *Vision and Visual Dysfunction*, **2**: 364–397.

Milner, B., Squire, L. R. and Kandel, E. R. (1998). Cognitive neuroscience and the study of memory. *Neuron*, **20**: 445–468.

Muntz, W. R. A. (1986). Short communications: The spectral sensitivity of *Nautilus pompilius*. *Journal of Experimental Biology*, **126**: 513–517.

Muntz, W. R. A. (2010a). A possible function of the iris groove of *Nautilus*. In *Nautilus: The biology and paleobiology of a living fossil*, 2nd edn. Saunders, W. B. and Landman, N. (Eds), pp. 245–247. New York, NY, USA: Springer.

Muntz, W. R. A. (2010b). Visual behavior and visual sensitivity of *Nautilus pompilius*. In *Nautilus: The biology and paleobiology of a living fossil*, 2nd edn. Saunders, W. B. and Landman, N. (Eds), pp. 231–244. New York, NY, USA: Springer.

Muntz, W. R. A. and Raj, U. (1984). On the visual system of *Nautilus pompilius*. *Journal of Experimental Biology*, **109**: 253–263.

Nixon, M. and Young, J. Z. (2003). *The brains and lives of cephalopods*. Oxford, UK: Oxford University Press.

O'Keefe, J. and Nadel, L. (1978). *The hippocampus as a cognitive map*. New York, NY, USA: Oxford University Press.

Packard, A. (1972). Cephalopods and fish: The limits of convergence. *Biological Reviews*, **47**: 241–307.

Pavlov, I. (1927). *Conditioned reflexes: An investigation of the physiological activity of the cerebral cortex*. Oxford, UK: Oxford University Press.

Pearce, J. M. (1987). A model for stimulus generalization in Pavlovian conditioning. *Psychological Review*, **94**: 61–73.

Pearce, J. M. (1994). Similarity and discrimination: A selective review and a connectionist model. *Psychological Review*, **101**: 587–607.

Pedreira, M. E. and Maldonado, H. (2003). Protein synthesis subserves reconsolidation or extinction depending on reminder duration. *Neuron*, **38**: 863–869.

Poucet, B., Chapuis, N., Durup, M. and Thinus-Blanc, C. (1986). A study of exploratory behavior as an index of spatial knowledge in hamsters. *Learning and Behavior*, **14**: 93–100.

Rescorla, R. A. and Wagner, A. R. (1972). A theory of Pavlovian conditioning: Variations in the effectiveness of reinforcement and nonreinforcement. *Classical Conditioning II: Current Research and Theory*, **2**: 64–99.

Ruth, P., Schmidtberg, H., Westermann, B. and Schipp, R. (2002). The sensory epithelium of the tentacles and the rhinophore of *Nautilus pompilius* L. (Cephalopoda, Nautiloidea). *Journal of Morphology*, **251**: 239–255.

Sanders, G. D. (1970). Long-term memory of a tactile discrimination in *Octopus vulgaris* and the effect of vertical lobe removal. *Brain Research*, **20**: 59–73.

Sangha, S., Scheibenstock, A., McComb, C. and Lukowiak, K. (2003). Intermediate and long-term memories of associative learning are differentially affected by transcription versus translation blockers in Lymnaea. *Journal of Experimental Biology*, **206**: 1605–1613.

Sasaki, T., Shigeno, S. and Tanabe, K. (2010). Anatomy of living *Nautilus*: Re-evaluation of primitiveness and comparison with *Coleoidea*. In *Cephalopods – present and past*. Tanabe, K., Shigeta, Y., Sasaki, T. and Hirano, H. (Eds), pp. 35–66. Tokyo, Japan: Tokai University Press.

Saunders, W. B. (1985). Studies of living *Nautilus* in Palau. *National Geographic Society Reseach Reports*, **18**: 669–682.

Saunders, W. B. and Landman, N. H. (1987). *Nautilus: The biology and paleobiology of a living fossil, reprint with additions*. New York, NY, USA: Springer.

Shettleworth, S. J. and Sutton, J. E. (2005). Multiple systems for spatial learning: Dead reckoning and beacon homing in rats. *Journal of Experimental Psychology: Animal Behavior Processes*, **31**: 125–141.

Shigeno, S., Sasaki, T., Moritaki, T., Kasugai, T., Vecchione, M. and Agata, K. (2008). Evolution of the cephalopod head complex by assembly of multiple molluscan body parts: Evidence from *Nautilus* embryonic development. *Journal of Morphology*, **269**: 1–17.

Shigeno, S., Takenori, S. and Boletzky, S. v. (2010). The origins of cephalopod body plans: A geometrical and developmental basis for the evolution of vertebrate-like organ systems. *Classical Conditioning II: Current Research and Theory*, **1**: 23–34.

Shillito, E. E. (1963). Exploratory behaviour in the short-tailed vole *Microtus agrestis*. *Behaviour*, **21**: 145–154.

Smith, B. H. (1997). An analysis of blocking in odorant mixtures: An increase but not a decrease in intensity of reinforcement produces unblocking. *Behavioral Neuroscience*, **11**: 57–69.

Smith, B. H. and Cobey, S. (1994). The olfactory memory of the honeybee *Apis mellifera*. II. Blocking between odorants in binary mixtures. *Journal of Experimental Biology*, **195**: 91–108.

Soucier, C. P. and Basil, J. A. (2008). Chambered *Nautilus* (*Nautilus pompilius pompilius*) responds to underwater vibrations. *American Malacological Bulletin*, **24**: 3–11.

Stork, O. and Welzl, H. (1999). Memory formation and the regulation of gene expression. *Cellular and Molecular Life Sciences*, **55**: 575–592.

Strugnell, J., Jackson, J., Drummond, A. J. and Cooper, A. (2006). Divergence time estimates for major cephalopod groups: Evidence from multiple genes. *Cladistics*, **22**: 89–96.

Strugnell, J., Norman, M., Jackson, J., Drummond, A. J. and Cooper, A. (2005). Molecular phylogeny of coleoid cephalopods (Mollusca: Cephalopoda) using a multigene approach; the effect of data partitioning on resolving phylogenies in a Bayesian framework. *Molecular Phylogenetics and Evolution*, **37**: 426–441.

Suboski, M. D., Muir, D. and Hall, D. (1993). Social learning in invertebrates. *Science*, **259**: 1628–1629.

Sutherland, N. S. (1963). The shape-discrimination of stationary shapes by octopuses. *American Journal of Psychology*, **76**: 177–190.

Teichert, C., Clarke, M. R. and Trueman, E. R. (1988). Main features of cephalopod evolution. In *The Mollusca*, Clarke, M. R. and Trueman, E. R. (Eds), pp. 11–79. San Diego, CA, USA: Academic Press.

Teichert, C. and Matsumoto, T. (2010). The ancestry of the genus *Nautilus*. In *Nautilus: The biology and paleobiology of a living fossil*, 2nd edn. Saunders, W. B. and Landman, N. (Eds), pp. 25–32. New York, NY, USA: Springer.

Teyke, T. (1985). Collision with and avoidance of obstacles by blind cave fish *Anoptichthys jordani* (Characidae). *Journal of Comparative Physiology A*, **157**: 837–843.

Teyke, T. (1988). Flow field, swimming velocity and boundary layer: Parameters which affect the stimulus for the lateral line organ in blind fish. *Journal of Comparative Physiology A*, **163**: 53–61.

Teyke, T. (1989). Learning and remembering the environment in the blind cave fish *Anoptichthys jordani*. *Journal of Comparative Physiology A*, **164**, 655–662.

Thein, T., Westbrook, R. F. and Harris, J. A. (2008). How the associative strengths of stimuli combine in compound: Summation and overshadowing. *Journal of Experimental Psychology: Animal Behavior Processes*, **34**: 155–166.

Tinbergen, N. (1963). On aims and methods of ethology. *Zeitschrift für Tierpsychologie*, **20**: 410–433.

Walters, E. T. (1991). A functional, cellular, and evolutionary model of nociceptive plasticity in Aplysia. *The Biological Bulletin*, **180**: 241–251.

Walters, E. T., Alizadeh, H. and Castro, G. A. (1991). Similar neuronal alterations induced by axonal injury and learning in Aplysia. *Science*, **253**: 797–799.

Ward, P. D., Carlson, B., Weekly, M. and Brumbaugh, B. (1984). Remote telemetry of daily vertical and horizontal movement of *Nautilus* in Palau. *Nature*, **309**: 248–250.

Ward, P. D. and Saunders, W. B. (1997). *Allonautilus*: A new genus of living nautiloid cephalopod and its bearing on phylogeny of the Nautilida. *Journal of Paleontology*, **71**: 1054–1064.

Welker, W. I. and Welker, J. (1958). Reaction of fish (*Eucinostomus gula*) to environmental changes. *Ecology*, **39**: 283–288.

Wells, M. J. (1964). Detour experiments with octopuses. *Journal of Experimental Biology*, **41**: 621–642.

Wells, M. J. (1978). *Octopus: Physiology and behaviour of an advanced invertebrate*. London, UK: Chapman and Hall.

Westermann, B. and Beuerlein, K. (2005). Y-maze experiments on the chemotactic behaviour of the tetrabranchiate cephalopod. *Marine Biology*, **147**: 145–151.

Woodhams, P. L. and Messenger, J. B. (1974). A note on the ultrastructure of the Octopus olfactory organ. *Cell and Tissue Research*, **152**: 253–258.

Young, J. Z. (1960). The failures of discrimination learning following the removal of the vertical lobes in Octopus. *Proceedings of the Royal Society. B: Biological Sciences*, **153**: 18–46.

Young, J. Z. (1961). Learning and discrimination in the octopus. *Biological Reviews*, **36**: 32–95.

Young, J. Z. (1964). *A model of the brain*. Oxford, UK: Clarendon Press.

Young, J. Z. (1965a). The central nervous system of *Nautilus*. *Philosophical Transactions of the Royal Society of London. Series B*, **249**: 1–25.

Young, J. Z. (1965b). The Croonian lecture, 1965: The organization of a memory system. *Proceedings of the Royal Society. B: Biological Sciences*, **163**: 285–320.

Young, J. Z. (1988). Evolution of the cephalopod brain. *The Mollusca*, **12**: 215–228.

Young, J. Z. (1991). Computation in the learning system of cephalopods. *The Biological Bulletin*, **180**: 200–208.

Young, J. Z. and Boycott, B. B. (1971). *The anatomy of the nervous system of Octopus vulgaris*. Oxford, UK: Clarendon Press.

Young, R. E. and Vecchione, M. (1996). Analysis of morphology to determine primary sister-taxon relationships within coleoid cephalopods. *American Malacological Bulletin*, **12**: 91–112.

Young, R. E., Vecchione, M. and Donovan, D. T. (1998). The evolution of coleoid cephalopods and their present biodiversity and ecology. *South African Journal of Marine Science*, **20**: 393–420.

3   Learning from play in octopus

Michael J. Kuba, Tamar Gutnick and Gordon M. Burghardt

3.1   Introduction

The brain of cephalopods rivals that of the vertebrates in relative size, being as large as or larger than the brains of many fish, although smaller than those of birds and mammals (Hochner, 2008). The elaborate sensory and neural system in many extant cephalopods enables them to exhibit complex types of adaptive behaviour (Wells, 1978; Hanlon & Messenger, 1996; Nixon & Young, 2003; Hochner, 2008, 2010). Of the many kinds of such complex behaviour, we focus here on exploration, play and cognition.

To adequately study exploration, or playful interaction, in cephalopods, we need to know a good deal about their behaviour, especially 'normal' or ethotypic behaviour, and have sufficient time and opportunities to observe changes to their behaviour across time and settings. This requires keeping animals in good condition in captivity or observing them in the wild in natural environments. This being said, most cephalopods live in the open waters of the deep sea and the majority are unavailable for systematic observation. Furthermore, most cephalopod species cannot be maintained regularly in laboratory conditions. For these reasons, most studies of the behaviour of individual cephalopods come from work on only three genera, *Octopus*, *Sepia* and *Loligo*, animals that live in coastal waters. These, and a few of their close relatives, are the only cephalopods that have been kept at all regularly in aquaria; *Octopus, Sepia* and, to some extent, *Sepiotheuthis* alone do sufficiently well under these conditions for their observed behaviour to be considered typical and natural (Wells, 1962; Sanders, 1975; Wells, 1978; Moynihan & Rodaniche, 1982; Hanlon & Messenger, 1996; Nixon & Young, 2003; Mather, Griebel & Byrne, 2010). Due to this lack of data on basic behaviours of these animals, it is often difficult to argue which observed playful behaviours might be considered exaggerations or modifications of normal behaviours. To date we are aware of only four papers, on two different species of octopus, dealing with exploration and play (Mather & Anderson, 1999; Kuba, Meisel, Byrne, Griebel & Mather, 2003; Kuba, Byrne, Meisel & Mather, 2006a, 2006b). In this chapter, therefore, we will focus on octopuses, probably the most studied group of all cephalopods.

Octopuses have fascinated observers for thousands of years and there is a wealth of anecdotal reports of their intelligence, cunning and curiosity. They are generalist predators and detect their prey both visually and by touch (Hanlon & Messenger, 1996). The loss of the external molluscan shell has been linked to their high behavioural plasticity for predator avoidance, an increase in brain size and the evolution of more effective sense organs, resulting in higher cognitive abilities (Packard, 1972; Hanlon & Messenger, 1996). The aim of the studies on octopus exploration and play is to describe the behavioural processes involved and to untangle the interplay between exploration, habituation and exploratory play in these animals. These studies show, for the first time, that an invertebrate does engage in playful interactions with objects (Burghardt, 2005).

3.2   Exploration

Exploration, in its most basic manifestation, can be defined as the acquisition of knowledge about animate or innate objects, the environment and its changes through sensory information gathering (Berlyne, 1966; Renner, 1990; Power, 2000). Exploration and sampling the surrounding environment is one of the most basic tasks each and every organism faces. It usually occurs when an animal is first exposed to an object or an environment. Yet, in spite of the above, defining and recognizing exploration is not easy. For example, exploration is not the only response to novel settings; it is affected by motivational and other internal states, and has often been conceptually dependent on recording easily measured changes in general behavioural activity (e.g. increased locomotion, alternation of search patterns or general contact with novel objects Renner, 1990). Renner (1990) criticized the fact that exploration was often treated as the animals' equivalent to Brownian random motion in molecules. Although early-learning theorists historically could not explain exploration (Burghardt, 2012), because it was not always associated with an obvious, primary biological need, evidence shows that there is a functional significance of exploration (Archer & Birke, 1983; Renner, 1990). The extraction of information from the surrounding environment (Hutt, 1966) can result in a learning process (Baldwin & Baldwin, 1997), which would allow for the establishment of a familiar area (territory or home range, see Russell, 1983) and the ability to monitor changes in it. For animals in the wild this means that the maintenance of familiarity with the environment necessitates regular inspections – i.e. exploration (Russell, 1983).

Exploration has been divided into two different types: extrinsic and intrinsic. Extrinsic exploration is exploration for obtaining information about a conventional reinforcer (Russell, 1983). Examples of this kind of motivated exploration include foraging for food when hungry or searching for conspecifics at times of reproduction (Toates, 1983). Due to the seemingly obvious motivational cause for this type of exploration, it has received little scientific attention. Laboratory research on birds and mammals has focused on intrinsic exploration (Archer & Birke, 1983; Huber, Rechberger & Taborsky, 2001; Gazzaniga & Heatherton, 2003). Intrinsic exploration is defined as a behaviour directed towards a stimulus of little biological importance (Russell, 1983). Early studies on intrinsic exploration in rats (see Toates, 1983) and later work on farm animals (Wood-Gush, Stolba & Miller, 1983; Day, Kyriazakis & Lawrence, 1994) focused on the effect of hunger or punishment on exploration. Most rats did not reduce or cease exploration when food deprived, and would even delay eating and endure physical stress for an opportunity to explore a Dashiell multi-arm maze filled with novel objects (Berlyne, 1960).

Captive aquatic animals typically face a lack of environmental variation and a rather stimulus-deprived setting; thus, novel, non-threatening stimuli may evoke exploration in intact animals of many phyla (see Archer & Birke, 1983). Therefore, stimulus seeking to avoid boredom is an important factor modifying intrinsic as well as extrinsic exploration (Toates, 1983). Early on, researchers (e.g. Craig, 1918; Harlow, 1953) looked into the motivational states behind exploratory behaviour and whether external stimuli or internal drives are more important for the manifestation of exploratory behaviours. Harlow (1950) showed that monkeys would try to solve a three-piece puzzle apparatus even if there was no extrinsic reward present.

Recent papers, influenced by learning theory (see Toates, 1983 for a review on theories affecting exploration), focus on the general linkage between learning and exploration (Toates, 1983; Renner, 1990; Renner & Seltzer, 1994; Heinrich, 1995). Learning during exploration has the potential to benefit the animal by reducing risk factors, such as susceptibility to predation and increasing the ability to incur positive outcomes like finding food. However, in order to study learning and memory through exploration the focus has to be on the form and function of the behaviour, rather than the more obvious performance methods used in classical learning studies. Octopuses, with their excellent learning abilities (Wells, 1978; Nixon & Young, 2003), foraging behaviour and semi-permanent home ranges (Mather, 1991a, 1991b) provide an appropriate subject for characterizing the behaviour in an invertebrate.

Kuba, Byrne, Meisel and Mather (2006b) divided the responses to an object dropped into the tank of a healthy octopus, into two levels of exploratory behaviour. At level 1 the animal used one or several arms to explore the object; at level 2 the animal brought the object to the mouth area under its interbrachial web (Figure 3.1a,b: levels 1 and 2 with objects). With non-food objects there were no significant differences in the number of level 1 or level 2 interactions; with food objects there were significantly more level 2 interactions. Food was essentially either eaten or ignored, resulting in more level 2 and lengthier interactions, and non-food items were explored with three to four times more contacts but with shorter interactions. When the same animals were tested 2 hours after feeding, the number of interactions with food items was significantly lower, but the number of interactions with non-food items remained the same (Figure 3.2a,b).

The results showed that the interaction with non-food items was not misplaced predation by an animal that cannot tell the difference between food and non-food items. Animals specifically chose to approach and manipulate the non-food item, and this intrinsic exploration did not change significantly under different feeding regimes. These results were consistent with those found in studies on intrinsic exploration in rats (see Toates, 1983 for a review), farm animals (Wood-Gush, Stolba & Miller, 1983; Day, Kyriazakis & Lawrence, 1994) and monkeys (Harlow, 1950).

How do other cephalopods fit into this picture? Despite the lack of laboratory studies, it seems certain that squids and cuttlefish as well as nautilus should show exploratory behaviour. There is evidence that spatial exploration in *Sepia* is based on visual clues

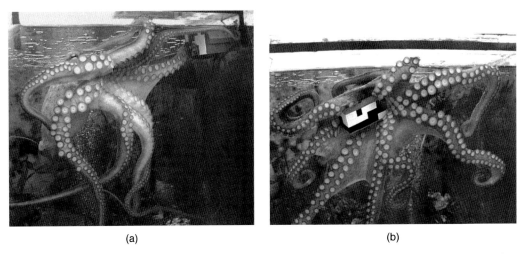

(a)   (b)

Figure 3.1 (a) Level 1 exploratory behaviour; the animal uses one or several arms to explore the non-food item. (b) Level 2 exploratory behaviour; the animal holds the objects in its interbrachial web. (From Kuba, Byrne, Meisel & Mather, 2006b.)

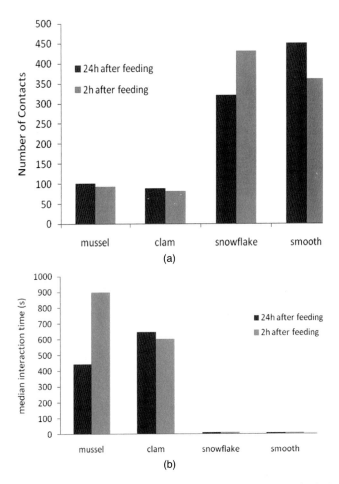

(a)

(b)

Figure 3.2 Difference in number and duration of contacts for food (a) and non-food (b) items. Black bars represent values 24 hours after feeding (hungry) and dark grey bars represent values 2 hours after feeding (satiated). (From Kuba, Byrne, Meisel & Mather, 2006b.)

(see, e.g. Alves, Chichery, Boal & Dickel, 2007). *Nautilus,* however, with a predominantly olfactory-based sensory world, would be an interesting future challenge for testing exploration in an evolutionary-old organism (Grasso & Basil, 2009). Despite their short lifespan, many cephalopods develop complex sensory and motor abilities and behaviours. This could be exploited to understanding the adaptiveness of behavioural and cognitive traits and the role of experience. Theoretically, this would enable researchers to conduct longitudinal studies throughout the lifespan of an individual to get an in-depth look at the change/progression of exploratory behaviour in that individual. An especially promising area could be the investigation of motivation for exploration, from looking for food and suitable home ranges in juveniles to looking for mates in adults.

3.3   Play

'Who would dare study play?' These were the first words in the introduction to a book on play and its evolution edited by Bruner, Jolly and Sylva (1976). In an effort to formalize the study of play, Fagan (1981) described three different types of play: locomotor-rotational play (typically solitary), object play and social play. However, these are not absolutely separate and all can occur together in spite of having, in some species, different developmental trajectories. Locomotor-rotational play consists of movements matching the traditional criteria for play activity (Byers & Walker, 1995) and includes playful running and twisting in ungulates to somersaulting in monkeys (Müller-Schwarze, 1984; Sommer & Mendoza-Granados, 1995). Object play, which may be either solitary or social, involves manipulating an object. This type of play has been linked to exploratory behaviour and is sometimes also referred to as diversive exploratory play (Berlyne, 1960; Hutt, 1966; Drickamer, Vessey & Meikle, 1996; Power, 2000). Social play involves chasing, wresting, sexual and other interactions, mostly performed by two or more conspecifics, but can occur across species (Bekoff & Byers, 1998; Pellis & Iwaniuk, 2004). Although octopuses, with their solitary lifestyle and opportunistic cannibalism (Hanlon & Messenger, 1996), cannot be expected to engage in social play, object and locomotor play may be more likely given their predatory lifestyle and capacity for an almost infinite array of movements employing their eight arms.

The last 20 years have seen a surge in identifying play in animals other than birds and mammals. This raises the crucial issue of quantitatively studying play as it is exhibited differently by a wide variety of animals. Burghardt (1999, 2005) formulated five criteria to standardize the research on play behaviour. These criteria were the first to offer scientists working on different groups of animals the opportunity to find a common guideline to compare their findings. The first criterion is that play behaviour is incompletely functional in the context in which it is expressed. The second criterion states that play behaviour is spontaneous and pleasurable ('done for its own sake'). To meet the third criterion, play has to differ from 'regular' behaviour in being exaggerated or modified. The fourth criterion says that play is repeatedly produced, but not stereotypical. According to the fifth criterion, play is observed in healthy subjects and in a stress-free condition.

One of the biggest problems when dealing with an animal that has such a radically different, and little understood, behaviour repertoire is to discern what might or might not be play. In the first paper to broach this subject, Mather and Anderson (1999) observed play-like behaviour in *Enteroctopus dofleini*. In a series of 10 daily trials over 5 days, they presented their octopuses with object stimuli and recorded their behaviour on a rising scale of object interaction. The most striking result was that two of the octopus used water jetting, through the exhalant funnel, to manipulate the object in a play-like manner. While jetting by octopus is used as a means of removing an unpleasant or unwanted stimulus from the body, such as food remains or annoying fish, in experiments it was used, in a modified way, to move an object around the aquarium. The extent of use, the 'out of context' circumstance and the modification of a purposeful behaviour met the criteria for play.

Kuba and colleagues (Kuba, Meisel, Byrne, Griebel & Mather, 2003; Kuba, Byrne, Meisel & Mather, 2006a) expanded this way of recognizing play by formulating a 'tree' of behaviours leading up to and including play (Figure 3.3). By presenting *Octopus vulgaris* with a variety of food and non-food objects under different feeding regimes, they defined interaction levels ranging from the more predatory/exploratory contacts to play behaviour. The intensity of each behaviour was manifested by a rise in levels (0–4) on a 'play scale'. Holding the object to the mouth was designated as level 0 interaction, this behaviour, if not for feeding, allowed for inspection by the very sensitive mouth area suckers. Level 1 exploratory interaction, when animals held the object with the distal suckers of one or several arms led to one of three further exploration methods, but also sometimes to a level 0 Web Over. The three different interactions defined in level 2 are the first out-of-context interactions. When these interactions were repeated or prolonged they were considered play-like interactions, level 3, and if repeated or prolonged further they were defined as level 4, play. So how did the octopuses play? The first mode of exploration-play was towing the objects on the water surface. Animals held the object with one or more arms and then started to move. Initially this behaviour was short and unidirectional (level 2a), but when it was towed in more than one direction (level 3a) it was play-like. Towing the object in more than one direction for over 30 seconds was play (level 4a). The second type of interaction was a simple, single action, where the animals pulled the objects closer or pushed them away, either horizontally or vertically (level 2b). When this action was repeated up to five times it was play-like (level 3b), and if repeated more than five times it was play (level 4b). The third mode was passing the object from one arm to another. If the object was passed once or twice between arms it was termed level 2c. When the object was passed three to six times between arms, it was play like (level 3c); seven or more of such passings were considered play (level 4c).

These two studies (Kuba, Meisel, Byrne, Griebel & Mather, 2003; Kuba, Byrne, Meisel & Mather, 2006a) showed that 11 out of 21 tested animals exhibited play behaviour. Similar to the findings of Mather and Anderson (1999), these behaviours followed a certain sequence across experimental days. They began engaging in longer and fewer exploratory contacts, followed by a period of boredom/habituation. When encountering food items, interactions never exceeded level 2; after exploring the object,

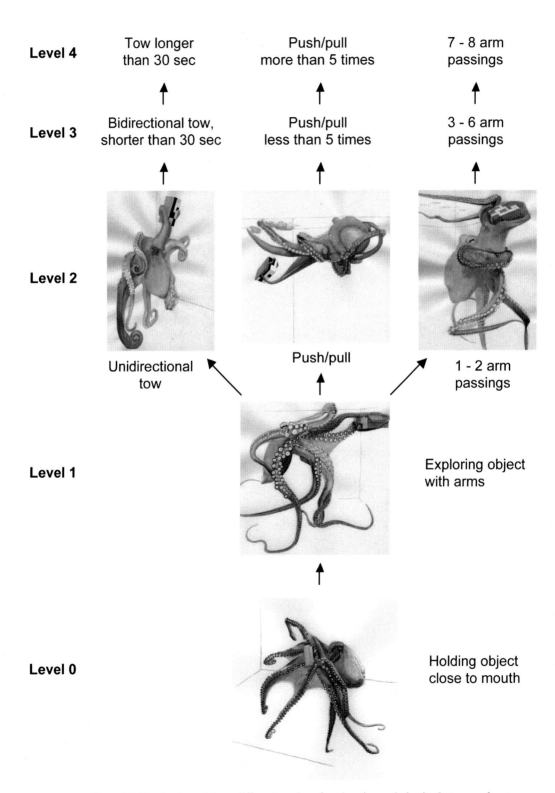

Figure 3.3 Five levels and three different modes of exploration and play in *Octopus vulgaris*. (From Kuba, Byrne, Meisel & Mather, 2006a.)

Table 3.1 The five play criteria as applied to octopuses

Criterion	Fit
The behaviour is incompletely functional in the context in which it is expressed	The use of water jets for object manipulation in the study by Mather and Anderson (1999) and level 3 and 4 interactions in the studies by Kuba and colleagues (Kuba, Meisel, Byrne, Griebel & Mather, 2003; Kuba, Byrne, Meisel & Mather, 2006b) are exhibits of natural behaviours that are incompletely functional in the context in which they were used
The behaviour is voluntary, spontaneous or rewarding	In all studies (Mather & Anderson, 1999; Kuba, Meisel, Byrne, Griebel & Mather, 2003; Kuba, Byrne, Meisel & Mather, 2006b) octopuses sought out the objects to interact with them
The behaviour differs from regular forms of behaviour (e.g. exaggerated)	Tossing, towing and push/pull behaviours (Kuba, Meisel, Byrne, Griebel & Mather, 2003; Kuba, Byrne, Meisel & Mather, 2006b) as well as water jets (Mather & Anderson, 1999) are modifications of regular behaviour
Repeatedly observed but not stereotypic	All studies (Mather & Anderson, 1999; Kuba, Meisel, Byrne, Griebel & Mather, 2003; Kuba, Byrne, Meisel & Mather, 2006b) show that contacts with the objects are repeated in a non-stereotypic way
The behaviour is performed in a stress-free condition	Only relaxed and healthy octopuses are curious and active and engaging in voluntary interactions with innate or food objects

it was either eaten or abandoned. In the case of non-food objects, interest in the object returned and in some instances led to more diversified interactions and to play (Table 3.1; Figure 3.4).

Any interactions exeeding level 2 that the animals made with objects were considered non-functional in the specific context. They differed from behaviours that animals show towards food objects. Food objects were always explored – either with one or several arms, or brought the web between the arms for further chemotactile exploration and subsequent rejection or consumption. The behaviour towards non-food items was spontaneous and repeated, and since behaviours in levels 0–2 could be considered 'normal' interactions, it was thus an exaggeration/modification of that behaviour. These behaviours, therefore, meet the five criteria set by Burghardt (1999, 2005). Additionally, the progression of the sequence of behaviours that all papers observed resembles the sequence preceding object-play in children (Mather & Anderson, 1999; Kuba, Meisel, Byrne, Griebel & Mather, 2003; Kuba, Byrne, Meisel & Mather, 2006b). Hughes (1983) suggested that a child starts exploration of an object asking the question 'What is this object?' and later transforms this to the question 'What can I do with this object?', which

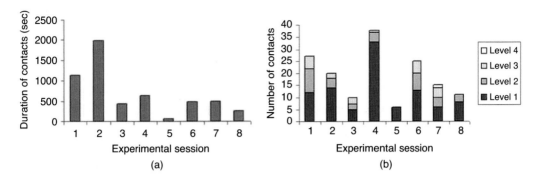

Figure 3.4 A representative graph showing the duration of contacts with the smooth Lego® block for the octopus 'Dorian' (a). Representative graph showing the number of different levels of interaction by 'Dorian' (b) for each experimental session. (From Kuba, Byrne, Meisel & Mather, 2006a.)

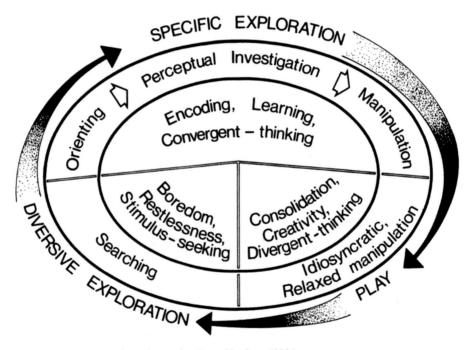

Figure 3.5 The exploration–play cycle. (From Hughes, 1983.)

leads to play (Figure 3.5). Similarly, the pattern of behaviours leads from learning to manipulate an object to playing with it.

Play and play-like behaviour in *O. vulgaris* differs from that reported for *E. dofleini* (Mather & Anderson, 1999), who used their funnels, rather than their arms, to manipulate objects. This difference in mode of play between the two species is not surprising – even closely related mammals such as rodents, carnivores and primates also show different types and amounts of play (Pellis, 1993; Burghardt, 2005). Apart from ecological differences, *O. vulgaris* is also a diurnal (Meisel et al., 2006), curious and agile species, spending most of the time during observational periods moving around in its tank. *Enteroctopus dofleini*, on the other hand, is a nocturnal cold-water species (Anderson & Wood, 2001). It is probably less agile and interacted less with the object when the object was moved towards the octopus by the water current. These differences aside, both species fulfilled the criteria for play or play-like behaviour.

Do octopuses have the necessary prerequisites to show such a complex behaviour? Aristotle was the first to report the curiosity displayed by the *Octopus*, which sparked an age-old speculation about their intelligence. Their ability to learn and perform complex tasks points towards a highly evolved cognitive capacity (Mather 1995; Hanlon & Messenger, 1996; Hochner, 2008, Mather 2008; Hochner, 2010; Gutnick, Byrne, Hochner & Kuba, 2011; Figure 3.4). Researchers have also demonstrated the existence of personalities (Mather & Anderson, 1993; Sinn, Perrin, Anderson & Mather, 2001) and, perhaps, even archaic forms of consciousness in octopuses (Mather, 2008; Edelmann & Seth, 2009), further indicators of complex behaviour. All these factors fit into the model on factors underlying primary process play formulated by Burghardt (2005; Table 3.1).

What might be the function of play in a cephalopod mollusc? If play has an adaptive (e.g. learning, training) function it should be more frequently observed in younger, smaller animals, as proposed by various theories on the importance of play in training and preparing animals for future behaviours (Byers & Walker, 1995; Bekoff & Byers, 1998; Spinka, Newberry & Bekoff, 2001). While there was no difference in play by smaller (potentially) younger versus larger (potentially) older animals (Kuba, Byrne, Meisel & Mather, 2006a), the standard concepts of juvenile and adult life found in vertebrates do not easily translate to cephalopods and, thus, need further scientific research. Presumably, play behaviour might not have the training, or practice, role for life in an octopus as it has in many vertebrates (Bekoff & Byers, 1998; Burghardt, 2004). In contrast to the view of play as a preparation for the future, Hall (1904) formulated the long neglected recapitulation theory of play. Hall (1904) stated that play is more a legacy from the past than a preparation for the future. Burghardt (1984, 1998, 2004, 2005, 2010; Graham & Burghardt, 2010) picked up some of the implications of Hall's theory in his Surplus Resource Theory (SRT) and his division of play into primary, secondary and tertiary processes. He claimed that primary process play is most likely to occur when behaviourally complex animals have some surplus resources including metabolic energy, time, minimal stress and a rich repertoire of behavioural movements to deploy (Burghardt, 1998, 1999, 2004, 2005, 2010; Graham & Burghardt, 2010). Burghardt (2004) formulated his theory on the evolutionary importance of primary process play (play without a direct selective benefit from the behaviour itself), claiming that it might not have adaptive functions, but can be useful to the individual if it is, to the extent it is heritable, transformed via selection to enhance survival and reproductive fitness. Additionally, it provides variation from which novel and complex behaviour can be derived more rapidly than through selection of the more fixed functional aspects of an animal's behavioural repertoire. In other words, play can indeed become an evolutionary pump. In this case, play might have additional functions not easily tested. Darwish, Korányi, Nyakas & Almeida (2001) showed that providing novel objects to aged rats reduced anxiety levels and that in both young and adult rats, play behaviour dampens the stress response as measured by the corticosterone level (Darwish, Korányi, Nyakas & Ferencz, 2001). In their case, play had the function of creating bolder animals with increased behavioural flexibility (Darwish, Korányi, Nyakas & Ferencz, 2001). As sensory deprivation tank experiments (Lilly & Shurley, 1961) showed that humans had visual sensations of sensory inputs (hallucinations) without stimulation, play might also be a way to keep a brain 'busy' in times of stimulus deprivation. Play could, therefore, be a by-product of a complex nervous system heavily depending on learning (Hanlon & Messenger, 1996; Hochner, 2008) and have the function of maintaining a status quo in times of lesser ecological pressure and lack of stimuli. Thus, play has been an important indicator for evaluating animal welfare in vertebrates (for a review, see Held & Spinka, 2011). This raises the issue of enrichment as an essential part of cephalopod welfare and, in that context, whether exploratory and play behaviour has to be considered as an indicator for welfare. All these questions provide important and interesting avenues for research into further underlying mechanisms in cephalopods.

What about cephalopod play in groups other than octopus? Certainly cuttlefish and squid might have the cognitive capacity to engage in playful interactions. However, due to the different nature of their body plan, life history and ecology, they might engage in other activities such as locomotor play or, to the extent they are social, rudimentary forms of social play. An especially promising candidate to study this would be cuttlefish or the Caribbean reef squid. Both groups show highly complex social interactions ranging from sneaker males (Hanlon, Naud, Shaw & Havenhand, 2005) to more or less complex communication using body shape and colour (Byrne, Griebel, Wood & Mather, 2003; Mather, Griebel & Byrne, 2010).

3.4   Conclusions

A true comparative approach to play was long neglected, as play was seen to be a trait unique to mammals. For example, the eminent brain researcher Paul MacLean (1985, 1990) stated that play behaviour was one of the 'signature behaviours' separating mammals from other vertebrates. However, his theories did not take into account reports on avian play already documented by Fagan (1981). Burghardt, Ward and Rosscoe (1996) reported play behaviour in a Nile soft-shelled turtle, and thereby stretched the 'phylogenetic boundaries' of play even further. To date animals as diverse as lizards, crocodilians, frogs, fishes (Burghardt, 2005), insects (Dapporto, Turilliazzi & Palagi, 2006) and, most recently, spiders (Pruitt, Burghardt & Reichert, 2012) have been reported to show at least some form of play behaviour. Due to the phylogenetic distance of the invertebrate octopus to other studied playful animals, a new window has opened for comparative studies on the evolution of not only play behaviour but also how play may impact the evolution and instantiation of other behavioural systems.

References

Alves, C., Chichery, R., Boal, J. G. and Dickel, L. (2007). Orientation in the cuttlefish *Sepia officinalis*: Response versus place learning. *Animal Cognition*, **10**: 29–36.

Anderson, R. C. and Wood, J. B. (2001). Enrichment for giant Pacific octopuses: Happy as a clam? *Journal of Applied Animal Welfare Science* **4**: 157–168.

Archer, J. and Birke, L. (eds) (1983). *Exploration in Animals and Humans*, Wokingham, Berks, UK: Van Nostrad Reinhold.

Baldwin, J. D. and Baldwin, J. I. (1997). *Behavioral Principles in Everyday Life*, Upper Saddle River, NJ: Prentice Hall.

Bekoff, M. and Byers, J. A. (1998). *Animal Play: Evolutionary, Comparative, and Ecological Perspectives*, Cambridge: Cambridge University Press.

Berlyne, D. E. (1960). *Conflict, Arousal, and Curiosity*, New York: McGraw-Hill.

Berlyne, D. E. (1966). Curiosity and exploration. *Science* **153**: 25–33.

Bruner, J. S., Jolly, A. and Sylva, K. (1976). *Play – Its Role in Development and Evolution*, New York: Basic Books.

Burghardt, G. M. (1984). On the origins of play. In *Play in Animals and Humans*, Smith, P. K. (ed.), London: Basil Blackwell.

Burghardt, G. M. (1998). The evolutionary origins of play revisited: Lessons from turtles. In *Animal Play: Evolutionary, Comparative, and Ecological Perspectives*, Bekoff, M., Byers J. A. (eds.), Cambridge: Cambridge University Press.

Burghardt, G. M. (1999). Conceptions of play and the evolution of animal minds. *Evolution and Cognition*, **5**: 115–123.

Burghardt, G. M. (2004). Play: How evolution can explain the most mysterious behavior of all. In *Evolution from Molecules to Ecosystems*, Moya, A., Font, E. (eds.), Oxford: Oxford University Press.

Burghardt, G. M. (2005). *The Genesis of Animal Play: Testing the Limits*, Cambridge, MA: MIT Press.

Burghardt, G. M. (2010). Play. In *Encyclopedia of Animal Behavior*, Breed, M., Moore J. (eds.) Oxford: Academic Press.

Burghardt, G. M. (2012). Play, exploration and learning. In *Encylopedia of Sciences of Learning*, Seel, N. M. (ed.), Heidelberg: Springer.

Burghardt, G. M., Ward, B. and Rosscoe, R. (1996). Problem of reptile play: Environmental enrichment and play behavior in a captive Nile soft-shelled turtle, *Trionyx triunguis*. *Zoo Biology*, **15**: 223–238.

Byers, J. A. and Walker, C. (1995). Refining the motor training hypothesis for the evolution of play. *The American Naturalist*, **146**: 25–40.

Byrne, R. A., Griebel, U., Wood, J. B. and Mather, J. A. (2003). Squid say it with skin: A graphic model for skin displays in Caribbean Reef Squid (*Sepioteuthis sepioidea*). *Berliner Palaeoontologische Abhandlungen*, **3**: 29–35.

Craig, W. (1918). Appetites and aversions as constituents of instincts. *The Biological Bulletin*, **34**: 91–107.

Dapporto, L., Turilliazzi, S. and Palagi, E. (2006). Dominance interactions in young adult paper wasps (*Polistes dominulus*) foundresses: A playlike behavior? *Journal of Comparative Psychology*, **120**: 394–400.

Darwish, M., Korányi, L., Nyakas, C. and Almeida, O. F. X. (2001). Exposure to a novel stimulus reduces anxiety level in adult and aging rats. *Physiology and Behavior*, **72**: 403–407.

Darwish, M., Korányi, L., Nyakas, C. and Ferencz, A. (2001). Induced social interaction reduces corticosterone stress response to anxiety in adult and aging Rats. *Klinikai és Kísérletes Laboratoriumi Medicina*, **28**: 108–111.

Day, J. E. L., Kyriazakis, I. and Lawrence, A. B. (1994). The effect of food deprivation on the expression of foraging and exploratory behavior in the growing pig. *Applied Animal Behavior Science*, **42**: 193–206.

Drickamer, L.C., Vessey, S.H. and Meikle, D. (1996). *Animal Behavior*, 4th edn. Dubuque, IA: William C. Brown.

Edelman, D. B. and Seth, A. K. (2009). Animal consciousness: A synthetic approach. *Trends in Neurosciences*, **32**: 476–484.

Fagan, R. (1981). *Animal Play Behavior*, New York: Oxford University Press.

Gazzaniga, M. S. and Heatherton, T. F. (2003). *Psychological Science: Mind, Brain and Behavior*, New York: W. W. Norton and Company.

Graham, K. L. and Burghardt, G. M. (2010). Current perspectives on the biological study of play: Signs of progress. *Quarterly Review of Biology*, **85**: 393–418.

Grasso, F. and Basil, J. (2009). The evolution of flexible behavioral repertoires in cephalopod molluscs. *Brain Behavior and Evolution*, **74**: 231–245.

Gutnick, T., Byrne, R. A., Hochner, B. and Kuba, M. (2011). *Octopus vulgaris* uses visual information to determine the location of its arm. *Current Biology*, **21**: 460–462.

Hall, G. S. (1904). *Adolescence, its Psychology and its Relation to Physiology, Anthropology, Sex, Crime, Religion, and Education*, New York: D. Appleton and Company.

Hanlon, R. T. and Messenger, J. B. (1996). *Cephalopod Behaviour*, New York: Cambridge University Press.

Hanlon, R. T., Naud, M.-J., Shaw, P. W. and Havenhand, J. N. (2005). Transient sexual mimicry leads to fertilisation. *Nature*, **430**: 212.

Harlow, H. F. (1950). Learning and satiation of response in intrinsically motivated complex puzzle performance by monkeys. *Journal of Comparative and Physiological Psychology*, **43**: 289–294.

Harlow, H. F. (1953). Mice, monkeys, men and motives. *Psychological Review*, **60**: 23–33.

Heinrich, B. (1995). Neophilia and exploration in juvenile common raven *Corvus corax*. *Animal Behaviour*, **50**: 695–704.

Held, S. D. E. and Spinka, M. (2011). Animal play and animal welfare. *Animal Behaviour*, **81**: 891–899.

Hochner, B. (2008). Octopuses. *Current Biology*, **18**: R897.

Hochner, B. (2010). Functional and comparative assessments of the octopus learning and memory system. *Frontiers in Biosciences*, **2**: 764–771.

Huber, L., Rechberger, S. and Taborsky, M. (2001). Social learning affects object exploration and manipulation in keas, *Nestor notabilis*. *Animal Behaviour*, **62**: 945–954.

Hughes, M. (1983). Exploration and play in young children. In *Exploration in Animals and Humans*, Archer J., Birke L. (eds.), Wokingham, Berks, UK: Van Nostrad Reinhold.

Hutt, C. (1966). Exploration and play in children. *Symposia of the Zoological Society of London*, **18**: 61–81.

Kuba, M. J., Byrne, R. A., Meisel, D. V. and Mather, J. A. (2006a). When do octopuses play? Effects of repeated testing, object type, age, and food deprivation on object play in *Octopus vulgaris*. *Journal of Comparative Psychology*, **120**: 184–190.

Kuba, M. J., Byrne, R. A., Meisel, D. V. and Mather J. A. (2006b). Exploration and habituation in intact free moving *Octopus vulgaris*. *International Journal of Comparative Psychology*, **19**: 426–438.

Kuba, M. J., Meisel, D. V., Byrne, R. A., Griebel, U. and Mather, J. A. (2003). Looking at play in *Octopus vulgaris. Berliner Paläontologische Abhandlungen*, **3**: 163–169.

Lilly, J. C. and Shurley, J. T. (1961). Experiments in solitude in maximum achievable physical isolation with water suspension of intact healthy persons. (Symposium, USAF Aerospace Medical Center, San Antonio, Texas, 1960.) In *Psychophysiological Aspects of Space Flight*, New York: Columbia University Press.

MacLean, P. D. (1985). Brain evolution relating to family, play, and the separation call. *Archives of General Psychiatry*, **42**: 504–517.

MacLean, P. D. (1990). *The Triune Brain in Evolution: Role in Paleocerebral Functions*, New York: Plenum Press.

Mather, J. A. (1991a). Foraging, feeding and prey remains in middens of juvenile *Octopus vulgaris*. *Journal of Zoology*, **224**: 27–39.

Mather, J. A. (1991b). Navigation by spatial memory and use of visual landmarks in octopuses. *Journal of Comparative Physiology A*, **168**: 491–497.

Mather, J. A. (1995). Cognition in cephalopods. *Advances in the Study of Behavior*, **24**: 317–353.

Mather, J. A. (2008). Cephalopod consciousness: Behavioral evidence. *Consciousness and Cognition*, **17**: 37–48.

Mather, J. A. and Anderson, R. C. (1993). Personalities of octopuses (*Octopus rubescens*). *Journal of Comparative Psychology*, **107**: 336–340.

Mather, J. A. and Anderson, R. C. (1999). Exploration, play and habituation. *Journal of Comparative Psychology*, **113**: 333–338.

Mather, J. A., Griebel, U. and Byrne, R. A. (2010). Squid dances: An ethogram of postures and actions of *Sepioteuthis sepioidea* squid with a muscular hydrostatic system. *Marine and Freshwater Behaviour and Physiology*, **43**: 45–61.

Meisel D. V., Byrne R. A., Kuba M. J., Mather J. A. Ploberger W. and Reschenhofer E. (2006). Comparing the activity patterns of two Mediterranean cephalopod species. *Journal of Comparative Psychology*, **120**: 191–197.

Moynihan, M. H. and Rodaniche, A. F. (1982). The behavior and natural history of the Caribbean reef squid *Sepioteuthis sepioidea* with a consideration of social, signal and defensive patterns for difficult and dangerous environments. *Advances in Ethology*, **25**: 1–151.

Müller-Schwarze, D. (1984). Analysis of play behaviour: What do we measure and when? In *Play in Animals and Humans*, Smith, P. K. (ed.), Oxford: Basil Blackwell.

Nixon, M. and Young, J. Z. (2003). *The Brains and Lives of Cephalopods*. Oxford: Oxford University Press.

Packard, A. (1972). Cephalopods and fish: The limits of convergence. *Biological Reviews*, **47**: 241–307.

Pellis, S. M. (1993). Sex and the evolution of play fighting: A review on the behavior of muroid rodents. *Play Theory and Research*, **1**: 55–75.

Pellis, S. M. and Iwaniuk, A. N. (2004). Evolving a playful brain: A level of control approach. *International Journal of Comparative Psychology*, **17**: 92–118.

Power, T. G. (2000). *Play and Exploration in Children and Animals*. Mahwah, NJ: Lawrence Erlbaum Associates.

Pruitt, J. N., Burghardt, G. M. and Riechert, S. E. (2012). Non-conceptive sexual behavior in spiders: A form of play associated with body condition, personality type, and male intrasexual selection. *Ethology*, **18**: 33–40.

Renner, M. J. (1990). Neglected aspects of exploratory and investigative behavior. *Psychobiology*, **18**: 16–22.

Renner, M. J. and Seltzer, C. P. (1994). Sequential structure in behavioral components of object investigations by Long–Evans rats. *Journal of Comparative Psychology*, **108**: 81–91.

Russell, P. A. (1983). Psychological studies of exploration in animals. In *Exploration in Animals and Humans*, Archer J., Birke L. (eds.), Wokingham, Berks, UK: Van Nostrad Reinhold.

Sanders, G. D. (1975). The cephalopods. In *Invertebrate Learning*, Corning, W.C. (ed.), New York: Plenum Press.

Sinn, D. L., Perrin, N. A., Anderson, R. C. and Mather, J. A. (2001). Early temperamental traits in an octopus (*Octopus bimaculoides*). *Journal of Comparative Psychology*, **115**: 351–364.

Sommer, V. and Mendoza-Grandos, D. (1995). Play as indicator of habitat quality: A field study of langur monkeys (*Presbytis entellus*). *Ethology*, **99**: 177–192.

Spinka, M., Newberry, R. C. and Beckoff, M. (2001). Mammalian play: Training for the unexpected. *Quarterly Review of Biology*,**76**: 141–168.

Toates, F. M. (1983). Exploration as a motivational and learning system. In *Exploration in Animals and Humans*, Archer J., Birke L. (eds.), Wokingham, Berks, UK: Van Nostrad Reinhold.

Wells, M. J. (1962). *Brain and Behavior in Cephalopods*, London: Heinemann.

Wells, M. J. (1978). *Octopus. Physiology and Behaviour of an Advanced Invertebrate*, London: Chapman and Hall.

Wood-Gush, D., Stolba, A. and Miller, C. (1983). Exploration in farm animals and animal husbandry. In *Exploration in Animals and Humans*, Archer J., Birke L. (eds.), Wokingham, Berks, UK: Van Nostrad Reinhold.

4   The neurophysiological basis of learning and memory in an advanced invertebrate: the octopus

Binyamin Hochner and Tal Shomrat

4.1   Introduction

It is commonly believed that invertebrates should be used for studying general questions in neurobiology only when their specific features, such as "a small number of large identifiable neurons" or their amenity to genetic manipulation, provide a special experimental advantage. We do not agree. We believe it is important to study octopuses and other modern cephalopods for totally different reasons. These invertebrates show behavioral repertoires comparable to those of higher vertebrates (Packard, 1972; Wells, 1978; Hochner, Shomrat & Fiorito, 2006; Hochner, 2008; Grasso & Basil, 2009), yet their brains maintain the much simpler invertebrate organization (Budelmann, 1995). This unique combination of simpler nervous system and complex behavior is especially advantageous for tackling the central question of how a nervous system controls complex behaviors and cognitive functions.

Although the subject of this book is cephalopod cognition, this chapter deals with the neurophysiological bases of learning and memory, which, in our opinion, is not necessarily a cognitive capacity. It is true that cognitive functions are usually thought (e.g. Wikipedia definition) to include learning and memory in addition to attention, association, language, problem-solving, decision-making, mental imagery and more. There is no doubt, however, that cognitive function cannot happen without learning and memory. Some cognitive functions may emerge from mutual high level processing of long-term stored memories and the current sensory information stored temporarily as short-term working memory. In this mechanistic scenario memory itself, especially in its more basic forms like associative and non-associative learning, would not be considered a cognitive function. It is worth noting that certain animals without obvious high cognitive abilities show excellent learning and memory, and humans with cognitive disorders may still possess an excellent memory.

As part of their sophisticated behavioral repertoire, the octopus and other modern cephalopods exhibit vertebrate-like learning and memory behaviors (Sanders, 1975; Wells, 1978; Fiorito & Scotto, 1992; Hanlon & Messenger, 1996; Hochner, Shomrat & Fiorito, 2006; Grasso & Basil, 2009). Analyzing the cellular processes and neuronal circuitry of their learning and memory systems and comparing the results with those

Cephalopod Cognition, eds A.-S. Darmaillacq, L. Dickel and J. Mather. Published by Cambridge University Press. © Cambridge 2014.

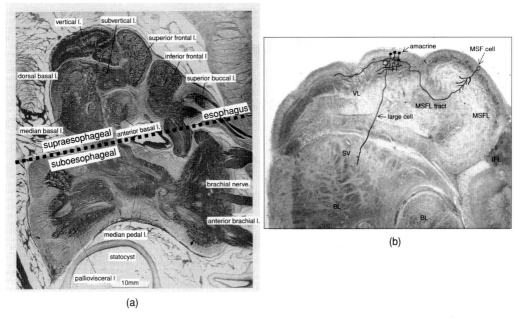

(a)

(b)

Figure 4.1 The morphological organization of the octopus central brain. (a) Sagittal section of the sub- and supraoesophageal lobes of *Octopus vulgaris* showing the dorsal location of the median superior frontal (MSFL)–vertical lobe (VL) system and the organization of the lobes which are discussed in the text. (Modified from Nixon and Young, 2003.) (b) Unstained median sagittal section through the dorsal part of the supraoesophageal brain mass with superimposed schematic drawing of the three types of neurons in this system and their connections. This area in the supraoesophageal lobes (see (a)) forms the main part of the VL-slice. (*BL*, basal lobes; *IFL*, inferior frontal lobe; *MSFL*, median superior frontal lobe; *SV*, subvertical lobe; *VL*, vertical lobe).

of other invertebrate and vertebrate systems may advance our understanding of their evolution and function. This comparative evolutionary approach can determine whether mechanisms subserving cognitive functions evolved convergent across widely diverse phyla or, alternatively, whether evolutionarily primitive mechanisms mediating simple forms of behaviors are conserved in more advanced animals to mediate complex behaviors.

The octopus central brain consists of ~40 lobes that maintain some simple organizational features of the central nervous system of simple mollusks (Figure 4.1). The neuron cell bodies lie in the outer region of each lobe, while their processes form the central neuropil (Figure 4.1a; Young, 1971).

Previous experiments have indicated that the vertical lobe (VL) is involved in higher brain functions. Stimulating it or the superior frontal lobes evoked no obvious effects, whereas stimulating other parts of the brain caused movements of some part of the body (Boycott, 1961; Zullo, Sumbre, Agnisola, Flash & Hochner, 2009). Removing the VL also did not appear to affect the animal's general behavior (Boycott & Young, 1955; Maldonado, 1965; Sanders, 1975). Thus, the VL and the superior frontal lobe do not seem to be engaged in simple motor functions. Deficiencies were revealed only when animals were required to learn new tasks. After removal or lesion of the VL, octopuses continued to attack crabs in spite of receiving electrical shocks, unless the intertrial interval was less than ~5 minutes (Boycott & Young, 1955). Thus, the VL appears to be specifically involved in long-term and more complex forms of memory.

Another complex form of learning demonstrated by octopuses is observational learning. A naive octopus learns to attack a previously positively rewarded target after only four observations of a trained octopus attacking the same target. This is much faster than it takes to train the demonstrator octopus (Fiorito & Scotto, 1992). Lesion study has demonstrated that the VL is important for this advanced form of learning (Fiorito & Chichery, 1995).

Finally, the morphological structure of the VL appears very simple, but its unique matrix-like organization led Boycott and Young (1955) to postulate that the median superior frontal lobe (MSFL)–VL and inferior frontal lobe (IFL) (Figure 4.1b) networks form associative networks for learning and memory. Wells (1978) and Young (1991) further suggested that the VL matrix is analogous to the mammalian hippocampus memory system and the insect mushroom body (Young, 1991, 1995; Hochner, 2010). The VL system is, thus, an exciting site for exploring the neuronal circuitry and physiological mechanisms involved in learning and memory.

4.2   The anatomy of the vertical lobe system

The octopus VL contains only two types of neuron, amacrine cells and large neurons, both of which are morphologically typical invertebrate monopolar neurons (Figure 4.2; Gray & Young, 1964; Gray, 1970; Young, 1971). Twenty-five million amacrine cells, which are the smallest neurons in the octopus brain (diameter 6–10 µm) converge onto only ~65 000 large neurons (diameter ~17 µm). The amacrine processes are confined within the VL (Figures 4.1b, 4.2), while the axons of the large neurons form the only output of the VL, leaving it in organized axons bundles or roots, which are easy to identify and record from (Figure 4.1b).

The VL receives inputs from the MSFL. This lobe is thought to integrate visual and taste information. It contains only one morphological type of neuron, whose 1.8 million axons project to the VL in a distinct tract running between the VL neuropil and its outer cell body layer (Figure 4.1a,b). This arrangement allows each MSFL axon to make *en passant* synapses with many amacrine neurons along the VL (Figure 4.2). Young (1971) also postulated a direct connection to the large neurons but this was not supported by Gray's (1970) electron microscopic study, and is also not supported by recent physiological results (see below and Shomrat et al., 2011). This special matrix-like organization of the MSFL–VL complex is shared by the inferior frontal lobe (Figure 4.1), which plays a role in chemotactile memory (Wells, 1978; Young, 1991).

Testing Boycott and Young's (1955) hypothesis that the VL and inferior frontal networks are associative networks for learning and memory clearly requires physiological characterization of these brain circuits and their plastic properties. The new experimental

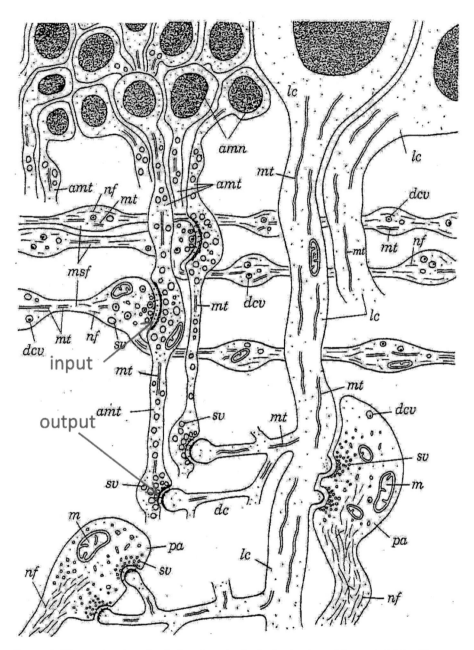

Figure 4.2 Digram showing what is thought to be the basic circuitry of the vertical lobe. The nature of the "serial synapse" of the amacrine cells is depicted by the arrows indicating input and output at the same amacrine dendrite. (*amn,* amacrine cells; *amt,* amacrine trunk; *dc,* dendritic collaterals of large cell; *dcv,* dense-core vesicle; *lc,* large cell; *msf,* median superior frontal axon; *mt,* microtubule; *nf,* neurofilaments; *pa,* possible "pain" axon input to the large cell; *sv,* synaptic vesicles.) (From Gray, 1970.)

preparations that have been developed now allow neurophysiological exploration of this anatomically unique system.

4.3   Neurophysiology of the vertical lobe

Most of the octopus brain shows a typical invertebrate form (see Bullock & Horridge, 1965), but the VL shows a greater resemblance to vertebrae brain organization, with its large numbers of neurons organized in layers and their processes aligned more or less in parallel. This organization, unlike the more random organization of typical invertebrate ganglia, generates a measurable external electric field near the active neurons. This field potential shows local field potentials (spontaneous, ongoing background activity), evoked potentials (EP) and event-related potentials (ERP), and a compound field potential similar to an electroencephalography (EEG) (e.g. Bullock & Basar, 1988). Bullock (1984) suggested that the existence of such a compound field potential indicates the high level of complexity of the octopus brain.

How does the anatomical organization allow us to record field potentials? The amount of current flowing in the extracellular space due to neuron activity, such as an action potential, is usually tiny and, as the extracellular impedance is very low (about 3–4 orders of magnitude lower than the neurons' input resistance), only summation of local field potentials generated by many neurons becomes large enough to be reliably monitored. Such summation accrues only if the neurons are synchronously active and their currents flow in the same direction, otherwise they cancel each other out. This condition is achieved only when the neurons have elongated morphology and they are organized in the same orientation. Such an arrangement occurs in the MSFL–VL system, where the MSFL axons input to the VL is organized in bundles. The cell bodies of the millions of amacrine neurons lie in the outer zone of the lobe, while their axons project in parallel into the lobe, perpendicular to the MSFL axons bundles (Figures 4.1, 4.2). Such an architecture would be expected to generate a significant local field potential (LFP), possibly similar to that generated close to the Schaeffer collaterals in the hippocampus.

The existence of such a local field potential was confirmed by physiological experiments. Stimulating the MSFL tract with a short current pulse evokes a typical field potential waveform (Figure 4.3). This is a tri-phasic (positive–negative–positive) tract potential (*TP*) generated by the volley of action potential propagating along the stimulated axons in the MSFL tract. The delay after the stimulus artifact (*stim.*) depends on the distance between stimulus and recording electrodes. A mainly negative field potential immediately follows the second positive wave of the TP. This potential is a postsynaptic field potential (fPSP) because it disappears in zero-calcium physiological solution (Figure 4.3a). In contrast to the action potential, which is generated by sodium and potassium ionic currents, the release of neurotransmitter depends on calcium ions and, therefore, removal of calcium blocks the part of the LFP, which is generated by postsynaptic response while leaving the TP unchanged. This fPSP is generated by opening of postsynaptic glutamate receptors because the fPSP is also blocked by

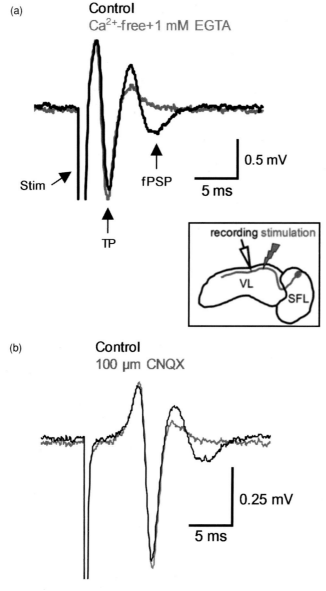

Figure 4.3 (a) Superimposed local field potentials (LFP) in control and after blocking postsynaptic field potential (fPSP) in Ca^{2+}-free EGTA ASW (artificial seawater) *fPSP*, postsynaptic field potential; *Stim,* stimulus artifact; *TP* tract potential). (b) Similar to (a), showing blockade of fPSP by AMPA-like glutamatergic receptor antagonists CNQX. *Inset*: Schematic depiction of median superior frontal (MSFL)–vertical lobe (VL) slice preparation with a possible electrodes placement for stimulation and recording of LFP.

AMPA (α-amino-3-hydroxy-5-methyl-4-isoxazolepropionic acid)-like antagonists such as CNQX (6-cyano-7-nitroquinoxaline-2,3-dione) (Figure 4.3b), DNQX (6,7-dinitroquinoxaline-2,3-dione) or kynurenate (Hochner, Brown, Langella, Shomrat & Fiorito, 2003).

The types of fast neurotransmitters in the invertebrate nervous system are more diversified than in vertebrates, and finding glutamate neurotransmission in the VL has hinted to the universality of this transmitter in learning neural networks. However, as will be shown below, this is not entirely true, because acetylcholine was found to be another fast transmitter in the VL. In vertebrates acetylcholine is a fast neurotransmitter mainly at the neuromuscular system. "Fast" neurotransmitters serve for fast transmission of information (at the range of a few milliseconds) between neurons and involves the opening of ionic channels, while "slow" neurotransmitters serve mainly in modulation of cell activity and their action involves activation of a special class of receptors that are coupled, via a biochemical cascade, to the activation of second messengers (e.g. cyclic adenosine monophosphate [c-AMP]).

The short latency between the peak negativity of the TP and the fPSP onset (~3 ms, Figure 4.3a,b) suggests a monosynaptic delay. The physiological results are thus in good agreement with Gray's scheme (Figure 4.2), in which the MSFL axon terminals synapse directly on the amacrine dendrites. The recent physiological results (Figure 4.3b), further suggest that the first synaptic layer of the VL is likely glutamatergic.

As expected from the anatomical organization, the local field potential in the VL (presynaptic TP followed by fPSP; Figure 4.3) is similar to that evoked at the stratum radiatum of the hippocampus by stimulating the Schaffer fiber collaterals in CA1. In both cases the collaterals/tract terminals make synapse *en passant* with the dendrites of the pyramidal/amacrine cells, respectively. However, because the amacrine cells are inexcitable as they don't generate regenerative action potentials (Hochner, Brown, Langella, Shomrat & Fiorito, 2003; Hochner, Shomrat & Fiorito, 2006), the fPSP has an amplitude-independent waveform with no population spikes, in contrast to the postsynaptic field potential of the hippocampal pyramidal neurons (Miyakawa & Kato, 1986).

The amacrine cells innervate the large efferent neurons via special "serial" synapses (Figure 4.2). This synapse is called serial because the dendrites of the amacrine cells are both the input site for the MSFL axonal terminals and the output site to the large cell (arrows in Figure 4.2). To investigate the nature of this input to the large cells, infrared differential interference contrast (DIC) microscopy was used to record intracellularly from their cell bodies, as well as recording their spiking activity extracellularly from their axon bundles. Figure 4.4a shows excitatory postsynaptic potential (EPSP) evoked by stimulating the MSFL tract and spontaneous EPSPs in a large neuron. Like most invertebrate neurons, the cell bodies of the large neurons are inexcitable, as demonstrated by the small non-overshooting spikelets (arrowhead). These decrease in size passively as they pass along the single neurite to the cell body from a distant spike initiation zone at the junction between the dendritic tree and the axon.

The synaptic input to the large neurons is cholinergic, since both evoked and spontaneous EPSPs were blocked by hexamethonium (Figure 4.4a), a muscarinic receptor antagonist that also blocks the synaptic potential at the neuromuscular junctions of the

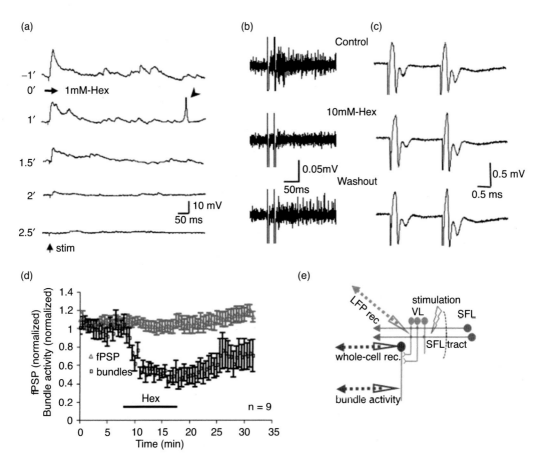

Figure 4.4 The synaptic inputs to the large cells are most likely cholinergic. (See (e) for the different recording modes.) (a) Hexamethonium blocked the spontaneous and SFL tract-evoked EPSPs recorded intracellularly from large cells (arrowheads point to example of spikelet). (b) Hexamethonium blocked the burst of action potentials recorded extracellularly from large cells axonal bundles. Note that twin stimuli (b,c) were used to obtain a clearly measurable bundle response. (c) Hexamethonium had no effect on the tract potential (TP) and postsynaptic field potential (fPSPs). Records were obtained simultaneously with bundle activity shown in (b). (d) Summary of nine experiments as exemplified in (b) and (c). Black curve, normalized integrated bundle activity; gray, fPSP amplitude. Here and in subsequent figures responses were normalized to the average of 3–10 test responses at the beginning of the experiments. (Modified from Shomrat et al., 2011.)

octopus arm (Matzner, Gutfreund & Hochner, 2000). Hexamethonium also blocked both spontaneous and evoked spiking activity recorded from the large neuron axon bundles (Figure 4.4b,d). As would be expected for glutamatergic synapses, the fPSP of the first synaptic layer was unaffected by cholinergic antagonists (Figure 4.4c,d). Thus, it must be the amacrine-to-large neuron synapse that is cholinergic.

Both cholinergic and glutamatergic antagonists blocked activity output of the large neuron axon bundles. This finding suggests that there is no strong direct connection from

MSFL input axons to the large neurons and that the main connections within the VL are the MSFL inputs onto the amacrine cells, which then innervate the large efferents neurons (Shomrat et al., 2011).

The VL system thus appears to be organized as a simple feed-forward fan-out fan-in network. This type of network architecture is frequently found amongst biological and artificial networks (e.g. a machine-learning algorithm; Vapnik, 1998) that learn to classify when endowed with the synaptic plasticity that creates learning ability. The first fan-out synaptic layer may create a neural representation of the incoming sensory information in a form suitable for further processing at the fan-in layer (Nowotny, Huerta, Abarbanel & Rabinovich, 2005; Shomrat et al., 2011). If the VL system possesses this architecture and functions as a learning and memory network, as shown above, then we would expect to find synaptic plasticity at one or more of its synaptic sites.

4.4   Synaptic plasticity in the vertical lobe

Examining the neurophysiological properties of synaptic transmission in the VL network revealed clear synaptic plasticity.

The local field potential recorded at the MSFL tract demonstrates a very robust activity-dependent plasticity. Tetanization led to a long-term potentiation (LTP) with a ~4-fold increase in fPSP amplitude without affecting the amplitude of the presynaptic TP (Figure 4.5, *inset top left*). The potentiation of the glutamatergic synaptic input to the amacrine neurons is long-term as it was maintained for at least 5 hours (Hochner, Brown, Langella, Shomrat & Fiorito, 2003). Tetanizing a second time showed that this LTP is a saturated phenomenon, because no additional long-term enhancement is obtained (Figure 4.5).

Does activity-dependent plasticity occur only at the fan-out glutamatergic connections (Figures 4.1, 4.5)? Tetanization, which induced LTP of the fPSP, also caused a long-term increase in the extracellular spiking activity of the large neuron axon bundles (Figure 4.6a,b). This result was not surprising; facilitation of the synaptic input to the amacrine cells (the fPSP) should increase their cholinergic input to the large neurons and thus to an enhancement of the large neurons output (i.e. increase bundle activity).

This result does not tell whether there is also synaptic plasticity at the input to the large neurons. However, analyzing the relationship between the amplitude of the fPSP and bundle activity showed a linear relationship that did not change after LTP induction (Figure 4.6c, gray labels; Shomrat et al., 2011). Because the same fPSP amplitude gave rise to the same level of bundle activity, irrespective of LTP, then LTP must occur only at the first, fan-out, synaptic layer.

This linear input–output relationship (Figure 4.6c) has important computational consequences. In a linearly operating network such as this, similar computation capacity is obtained regardless of whether the plasticity is localized at the fan-out or the fan-in layer (see Shomrat et al., 2011).

The cuttlefish (*Sepia officinalis*) and the octopus show opposite plasticity sites in their otherwise similar network synaptic connectivity arrangements. The cuttlefish shows

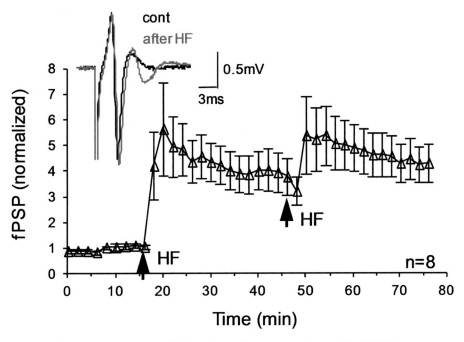

Figure 4.5 Long-term potentiation (LTP) at the median superior frontal lobe (MSFL) to amacrine cells synaptic connection. Summary of eight experiments in octopus: the development, maintenance and saturability of LTP in octopus. LTP was induced by four high frequency (HF) trains (20 pulses, 50 Hz, 10 s interval), postsynaptic field potentials (fPSP) were normalized to the averages of 10 test fPSP at the beginning of the experiments. The insets show a superimposition of LFP traces before (black) and after HF stimulation (gray). See explanation in the text. (Modified from Shomrat et al., 2011.)

synaptic plasticity at the fan-in and not at the fan-out layer, whereas the octopus has plasticity in the fan-out and not the fan-in layer. This led to suggest that evolutionary or self-organizational processes, which shape nervous systems organization, select for the network's computational properties rather than for its specific neuronal properties (Shomrat et al., 2011).

4.5   Mechanism of LTP induction in the octopus vertical lobe

Is activity-dependent synaptic plasticity mediated by associative or non-associative mechanisms? That is, does the synaptic plasticity in the VL fulfill Hebb's rule for associative plasticity, which postulates that the synaptic connection between the pre- and postsynaptic cells strengthens only when both are simultaneously and sufficiently active. The N-Methyl-D-aspartate (NMDA) channel, whose discovery was one of the most exciting breakthroughs in modern neuroscience, shows such a coincidence-detecting gating property. Therefore, the possible involvement of such a Hebbian mechanism in the octopus LTP has been explored. Direct tests for the involvement of an NMDA-like receptor

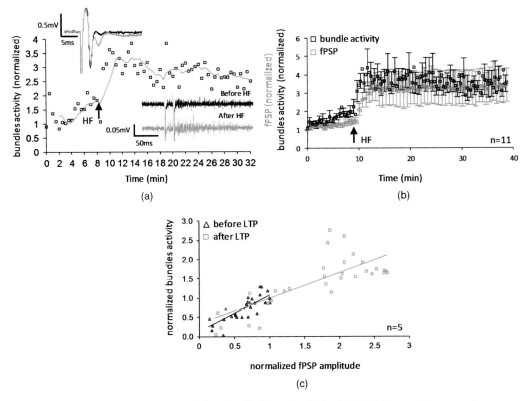

Figure 4.6 Input–output relationships in the vertical lobe (VL). (a) Extracellular recordings from the large cells axon bundles show long-term potentiation (LTP) of the VL output. The development and maintenance of LTP as measured by the median superior frontal lobe (MSFL) tract-evoked integrated bundles activity (gray line is a moving average of five test pulses). Upper insets, superimposition of LTP before (black) and after (gray) high frequency (HF). Lower insets, activity of the large cells axon bundles before (black) and after (gray) HF. (b) Summary of the experiments of the type shown in (a). (c) The VL input–output relationship before (black) and after (gray) LTP induction. The relationship is expressed as the correlation between the integrated activity in large cells axon bundles and the postsynaptic field potential (fPSP) amplitude generated by various stimulus intensities. The fPSP amplitudes and the bundles activity were normalized to those obtained in controls by a test pulse at the intensity used for LTP induction. (Modified from Shomrat et al., 2011.)

in the postsynaptic current (fPSP) or in LTP induction gave negative results; neither APV ((2R)-amino-5-phosphonovaleric acid), which blocks NMDA-like current in cephalopod chromatophore muscles (Lima, Nardi & Brown, 2003), nor MK-801 blocked these phenomena (Hochner, Brown, Langella, Shomrat & Fiorito, 2003; T. Shomrat & B. Hochner, unpublished data).

The crucial experiment to test whether the octopus VL evolved an NMDA-independent Hebbian plasticity is to completely block the postsynaptic response and then check whether tetanization leads to LTP induction after washing out the antagonists. The results from such experiments (summarized in Figure 4.7) show that the LTP in the octopus VL

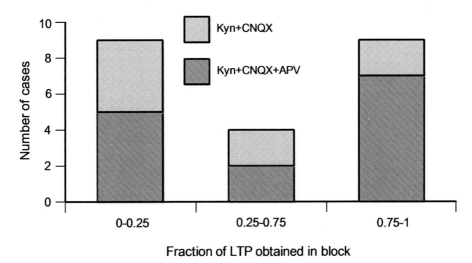

Figure 4.7 Dependence of long-term potentiation (LTP) induction on postsynaptic response. Summary of 22 experiments where the response during high frequency (HF) tetanization was completely blocked by a mixture of 20 mM kynurenate plus 200 µM CNQX and in some experiments also 200 µM APV. The histogram categories depict three ranges of LTP (expressed as the percent of total LTP) induced in the presence of the blocking mixture. The distribution shows a higher proportion of either largely blocked (0–25%) or hardly blocked (75–100%) LTP. (From Hochner, Brown, Langella, Shomrat & Fiorito, 2003.)

uses both associative and non-associative induction mechanisms. In somewhat less than half of the experiments, LTP induction was largely blocked by glutamatergic antagonists (*left bar*); in the other experiments there was hardly any blocking effect and LTP appears to have occurred in the absence of a postsynaptic response. Thus, if the two processes revealed were evenly distributed among the different synaptic connections in the VL, we would expect a normal distribution of the results. The bimodal distribution in Figure 4.7 can only be explained by the two types of plasticity being segregated in anatomically different regions, as in the hippocampus (CA3 vs. CA1; Kandel, Schwartz & Jessel, 2000). Such morphological differentiation has not yet been demonstrated in the octopus VL.

Characterizing associative/Hebbian type activity-dependent synaptic plasticity requires determining whether LTP results from an increase in the amount of transmitter released, or an increase in postsynaptic response, or both, an issue that is yet not completely resolved in the various hippocampal synapses. Detailed analysis of the changes in the properties of synaptic transmission accompanying LTP induction in the VL suggested that the expression of LTP is mainly, if not exclusively, presynaptic. That is, it occurs in the MSFL neuron terminals at their synapses with the amacrine neurons (Hochner, Brown, Langella, Shomrat & Fiorito, 2003).

This raises a mechanistic question regarding presynaptic expression of LTP as a result of strong enough postsynaptic response – the essence of associative/Hebbian plasticity. The prevailing hypothesis to explain such association is by a retrograde message that is transmitted from the postsynaptic to the presynaptic site, the most popular candidate has been nitric oxide (NO). Because of its gaseous nature NO can cross membranes readily and rapidly and activates biochemical processes in the presynaptic terminals. Although the involvement of NO in the induction of presynaptic LTP in mammals is supported by several experimental results (Garthwaite, 2008), it is still not a completely resolved issue. It is interesting that although NO was implicated first in mammalian synaptic plasticity, including LTP, it has become apparent that NO is an important modulator of invertebrates learning and memory (Susswein & Chiel, 2012), and NO was even implicated in the octopus learning and memory (Robertson, Bonaventura & Kohm, 1994; Robertson, Bonaventura, Kohm & Hiscat, 1996). It is conceivable, therefore, that the synapse that shows that the Hebbian type of LTP induction in the VL (Figure 4.7) may involve a retrograde messenger, such as nitric oxide, which would transfer the association signal from the postsynaptic cell to the presynaptic terminals to induce the LTP.

4.6   Neuromodulation in the vertical lobe

The highly dynamic properties of neural networks mediating learning and memory are not only achieved by the various types of activity-dependent plasticity but also by neuromodulators. Neuromodulators may feed back negative or positive heterosynaptic reward or punishment signals that facilitate or inhibit, respectively, the activity-dependent (homosynaptic) processes (Bailey, Giustetto, Huang, Hawkins & Kandel, 2000). The involvement of neuromodulators in associative learning is well documented in insects (Keene & Waddell, 2007), molluscs (Kemenes, O'Shea & Benjamin, 2011) and vertebrates (Schultz, 2007), and thus has most likely a universal role in complex neural function.

The search for neuromodulators in the octopus VL started by testing whether serotonin plays a role in VL function. Serotonin is a well known neuromodulator in mollusks, involved in both short- and long-term facilitation of the sensory-motor synapse in the defensive reflex of *Aplysia californica* (Kandel, 2001). Immunohistochemistry showed serotonin reactivity in nerve terminals in the VL neuropil but not of cell bodies, indicating that serotonin indeed may convey signals to the VL from other brain areas (Shomrat, Feinstein, Klein & Hochner, 2010).

The short-term modulatory effects of serotonin on VL function are shown in Figure 4.8a,b. A dose of 100–200 μM 5-hydroxytryptamine (5-HT) caused an average of ~3.5-fold facilitation of the fPSP. This facilitation involves presynaptic modulation of transmitter release, as it was accompanied by a reversible reduction in twin pulse facilitation (i.e. reduction in the ratio of the second fPSP amplitude to that of the first in twin pulse stimulation; Figure 4.8a,c). Repeated exposure to 5-HT did not lead to long-term modulation in the octopus VL, unlike its long-term effects on the *Aplysia* sensory-motor synapse. Also in contrast to *Aplysia*, c-AMP does not appear to be a major second messenger in 5-HT induced fPSP facilitation in the octopus VL (Shomrat, Feinstein, Klein & Hochner, 2010).

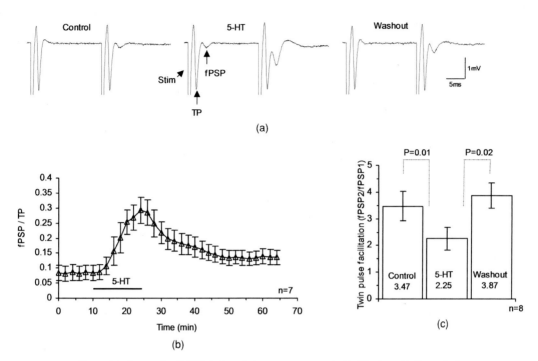

Figure 4.8 Serotonin (5-HT) induced short-term synaptic facilitation. (a) Records from one experiment. Responses to stimulation by twin pulses. *fPSP*, postsynaptic field potential; *Stim*, stimulation artifact; *TP*, tract potential.) (b) Summary of seen experiments demonstrating the facilitatory effect of 100–200 μM 5-HT and its reversal on washout. Test stimuli were applied every 10 or 20 seconds. (c) 5-HT reversibly reduced the level of paired–pulse facilitation measured as the ratio of the second to the first fPSP amplitudes. Unlike the example shown in (a), the histogram in (c) includes only experiments in which the first fPSP was apparent. (From Shomrat, Feinstein, Klein & Hochner, 2010.)

It is intriguing that serotonin has only a short-term robust facilitatory effect on a synaptic connection that undergoes long-term activity-dependent facilitation. Therefore, the serotonergic system in the octopus VL may have been adapted to provide a modulatory signal to the VL rather than inducing long-term plasticity changes as in *Aplysia*. The reinforcement effect of 5-HT on LTP induction (Shomrat, Feinstein, Klein & Hochner, 2010) suggests such a mechanism.

The reinforcement effect of 5-HT was proposed on the basis of the experiment shown in Figure 4.9. Here, instead of using 4 tetanization trains of 20 pulses (50 Hz), trains of only 3 pulses were applied. This reduced tetanization intensity induced only a partial and very modest LTP (19% of the final LTP; Figure 4.9a *triangles* and 4.9b *control*). In contrast, similar triplet stimulation in the presence of 5-HT, which caused a robust short-term fPSP facilitation, induced a much higher LTP (60.7%) (Figure 4.9a *squares* and 4.9b *5-HT*). Since LTP induction depends on the postsynaptic response or the presynaptic release processes (Figure 4.7; Hochner, Brown, Langella, Shomrat & Fiorito, 2003), the simple explanation is that 5-HT augments LTP indirectly by enhancing synaptic activity.

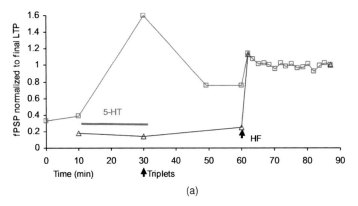 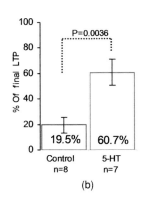

Figure 4.9 Serotonin (5-HT) reinforced activity-dependent long-term potentiation (LTP) induction. (a) Partial LTP was induced by the triple-pulse stimulation protocol. 5-HT (gray trace, open squares) caused large short-term facilitation (measuring the first postsynaptic field potential [fPSP] in the triple-pulse at ~30 min). After 30 min washout (60 min), high frequency (HF) stimulation revealed the residual LTP. HF stimulation gave rise to greater facilitation of the fPSPs in the control experiments (black trace, open triangles), indicating less recruitment of LTP than in the presence of 5-HT. (b) Summary histogram showing the percentage of the final LTP measured at the end of the experiments exemplified in (a). LTP was induced by the triplet stimulation protocol with and without 5-HT. (From Shomrat et al., 2010).

That is, the serotonergic system of the VL appears to reinforce the induction of activity-dependent plasticity and, thus, serotonin may convey reward signals to the learning and memory network in the VL, as do dopamine in mammals (Schultz, 2007) and octopamine in insects (Cassenaer & Laurent, 2012).

4.7   Are the vertical lobe and its LTP involved in behavioral learning and memory?

The octopus VL may be the preparation of choice to investigate how neurons store memories and how these memories are retrieved or forgotten. The simple VL circuitry may allow us to clarify how neurophysiological processes are utilized to build a behaviorally related neural system. Pioneering steps in this direction were made by Young, Boycott, Wells and their colleagues during the second half of the previous century. Their behavioral, morphological and lesion experiments showed that the octopus VL is important for learning and memory, but that it is not the sole brain lobe involved in these functions. The discovery of activity-dependent long-term plasticity and its neuromodulation in the VL provided physiological support for a VL function in learning and memory. However, a direct experimental test was required to confirm the involvement of these physiological processes in learning behavior.

To test the involvement of the LTP in the VL in learning and memory, Shomrat, Zarrella, Fiorito and Hochner (2008) followed the experiments of Moser, Krobert, Moser and Morris (1998). These showed that artificial saturation of LTP induced in the rat hippocampus by tetanization impaired spatial learning when tetanization was applied prior to learning. This technically challenging experiment in the rat is much simpler in the octopus, as the VL lies most dorsally in the brain and is relatively easily accessible to a large electrode for global tetanization. Such tetanization induced on average 56% of the available LTP.

Now Shomrat, Zarrella, Fiorito and Hochner (2008) could test whether this reduction in the available LTP induced by the tetanization affected a learning task. This was tested after 75 minutes of recovery from anesthesia used during the tetanization. The learning task was a passive avoidance task in which a mild electric shock to the arms "taught" the octopus to stop attacking a red ball. The results of LTP saturation by the tetanization were contrasted with the effects of transecting the MSFL tract to the VL, which disconnects the VL system from its sensory input. In contrast, inducing strong LTP of the synaptic connection between the MSFL axons terminals and the amacrine cells may be viewed as "short-circuiting" the VL, because after LTP the same MSFL input will lead to a stronger VL output via the large cells axonal bundles (see VL circuitry Figure 4.4e and Figure 4.6).

Neither tetanization nor transection eliminated the ability of the octopuses to learn the task; however, they both affected the rate of learning (Figure 4.10). Transection slowed the learning rate relative to sham-operated animals (Figure 4.10a). Unexpectedly, saturating the LTP had the opposite effect, enhancing the learning process relative to non-tetanized animals (sham controls). Thus, LTP of specific synaptic connections in the VL do not appear to be involved in short-term learning. The VL output most likely controls the process mediating short-term learning that occurs outside the VL, with transection reducing and LTP enhancing the rate of learning by respectively modulating the VL output.

Testing for long-term memory 24 hours after training produced more easily under-standable results. Both treatments severely impaired the long-term memory (Figure 4.11). Sham-operated and control animals did not demonstrate perfect memory of the task, with about 70% of the animals attacking the ball on their first trial. However, they demonstrated a robust saving or recollection, as they stopped attacking the ball in the following test trials (Figure 4.11a,b; open symbols). The transected animals (Figure 4.11a) remembered almost nothing of the avoidance task they had learned the day before, while the tetanized animals showed severe impairment (Figure 4.11b). This difference was probably due to the tetanization not completely saturating the LTP (see Shomrat, Zarrella, Fiorito & Hochner, 2008). However, memory acquired before tetanization or transection, such as to attack a crab or a white ball (associated with positive reward in pre-training), was not impaired (Shomrat, Zarrella, Fiorito & Hochner, 2008). This experiment demonstrated clearly that the VL and its LTP are not important for long-term memory storage, confirming previous experiments showing that previous memories were not affected by lesions of the VL; similarly to results obtained in mammals and even humans (Corkin, 2002; Stellar, 1957) with a severed hippocampus.

This finding adds support to the suggestion that short- and long-term memory traces are stored outside the VL, possibly in the circuitry mediating the attack behavior, and that the VL plays an important role in controlling the processes involved in the consolidation of short-term memory occurring elsewhere.

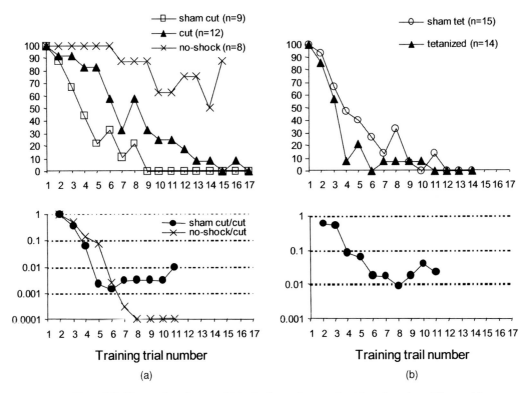

Figure 4.10 Transection slows and tetanization enhances short-term learning of the avoidance task. (a) The median superior frontal lobe (MSFL)-transected animals show significantly slower learning curves than the sham-controls, with a significant difference from the fourth testing trial (*lower panel*). Nevertheless, the transected animals stopped touching the red ball significantly faster than no-shock controls (*lower panel*). (Lower panels show cumulative Fisher tests between the different experiments. *P* in the nth trial was calculated by Fisher's exact test of a 2 × 2 contingency table (two groups versus two outcomes), in which outcome 1 is the sum of touches and outcome 2 is the sum of no-touches made by the group from the second to the 'n'th trials.) (b) Tetanized animals learn faster than the sham-operated animals; by the eighth trial the level of cumulative Fisher's test fell to <0.01 (= 0.0094) (*lower panel*). (From Shomrat, Zarrella, Fiorito & Hochner, 2008.)

4.8   Conclusion: a system model for the octopus learning and memory

We conclude by proposing a tentative model for the octopus learning and memory system that incorporates the physiological and behavioral findings presented here (Figure 4.12). The rationale behind this model is as follows:

1. **Sensory inputs feed in parallel to the VL system and to the circuits controlling behavior.** Transection and tetanization did not affect the behavior; the octopuses still showed their stereotypical attack behavior.
2. **Long-term memory is stored outside the VL.** Both tetanization and transection did not erase old memories.

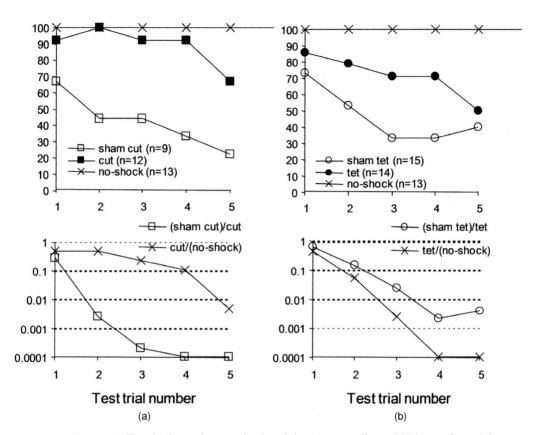

Test trial number

(a)

Test trial number

(b)

Figure 4.11 Tetanization and transection impair long term recall tested 24 hours after training. The animals were given five test trials without electric shock. Testing revealed no significant difference in long-term memory but impairment in recall in consecutive tests both in transected (a) and tetanized (b) animals. By the fifth test trial, the experimental animals showed some retention. Cumulative Fisher's exact test between the treated and the sham groups and the treated groups and the non-contingent controls are shown in the lower panels (see explanation in Fig. 4.10). (From Shomrat, Zarrella, Fiorito & Hochner, 2008.)

3. **The output of the VL modulates the rate of short-term learning that takes place outside the VL-system, possibly by inhibiting the attack mediating circuit.** Tetanization accelerated learning (inhibited the tendency to attack) and transection slowed learning (increased the tendency to attack). However, both treatments did not prevent the attack behavior.

4. **The LTP in the VL system is crucial for the consolidation of long-term memory outside the VL system.** Both treatments prevented the consolidation of short-term into long-term memory.

5. **Serotonin conveys the reward/punishment signal to the VL which reinforces LTP of specific synapses active during the signal.** Serotonin reinforced LTP induction.

We use the passive avoidance task employed by Shomrat, Zarrella, Fiorito and Hochner (2008) to illustrate how the model functions. In this task the octopus learns to refrain from

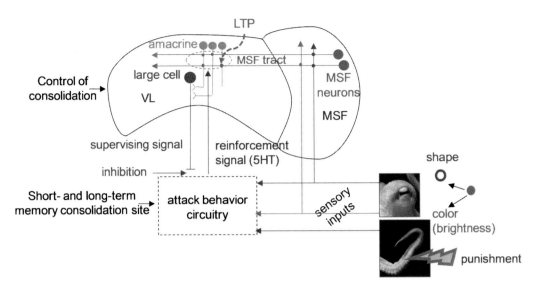

Figure 4.12 A tentative model for the octopus learning and memory system. See explanation in text. See plate section for color version.

attacking a red ball (actually dark, because the octopus is color-blind) by receiving an electric shock to its arms when it attacks. The visual information on *shape* and *brightness* is fed into yet to be delineated *attack behavior circuitry* that activates the natural attack behavior. This information is fed in parallel into the MSFL. Each quality (*brightness, shape*) is then transferred by different sets of MSFL neurons to the VL, most likely creating a sparse representation of each sensory quality in the matrix-like connections of the MSFL neurons with the amacrine interneurons. Those amacrine cells receiving inputs from both qualities are more likely to undergo LTP due to their higher level of activity. The "dark-round" association is highly *reinforced* if they are conjugated with the *pain* signal possibly conveyed to the VL by the *serotonergic* system. The strengthening of this association during training creates in turn a long-term enhancement of the amacrine cells input to the set of large neurons driven by this mutual sensory representation. The VL output generally inhibits the tendency to attack and can be regarded as an inhibitory *supervising* signal. The enhancement of the output generated by the *red ball* representation alone in the VL is now enough to specifically inhibit attacking the red ball.

It is not yet clear whether similar mechanisms mediate positive-reward learning, e.g. by decreasing the inhibitory drive of the VL.

Acknowledgments

The HUJI Octopus Group is supported by the Smith Family Laboratory in the Hebrew University, the United States–Israel Binational Science Foundation (BSF), the Israel Science Foundation (ISF) and the European Commission EP7 projects OCTOPUS and

STIFF-FLOP. We would also like to thank Jenny Kien for editorial assistance and suggestions.

References

Bailey, C. H., Giustetto, M., Huang, Y. Y., Hawkins, R. D. and Kandel, E. R. (2000). Is heterosynaptic modulation essential for stabilizing Hebbian plasticity and memory? *Nature Reviews Neuroscience*, **1**(1): 11–20.

Boycott, B. B. (1961). The functional organization of the brain of the cuttlefish *Sepia officinalis*. *Proceedings of the Royal Society. B: Biological Sciences*, **153**: 503–534.

Boycott, B. B. and Young, J. Z. (1955). A memory system in *Octopus vulgaris* Lamarck. *Proceedings of the Royal Society. B: Biological Sciences*, **143**(913): 449–480.

Budelmann, B. U. (1995). The cephalopods nervous system: what evolution has made of the molluscan design. In *The nervous system of invertebrates: an evolutionary and comparative approach*, Breidbach, O. and Kutsch, W., (eds). Basel: Birkhäuser Verlag, pp. 115–138.

Bullock, T. H. (1984). Ongoing compound field potentials from octopus brain are labile and vertebrate-like. *Electroencephalography and Clinical Neurophysiology*, **57**(5): 473–483.

Bullock, T. H. and Basar, E. (1988). Comparison of ongoing compound field potentials in the brains of invertebrates and vertebrates. *Brain Research*, **472**(1): 57–75.

Bullock, T. H. and Horridge, G. A. (1965). *Structure and function in the nervous systems of invertebrates*, San Francisco: W. H. Freeman.

Cassenaer, S. and Laurent, G. (2012). Conditional modulation of spike-timing-dependent plasticity for olfactory learning. *Nature*, **482**(7383): 47–52.

Corkin, S. (2002). What's new with the amnesic patient H. M.? *Nature Reviews Neuroscience*, **3**(2): 153–160.

Fiorito, G. and Chichery, R. (1995). Lesions of the vertical lobe impair visual discrimination learning by observation in *Octopus vulgaris*. *Neuroscience Letters*, **192**(2): 117–120.

Fiorito, G. and Scotto, P. (1992). Observational learning in *Octopus vulgaris*. *Science*, **256**(5056): 545–547.

Garthwaite, J. (2008). Concepts of neural nitric oxide-mediated transmission. *European Journal of Neuroscience*, **27**(11): 2783–2802.

Grasso, F. W. and Basil, J. A. (2009). The evolution of flexible behavioral repertoires in cephalopod molluscs. *Brain Behavior and Evolution*, **74**(3): 231–245.

Gray, E. G. (1970). The fine structure of the vertical lobe of octopus brain. *Philosophical Transactions of the Royal Society of London. Series B*, **258**: 379–394.

Gray, E. G. and Young, J. Z. (1964). Electron microscopy of synaptic structure of octopus brain. *Journal of Cell Biology*, **21**: 87–103.

Hanlon, R. T. and Messenger, J. B. (1996). *Cephalopod behaviour*. Cambridge: Cambridge University Press.

Hochner, B. (2008). Octopuses. *Current Biology*, **18**(19): R897–R898.

Hochner, B. (2010). Functional and comparative assessments of the octopus learning and memory system. *Frontiers in Bioscience*, **2**: 764–771.

Hochner, B., Brown, E. R., Langella, M., Shomrat, T. and Fiorito, G. (2003). A learning and memory area in the octopus brain manifests a vertebrate-like long-term *Journal of Neurophysiology*, **90**(5): 3547–3554.

Hochner, B., Shomrat, T. and Fiorito, G. (2006). The octopus: a model for a comparative analysis of the evolution of learning and memory mechanisms. *The Biological Bulletin*, **210**(3): 308–317.

Kandel, E. R. (2001). The molecular biology of memory storage: a dialogue between genes and synapses. *Science*, **294**(5544): 1030–1038.

Kandel, E. R., Schwartz, J. H. and Jessel, T. M. (2000). *Principles of neural science*, New York: McGraw-Hill.

Keene, A. C. and Waddell, S. (2007). Drosophila olfactory memory: single genes to complex neural circuits. *Nature Reviews Neuroscience*, **8**(5): 341–354.

Kemenes, I., O'Shea, M. and Benjamin, P. R. (2011). Different circuit and monoamine mechanisms consolidate long-term memory in aversive and reward classical conditioning. *European Journal of Neuroscience*, **33**(1): 143–152.

Lima, P. A., Nardi, G. and Brown, E. R. (2003). AMPA/kainate and NMDA-like glutamate receptors at the chromatophore neuromuscular junction of the squid: role in synaptic transmission and skin patterning. *European Journal of Neuroscience*, **17**(3): 507–516.

Maldonado, H. (1965). The positive and negative learning process in *Octopus vulgaris* Lamarck. Influence of the vertical and median superior frontal lobes. *Zeitschrift für vergleichende Physiologie*, **51**: 185–203.

Matzner, H., Gutfreund, Y. and Hochner, B. (2000). Neuromuscular system of the flexible arm of the octopus: physiological characterization. *Journal of Neurophysiology*, **83**(3): 1315–1328.

Miyakawa, H. and Kato, H. (1986). Active properties of dendritic membrane examined by current source density analysis in hippocampal CA1 pyramidal neurons. *Brain Research*, **399**(2): 303–309.

Moser, E. I., Krobert, K. A., Moser, M. B. and Morris, R. G. M. (1998). Impaired spatial learning after saturation of long-term potentiation. *Science*, **281**(5385): 2038–2042.

Nixon, M. and Young, J. Z. (2003). *The brain and lives of cephalopods*, Oxford: Oxford University Press.

Nowotny, T., Huerta, R., Abarbanel, H. D. and Rabinovich, M. (2005). Self-organization in the olfactory system: one shot odor recognition in insects. *Biological Cybernetics*, **93**(6): 436–446.

Packard, A. (1972). Cephalopods and fish: the limits of convergence. *Biological Reviews*, **47**: 241–307.

Robertson, J. D., Bonaventura, J. and Kohm, A. P. (1994). Nitric oxide is required for tactile learning in *Octopus vulgaris*. *Proceedings of the Royal Society. B: Biological Sciences*, **256**(1347): 269–273.

Robertson, J. D., Bonaventura, J., Kohm, A. P. and Hiscat, M. (1996). Nitric oxide is necessary for visual learning in *Octopus vulgaris*. *Proceedings of the Royal Society. B: Biological Sciences*, **263**(1377): 1739–1743.

Sanders, G. D. (1975). The cephalopods. In *Invertebrate learning. Cephalopods and Echinoderms*, Vol. 3, Corning, W. C., Dyal, J. A. and Willows, A. O. D., (eds). New York: Plenum Press, pp. 139–145.

Schultz, W. (2007). Behavioral dopamine signals. *Trends in Neurosciences*, **30**(5): 203–210.

Shomrat, T., Feinstein, N., Klein, M. and Hochner, B. (2010). Serotonin is a facilitatory neuromodulator of synaptic transmission and "reinforces" long-term potentiation induction in the vertical lobe of *Octopus vulgaris*. *Neuroscience*, **169**(1): 52–64.

Shomrat, T., Graindorge, N., Bellanger, C., Fiorito, G., Loewenstein, Y. and Hochner, B. (2011). Alternative sites of synaptic plasticity in two homologous "fan-out fan-in" learning and memory networks. *Current Biology*, **21**(21): 1773–1782.

Shomrat, T., Zarrella, I., Fiorito, G. and Hochner, B. (2008). The octopus vertical lobe modulates short-term learning rate and uses LTP to acquire long-term memory. *Current Biology*, **18**(5): 337–342.

Stellar, E. (1957). Physiological psychology. *Annual Review of Psychology*, **8**: 415–436.

Susswein, A. J. and Chiel, H. J. (2012). Nitric oxide as a regulator of behavior: new ideas from *Aplysia* feeding. *Progress in Neurobiology*, **97**(3): 304–317.

Vapnik, V. N. (1998). *Statistical learning theory*, New York: John Wiley and Sons, Inc.

Wells, M. J. (1978). *Octopus*, London: Chapman and Hall.

Young, J. Z. (1971). *The anatomy of the nervous system of Octopus vulgaris*, Oxford: Clarendon Press.

Young, J. Z. (1991). Computation in the learning-system of cephalopods. *The Biological Bulletin*, **180**(2): 200–208.

Young, J. Z. (1995). Multiple matrices in the memory system of octopus. In *Cephalopod Neurobiology,* Abbott, J. N., Williamson, R. and Maddock, L., (eds). Oxford: Oxford University Press, pp. 431–443.

Zullo, L., Sumbre, G., Agnisola, C., Flash, T. and Hochner, B. (2009). Nonsomatotopic organization of the higher motor centers in octopus. *Current Biology*, **19**: 1632–1636.

5   The octopus with two brains: how are distributed and central representations integrated in the octopus central nervous system?

Frank W. Grasso

5.1   The relationship between cognition and neuroscience in cephalopod cognition

~Ο δε. πολυ, πουσ αννο, ητον με, ν ενστι και. γα.ρ προ.σ τη.ν χει/ρα βαδι, ζει του/ αννθρω, που καθιεμε, νην καθιεμε, νην.

The octopus is a stupid creature, for it will approach a man's hand if it be lowered into the water.
   Aristotle, *The History of Animals*, Book IX, translated by D'Arcy Wentworth Thompson (2013).[1]

Today, two-and-a-quarter millennia after Aristotle denigrated octopuses' intelligence for behaviors that might be called "curiosity," this volume reflects the attitudes and accumulated evidence of our time in asserting that cephalopods possess cognition. And perhaps, with all due respect to the great philosopher whose writings were the foundation for the *scala naturae* behind medieval scholasticism, his definition of cognition would be too anthropomorphic to admit an intelligence that did not agree with the typical social conceptions of intelligence in humans. The definition of cognition that I will use in this chapter is broader: any adaptive process which connects sensing in the world to action in the world. The word *adaptive* in this definition requires some elaboration. I use adaptive in the sense that it is used in the field of cybernetics: that of a process that changes with experience. It is not the intergenerational sense of adaptation from evolution but something that happens within the individual during its lifetime.

   In the field of cybernetics a non-adaptive or fixed control system reliably produces the same output every time the same input is provided. The behavior is "machine-like." In biological neural systems there are four types of processes that lead to adaptive behavior. First are developmental processes in which new components, like limbs, muscles and neurons via neurogenesis and neural systems are added as the animal ages. The other three change the state of the central nervous system (CNS) without the addition and integration (or maturation) of new parts. Hormonal systems modify the performance

---

[1] I am indebted to Dimitris Tsakiris for drawing my attention to this passage and translation.

Cephalopod Cognition, eds A.-S. Darmaillacq, L. Dickel and J. Mather. Published by Cambridge University Press. © Cambridge 2014.

of targeted functional groups of neurons in activational and organizational modes. In octopus the action of hormonal systems on brain operation and the development of neural systems are areas in need of a large amount of basic research. The other two have better developed methods and a larger knowledge-base. Synaptic plasticity changes the strength of connections between neurons. This is what is classically[2] termed learning and its product is classical "memory." And, finally, there are internal recurrent connections (feedback loops) between neurons which cause inputs received some time in the past to persist in influencing behavior after the stimulus is no longer present. The cybernetics sense of adaptive systems has focused on the latter two, synaptic plasticity and recurrent connections. Broadly speaking, synaptic adaptation is a mechanism for long-term memory while recurrent connections are a mechanism for short-term memory. This chapter emphasizes the role of recurrent connections in the octopus.

This definition of cognition may seem too broad at first but it has several advantages when attempting to apply the concept to invertebrate behavior. First, the use of the word "process" makes clear that cognition is about information processing, for which we have many useful concepts and tools. In dealing with non-human species we are not concerned with the refined discriminations from human social and cultural systems found in the study of human psychology but with the biological foundations of intelligent behavior. So secondly, the definition relates to behavior directly and not to inferred internal states. Further, the effective adjustment of behavior is an effective selection force in the evolution of cognitive systems and such internal states are only a means to that end. In this chapter the term *adaptive* indicates that cognition is about the role of individual experience in shaping behavior.

Perhaps the most important aspect of this definition is that it usefully points us towards mechanism. This follows from the paragraph above, which identified development, hormones, plasticity and recurrent network architecture as defined biological processes that could change the brain in ways which might result in adjusting individual behavior based on experience. In an individual line of research, instances of these mechanisms may be profitably traced in the brains of real cephalopods to their influence on the unfolding of the behavior of the individual animal over its lifespan. Any explanation which cannot account for (or exclude) the contributions of these will be partial.

The study of mechanism is the bridge between cognitive processes as we conceive them and the neurobiological reality. Many theoretical mechanisms may reasonably reproduce a description of behavior. For this volume's stated purpose of understanding cognition in cephalopods we should be interested in discovering *the* mechanism not just *a* mechanism that fits a description of behavior. To do this cephalopod cognition studies are best served when the theories of cognitive processing can be excluded or retained based on neurobiological facts. Discovery of the unique cognitive innovations of cephalopods depend critically on such well-constrained approaches.

---

[2] Adaptive processes are those that might be construed loosely as "memory" processes. They all result in changes in behavior as a result of experience. The psychological literature uses the term narrowly in that memory has come to be used almost exclusively for processes associated with synaptic plasticity. Cybernetics uses the definition that changes to the system that produce different responses to the same input at different times are adaptive. My inclusion of hormonal and developmental processes is broader still.

Research in recent years has uncovered valuable insights into the synaptic plasticity of octopus that dovetails with research in other simpler-brained mollusks, like *Aplysia* and gastropods, and with learning mechanisms in primitive cephalopods, like *Nautilus*. And we possess an abundance of detailed neuroanatomical data that continues to grow with new techniques. This chapter will use some of that architectural knowledge to argue for a unique, decentralized information processing mechanism in octopus.

5.2   The problem of soft bodies controlled by complex brains

The neural representations that control and coordinate the behavior of cephalopods are great scientific value. Their soft bodies, in contrast to those of vertebrates and arthropods, which effect movement through the control of rigid (endo- or exo-) skeletons, suggest that cephalopods have new things to teach us about ways that brains produce action on the world that is useful to the animal. This chapter will not explain those principles because much research is required before they become known. It will, however, frame the problem of understanding neural representations in cephalopods and suggest one idea on how a special balance of centralized and distributed processing might occur in octopus.

Octopuses offer an important group for direct functional comparisons between soft-bodied and rigid-bodied creatures. They use and coordinate their eight arms in tasks involving dexterous manipulation that are functionally similar to tasks performed by rigid-bodied species. They can learn to open jars and uncork bottles (Fiorito, Von Planta & Scotto, 1990; Hanlon & Messenger, 1996), they naturally open bivalve shells (Fiorito & Gherardi, 1999; Anderson & Mather, 2007), and touch and fetch objects within reach of their arms (Sumbre, Gutfreund, Fiorito, Flash & Hochner, 2001; Sumbre, Fiorito, Flash & Hochner, 2006). The biomechanics that support these and other behaviors are suitably different from those of rigid-bodied species (Hochner, Shomrat & Fiorito, 2006; Grasso & Basil, 2009), but are the central representations that the octopuses use convergent on a common solution or, also, uniquely cephalopod in character? The bodies of cephalopods are markedly different from those of arthropods and vertebrates, but what of their CNS? The common ancestors of cephalopods, vertebrates and arthropods possessed muscles, specialized sensory receptor, specialized motor neurons and central interneurons between the sensory receptors and motor neurons. The common ancestors of vertebrates and mollusks used neurons for the control and coordination of behavior. Cephalopods are mollusks that separated from the molluscan line about 505 million years ago. So, when compared with arthropods and vertebrates, cephalopods offer an opportunity to evaluate the interplay of convergent selection pressures and phylogenetic inertia on the evolution of brains as information processing systems.

5.3   Representations and connectivity

David Marr specified three levels of analysis that needed to be understood in order to understand a cognitive process (Marr, 1982). They are theory, or what is being computed by the system; representation and algorithm, or a specification of the building blocks of the theory and rules as to how they can interact; and implementation, or the actual physical apparatus in which the process could be realized in the world. He pointed out that confusing these levels was a path to faulty understanding and that without a clear idea of the theory neither the representation nor the implementation could be realized. So it is essential, in this chapter on representation in the octopus CNS that we have our architectural components well defined.

In describing neural architecture, neurobiologists identify three classes of neuron: primary sensory neurons which transform environmental stimulus energy into neural information (e.g. spikes), motor neurons which transmit control signals to muscle fibers via neuro-muscular junctions to produce behavior and interneurons which lie in between and process information. Figure 5.1 provides a primer on these concepts and a graphical way of representing neural system architecture.

Figure 5.1a shows a complete wiring diagram for a simple system containing primary receptor neurons and no interneurons or motor neurons. On the left side is a sketch of an abstracted animal body showing a physical arrangement of muscles and sensors. To the right of this sketch is the corresponding neural connectivity diagram (Anastasio, 2010). Assume that activation of muscles on the left and the right sides of the animal are competent to steer the animal left or right or propel it forward depending on the level of left or right muscle activation. The primary sensory receptors (gray soma) each form a single neuromuscular junction on their respective muscles. The direction of information flow is indicated by the arrow beside the soma. It is interesting to note that this simple mechanism is competent to produce a taxis behavior (e.g. phototaxis, chemotaxis, phonotaxis, etc.) as noted by Braitenberg (1984) by virtue of the crossed connections which would produce more "propulsion" on the side opposite that with greater stimulation. When the input from the two sides is equal then forward movement would result instead of steering.

Figure 5.1b shows an imaginary animal of slightly greater neural complexity that adds committed motor neurons (gray soma), internal synapses between the primary sensory neurons and the motor neurons. Note the convention in the wiring diagram on the right of orienting progressive layers of neurons at right angles. The synapses are noted as circles at the intersection of output lines (i.e. axons) and input lines (i.e. dendrites). The absence of a synapse marker indicates a potential connection that is not made, a zero-valued connection. Note that this architecture also results in a mechanism that can competently produce a taxis behavior without any central representation. The only difference in behavior between Figure 5.1b and that in Figure 5.1a would be a delay in response to the input owing to the delay in signal transmission through the synapses. Otherwise the taxis behavior would be comparable.

Figure 5.1c is a simple configuration which, perhaps debatably,[3] includes a central representation. It is not a brain but this single layer of two interconnected interneurons (gray soma) is the closest thing that this imaginary animal has to a brain occupying, as

---

[3] As this was just an introduction for the specific treatment of octopus arm connectivity that follows, I've not mentioned the important issue of the strength of the connections, or *synaptic weight*. This is a key component of neural network performance which has received a large amount of theoretical consideration. For a thorough general introduction see Anastasio (2010).

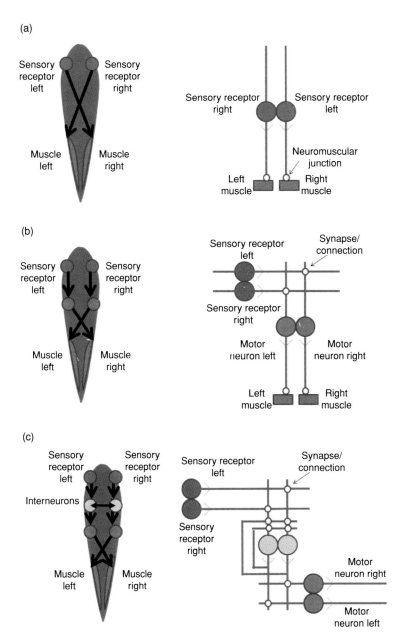

Figure 5.1 Schematic representation of behavioral control schemes for an abstracted bilateral creature. In each panel the left side shows the arrangement of neurons and muscles in the body, the right the central nervous system connectivity pattern following the conventions used in this chapter. (a) A hypothetical bilateral creature with sensory receptor cells connected directly to muscles via a neuromuscular junction. The connections crossing at the midline cause the side of the body with greater stimulation to stimulate greater activation on the contralateral side. This is sufficient to produce a taxis behavior. (b) The addition of motor neurons requires the addition of synapses, connections, between the neurons in the network. There will be no difference in taxis behavior. (c) The addition of interneurons – neurons that are neither sensory neurons nor motor neurons. The interneurons are interconnected. This is evident in the right connectivity schematic, which shows feedback connections from the interneurons to each other and themselves. These feedback connections cause past inputs to persist in the network. The network will produce taxis behavior but that behavior will depend more on the state of the entire network and its history (memory) of inputs.

it does, the brain's position between the primary sensory and the motor neurons. The addition of the interneurons changes the character of the network performance and the behavior of the imaginary animal because of the recurrent connections. Note the four additional synapses (compared with Figure 5.1b) on the connections that loop back from the outputs of each interneuron. These supply each interneuron with the new, additional, inputs of a copy of its own output and with the output of the other interneuron. This is a recurrent form of "memory," in the mathematical sense of hysteresis, which is not in agreement with classic psychological definitions of memory. This computational architecture corresponds to the neurobiological structure of a neuropil where neurons in the CNS interconnect. In the neuropil the previous (historical) past activity patterns are carried through loops to "reverberate" between them, maintaining patterns of activity after the stimulus has ceased to activate receptor(s). Thus, the output of the interneurons to the motor neurons and, therefore, the behavior of the hypothetical animal will depend, in part, on the past pattern of inputs and in part on the current inputs. Brain complexity grows (in the developmental and evolutionary sense) from the kernel of a single neuropil, through the multiplication of neuropils, their specialization and organization. This is one of the key building blocks of brain organization.

It is important to note that that in the third imaginary animal the change in behavior with experience does not depend on synaptic plasticity. So, in a larger network with proper arrangement of connectivity and connection strengths a "memory" (again in the mathematical, reverberating sense) can be produced in the interneurons, which will bias the performance of the network and, therefore, the behavior of the animal with experience. The permanent changes in synaptic strength that are considered in classical learning, when applied to these recurrent networks, could tune, adjust or even obliterate these reverberating memories, but the parallel existence of both forms of experience-derived performance modification indicates that an understanding of behavior must take both into account.

It is commonly accepted that interneurons are the elementary biological units for representing the world in the CNS of animals for the control and for the coordination of the behavior of animals. Removed as they are from primary sensory neurons, interneurons can potentially meet the important requirement of a representation in that their activity persists after a stimulus has ceased to be present. With a recurrent connectivity pattern between them or synaptic plasticity in the connections, interneurons can acquire representations with experience of the world that can be stored nervous systems. The nature of the representation depends on which mechanism is used to form the representation. Another key question is whether the representations formed in a nervous system are localized or distributed. Interneurons can be arranged to do either based on their connectivity and so, for clarity, I will review the organization of the CNS of the octopus as it pertains to the question of neural representations to control soft-bodied animals.

5.4 The organization of the octopus central nervous system

By invertebrate standards the CNS of cephalopods is enormous. The octopus CNS contains on the order of 5×10^8 neurons (Young, 1971). This number excludes the number of peripheral neurons in glandular, sensory, chromatophore, digestive and respiratory systems, which is larger still in number. This size is orders of magnitude larger than that of the next-largest mollusks. This quantum leap in size is undoubtedly responsible in part for the huge, individually adaptable behavioral repertoire of cephalopods.

5.4.1   The cerebral ganglia

The large size of the brain might reflect the complex requirements of controlling a soft body. Rather than having muscles that control a finite and fixed set of joints, cephalopods must operate muscles that overlap to reshape body surfaces at arbitrary location – to effectively form joints where they are needed. This increased complexity would be expected to require larger numbers of motor neurons and more motor control nuclei and lobes in the brain. This special demand for motor control circuitry, compared to rigid-bodied animals appears to contribute to the size of the brain as it does in vertebrates (Finlay, Darlington & Nicastro, 2001; Herculano-Houzel, Collins, Wong & Kaas, 2007). However, it does not account for the whole of the brain which is of considerable complexity with 35 lobes (Young, 1971; Grasso & Basil, 2009), only some of which are directly responsible for motor control. It appears that learning, in the classical psychological sense, is a specialty of the octopus brain.

The exceptional learning abilities of the octopus (in the classical psychological sense) are well documented (Wells & Wells, 1957b; Mackintosh & Mackintosh, 1963; Wells, 1964; Mackintosh, 1965; Fiorito & Scotto, 1992; Fiorito, Agnisola, D'Addio, Valanzano & Calamandrei, 1998). Among the 35 lobes of the octopus brain the vertical lobe, for example, is considered a committed central memory system. It has been the subject of focused studies of learning (Wells & Wells, 1957b) and recently in neurophysiological studies (Shomrat, Zarrella, Fiorito & Hochner, 2008; Shomrat et al., 2011; Zullo & Hochner, 2011). It has been demonstrated to be a site of long-term potentiation (LTP) and synaptic facilitation in both octopuses and cuttlefishes (Shomrat et al., 2011). The brains of octopuses are sophisticated cognitive systems, which have led some researchers to suggest the species as a model system for the study of consciousness (Edelman & Seth, 2009).

The neurons in the higher order neuropils of the brain, those that have no obvious impact on behavior, appear to serve the acquisition of new behaviors – classical learning and memory systems (Wells & Wells, 1957b). These findings and analysis suggest strong analogies with the centralization of neural representation such as the presence of cognitive maps in the brains of vertebrates and function in the "brains" of the cephalopods. Yet efforts to discover a somatotopic representation or other maps in the brains of octopuses have found none (Zullo, Sumbre, Agnisola, Flash & Hochner, 2009; Zullo & Hochner, 2011). Neurons in those areas seem to be strongly multimodal compared to their vertebrate and arthropod counterparts. A different overall brain representation of the world and of motor control compared to vertebrates is suggested (Zullo & Hochner, 2011).

An indication of the source of this difference is found in the fact that three-fifths ($\sim 3.5 \times 10^8$) of the neurons in the octopus CNS are located outside the central brain, or cerebral ganglia as it is called. These neurons are located in the brachial ganglia that extend down the length of the arm and in the plexus of interconnections between the arms. This large collection of neurons undoubtedly contributes locally to motor control in the arms but the organization of the ganglia suggests that these extracerebral portions of the CNS are serving other functions as well.

5.4.2   The brachial plexus and sucker ganglia

The CNS in the arms is organized to support the functions of the $\sim$300 suckers of the arm and the muscles of the arms. There is a central nerve cord running the length of each arm and interconnecting the arms. It contains nerve fibers originating outside the arm in the brain and interarm plexus, as wells as cells and neuropil throughout its length; however, there is a significant expansion of the cord, or ganglion, associated with each sucker, delineated by an increase in the number of neurons and the size of the neuropil. Technically, when a set of ganglia is interconnected, it is called a plexus. So I will refer to the interconnected nerve cords of the eight arms as the brachial plexus, and use the shorthand term of brachial ganglion when referring to portions of it such as a whole arm or portion or a selection of ganglia within an arm. Four smaller nerve cords that run the length of the arm and are more eccentrically located are important for motor control of the arm, but their role will not be discussed in this chapter which focuses on sensory representations. Outside each brachial ganglion there is a sucker ganglion associated with each sucker that lies eccentric from the central nerve cord just over each sucker and outside the main arm muscle mass (Graziadei, 1971).

The connectivity of the arm CNS structure is summarized in Figure 5.2. Sensory input to the arm CNS comes from the rims of the suckers and proprioceptors embedded in the muscular tissues of the arm and sucker. The rim of each sucker houses on the order of 10^4 chemo- and mechanoreceptors (Graziadei & Gagne, 1976). The axons from these receptors pass from the sucker rim to the sucker corresponding sucker ganglia. The proprioceptors of the sucker also pass in nerves to the sucker ganglia. The sucker ganglia contains motor neurons so local reflex arcs can result from information processing there. Each sucker ganglion is associated with a single sucker. It makes reciprocal connections with its corresponding brachial ganglion. At present the mode of operation of the sucker ganglia is not well investigated.

Sucker ganglia do not communicate directly with one another. Connections between brachial ganglia exist to channel the information from one sucker to its neighbors. Another role of the brachial ganglia is to control and coordinate the muscles of the arm and thereby effect arm movements by means of intrinsic motor neurons. Motor neurons in the brachial ganglia and sucker ganglia innervate muscle fibers in the arm and sucker respectively (Graziadei, 1971; Rowell, 1966). Proprioceptors embedded in the main arm (outside the suckers) send processes to the four smaller, eccentric nerve cords and the central nerve cord (Graziadei, 1965). These four eccentric nerve cords contain motor neurons of their own but their role is not well studied. Somehow the processing in the brachial ganglia and the four eccentric ganglia produce the reshaping of the arm, which provides it with its functional flexibility.

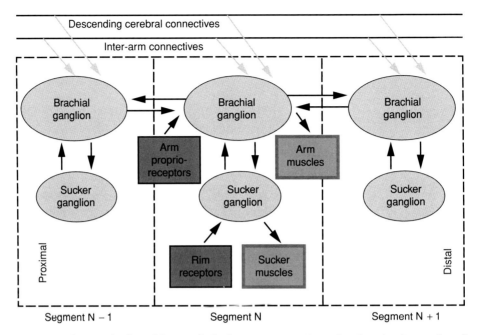

Figure 5.2 The organization of the ganglia in the octopus arm. Around each sucker is a section of the arm whose neural and muscular structure repeats along the length of the arm. The central segment, N, shows the complete set. Sensory inputs (gray) in the form of chemo-receptors on the sucker rim and propioceptors embedded in the tissues of the arm provide input to the sucker and brachial ganglia respectively. The brachial ganglion also receives inputs from the sucker ganglion in its segment, descending inputs from the cerebral ganglia, inputs from the other arms and several proximally and distally positioned brachial ganglia. The brachial ganglia process these sources of input and produce motor commands to the muscles of the arm. A shorter sensory motor loop exists from the sucker ganglia (which also processes input from the brachial ganglia in its segment) to the sucker muscles. The proximal and distal segments (delineated by dashed boxes) are included to illustrate the continuum nature of this organization proximally and distally down the arm.

The summary shown in Figure 5.2 makes clear the modular nature of the arm connectivity. I refer to these modules as local brachial modules (LBM) and they contain the neural components of each sucker–ganglion/brachial–ganglion pair (i.e. the primary receptors [chemo-, mechano- and proprioceptive], the motor neurons and the interneurons). In Figure 5.2 and the following text I use the term *segment* to refer to a section of the arm (i.e. muscle, connective tissue, non-CNS neural-components) associated with a given LBM. This basic organization repeats down the length of the arm, one module for each sucker. It is likely that the circuitry for controlling the arm movements forms a continuum down the arm that matches the continuum of tissue. The continuous connectivity of the brachial ganglia in the arm naturally reflects this. Evidence for arm-sucker coordination supports suggests that a modular view of the functional organization of the arm might be appropriate for even considering the circuitry responsible for the movement of the arm.

Table 5.1 Rowell's (1966) summary of the numbers of fibers originating from and entering into the brachial ganglia in one module

Neuron type	No. of fibers
Motor neurons	2000
Sensory cells	3000
Afferent axons in the axial cord	18 000
Efferent, chromatophore fibers	2300
Efferent, non-chromatophore fibers	2000

There are on the order 10^5 central neurons in each segment module. This seems a very large number of neurons when one reflects on the fact that this figure excludes the larger numbers of peripheral neurons that contribute to the chromatophore, circulatory and secretory systems and the primary sensory receptors. There are more neurons present in one segment of an octopus arm than exist in the whole of successful invertebrate animals such as the medicinal leech or *Aplysia*. In terms of the numbers of neurons, a module is on a comparable scale to the size of an arthropod brain. What requirement could produce such a commitment of neural resources?

Table 5.1 gives an indication. It lists Rowell's (Rowell, 1966) summary of the numbers of fibers originating from and entering into the brachial ganglia in one module. This makes clear that ~75% of the signal lines in a given module carry neither primarily sensory, nor primarily motor, nor chromatophore signals in nature; rather the majority of fibers carry information to and from other interneurons. Not only are the numbers of neurons in a module comparable to those of a whole organism, each segment is organized like the brain of a living organism (in at least the sense of Figure 5.1), with a diversity of sensory modalities, motor neurons effecting different motor systems and large central neuropils, which are processing centers for large amounts of information.

Yet, while a segment may resemble a brain functionally it is not a brain because by definition brains contain anatomically delineated areas of specialized function, such as the 35 lobes of the octopus brain. This in fact is an approximate definition of a ganglion: a collection of interconnected interneurons. In this sense the module compares to a segment in the vertebrate spinal cord. A recent quantitative analysis of the spinal cord of the Red Eared turtle found that one spinal cord segment (D3) contained on the order of 10^4 neurons, an order of magnitude fewer than in the octopus arm module, of which about 75% were interneurons and 25% were motor neurons (Walløe, Nissen, Berg, Hounsgaard & Pakkenberg, 2011). And, like the vertebrate spinal cord, the chain of brachial ganglia form a linear series. The important structural difference is that there are about 10 times more brachial ganglia in the arm of an octopus than there are spinal segments in a vertebrate like a human (31 versus 300), and that the chain of brachial ganglia in one octopus arm is connected through the brachial plexus to form a single continuous system with the other seven arms. It is also important to note that this huge investment in neurons and connectivity forms a *network of ganglia* of a more or less homogeneous type.

5.5   The computational roles of the arm module

One way to think about the arms of octopuses is as a device for delivering suckers to a work surface. In object manipulation and benthic locomotion the suckers play a key role. Arms are used for other behaviors such as swimming, anchoring, sensory exploration (Mather, 1998) and display (Packard, 1961), but I will omit a complete discussion of the uses of the arms here. The wrapping the arm around an object without sucker attachment has rarely, perhaps never, been seen. Generally, when an octopus uses its arms for manipulation of objects or for locomotion the suckers are attached to a surface and coordinated movements of the arm effect a movement of the object relative to the animal's body (small objects) or of the animal's body relative to the surface (objects more massive than the animal).

The coordination of the sucker attachment and orientation with arm movement, which is essential for proper locomotion and object manipulation, must be a part of what the brachial ganglia do. There is good evidence for intersucker coordination (Rowell, 1963, 1966; Altmann, 1971; F. W. Grasso, S. Nair, J. Barocas & S. Hadjisolomou, unpublished data) and for arm–sucker coordination (Grasso, 2008), both of which must be mediated by the brachial ganglia for the anatomical reasons stated above. Suckers themselves are not passive agents. They have the ability to rotate and extend relative to the arm in addition to attaching to surfaces, thanks to their extrinsic muscles (Kier, 1982). Doubtless, this is part of the computational load of the sucker ganglia and the brachial ganglia in combination.

In addition to the local information processing that anatomy and behavior demonstrate, descending influences from the cerebral ganglia contribute to the coordination of arm movement. Visual information has been shown to guide reaching and manipulation tasks (Gutfreund, Flash, Fiorito & Hochner, 1998; Grasso, 2008; Gutnick, Byrne, Hochner & Kuba, 2011). Integrating these and other descending influences to guide the activity of the arms must form part of the computational load borne by the local brachial module.

But this is a condition of influence and not a necessary condition for behavior. Various studies show that blind and even decerebrated octopuses can perform tactile discrimination and manipulation tasks (Wells, 1964; Wells & Wells, 1957a, 1957b) and that much of the postural and feeding behavior of the animal appears "normal" in the decerebrate condition (Wells, 1978). Figure 5.3 shows an intact *Enteroctopus dofleini* solving a tactile Y-maze task to obtain food. In this case the maze is opaque and the animal cannot see inside. It has to rely on the information provided by the sucker receptors and the coordination of the local brachial modules to solve the maze (F. W. Grasso, unpublished observations). These results indicate that the network of local brachial modules can operate independently from visual and perhaps all descending influence. It is known that local accept and reject reflexes persist in the suckers of a disconnected octopus arm (Altmann, 1971).

Perhaps, in light of the number of computational roles served by the LBM, it is unsurprising that the investment in neural resources in a single LBM is comparable to arthropod brain or vertebrate spinal cord. However, there is perhaps, an additional and cognitive role that a network of ganglia such as the LBM can perform in the octopus:

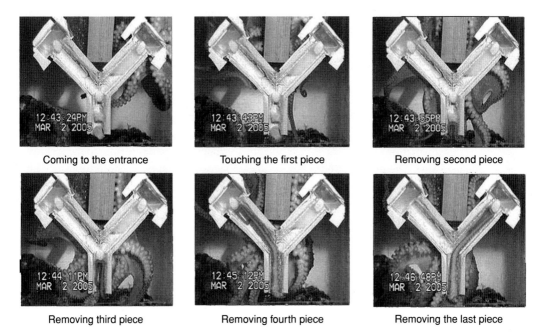

Coming to the entrance	Touching the first piece	Removing second piece
Removing third piece	Removing fourth piece	Removing the last piece

Figure 5.3 Flexible grasping and object manipulation by an octopus arm. The octopus in this series cannot see inside the Y-maze and must rely on touch and taste sensors in its arm to locate the five food items (pieces of shrimp abdomen) inside. The progression of slides shows the reshaping of the arm to produce bends at different orientations and at different positions along the arm as needed to achieve the grasping and retrieval task.

The network of LBMs may be capable of forming representations of the external world. This proposal is made based on two facts. First, that the sensory information about the external world that is available to an LBM comes from the sucker rims. And second that the sucker rims necessarily form a topologically-ordered spatial array. Surface contact is required for the chemical or mechanical information to be transmitted so a given LBM is excluded from sampling the same location as another and the sequence of suckers from proximal to distal ensures an orderly (though not necessarily Cartesian) arrangement of sample points.

5.6   A network of homogeneous ganglia

5.6.1   An analysis of ganglia network functions

The proposal of a representation outside the cerebral ganglia presented above poses a daunting technical challenge: where amongst the approximately 3.5×10^8 neurons associated with the arms should we look for this chemical or tactile representation of space? The organizing principle of the LBM helpfully narrows the focus to about 50 000 neurons but this does not help much when we remember that there are about 2400 LBMs in a typical octopus. The literature does not presently contain the types of simultaneous multisite recordings from octopus brachial ganglia that would inform us on this (though Altmann, 1971; Rowell, 1963, 1966, and Young, 1991 give useful indications). Instead a mathematical analysis grounded in the specifics of the system can provide a demonstration of the concept and supply predictions for what we might look for in future empirical studies.

Figure 5.4 is a connectivity diagram using the same conventions employed in Figure 5.1. It shows three LBMs interconnected in an ordered series. It could be mathematically extended to the 300 LBMs found in an octopus arm, but three will suffice for this illustration. The labels N–1, N and N+1 throughout the figure refer to the identity of the LBM. The network nodes labeled sucker sensory input N, the propriosensory input N, the sucker ganglion N and the brachial ganglion N, all constitute the same LBM (N) as appears in Figure 5.2.[4] The same applies for N–1 and N+1, which are, respectively, one LBM proximal and one LBM distal to N. The aim of this depiction, which rearranges the clear organization of an LBM shown in Figure 5.2, is to make clear the nature of this network as a short-term memory system, which will unfold in a series of steps in the following paragraphs.

First, note that each node in the network represents a group of neurons and not actual single neurons as implied in the same sort of diagram in Figure 5.1. For the purpose of this chapter the same network principles apply for a node whether it represents a neuron or a collection of neurons. Thus for LBM N the sucker sensory inputs (S_s) represent *all* the sensory neurons on the rim of sucker N, as similarly all the propriosensory inputs (S_a) represent all of the proprioceptors in the LBM N. These sensory units supply inputs to the sucker ganglia and brachial ganglia, respectively. The groups of neurons in these ganglia are represented as single units as well. Thus, this figure and analysis are of a network of pools of neurons or *ganglia*.

The interpool connections between the sensors and the ganglia are placed on gray background fields to suggest the two separate neuropils in which these synapses exist in the octopus. Mathematically, both types of sensors are at the same level of processing (primary receptors) so their neuropils are represented as a single connectivity (or *w*eight) matrix W_{sg}, which represents the connections between the sensors and the ganglia.

The connections in the Figure 5.4 for W_{sg} are presented in Table 5.2 in matrix form where the rows represent the source of the signal (from) and the columns represent the target of the signal (to) thus from *s*ensors to *g*anglia is W_{sg}.

In Table 5.2, a value of 0 indicates no connection. The letters **a** and **b** indicate connections of two different strengths with values other than zero. The values of these connections will be discussed below. Note that each sucker sensor (S_s) provides input to just one ganglion (in its own LBM). The off-diagonal matrix entries labeled **h** for the arm inputs reflect the fact that proprioceptors located between given brachial ganglia

---

[4] The motor output units could have been arranged according to this convention. Since the motor units are not essential to the representation question they were not enumerated in order to simplify the diagram. Matrix mathematics aficionados will see that the equations represent them as vector outputs to preserve the LBM identity.

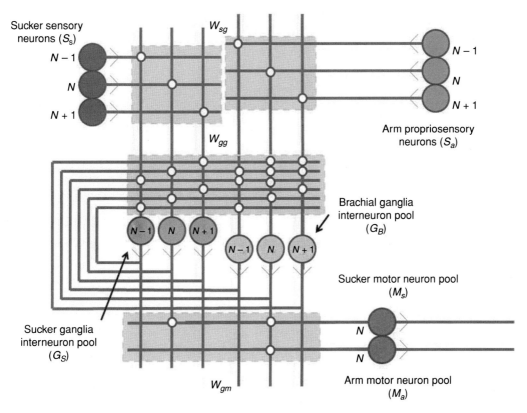

Figure 5.4 A schematic network representation of the segmental organization of the octopus arm. This figure represents the components of three segments of the arm as N–1, N and N+1 for the segment of interest and two adjacent suckers. The diagram could be extended to the 300 suckers of the arm but is reduced to this for convenience of illustration. Two sources of sensory input (s) are represented the chemo- and mechano-sensory inputs from the sucker rim are represented pooled as s_s and the proprioceptive sensory inputs of the arm as S_a. The motor outputs are schematized as arm M_a and sucker motor outputs M_s. The key feature in this diagram is the feedback matrix, W_{gg}, through which past network states and activations my continue to affect the output of the system (movements of the arms and suckers) at times after the application of the stimulus. Circles at the intersection of neuron inputs and outputs indicate a connection. The sign and magnitude are not indicated. The connectivity between, in the weights matrices (W's: W_{sg}, W_{gg} and W_{gm}) follows that described by Graziadei in Young (1971). In this diagram neurons are represented as polarized with an input (dendritic) line with connections, an integrating unit (soma) and output (axon) marked with an arrow. The sum of the input lines is assumed to be computed at the integrating unit and transmitted through the output.

provide input to both. The influence is known to spread farther than adjacent LBMs, but for the purpose of this analysis a single LBM lateral connectivity will not detract from illustrating the principles.

Each sucker ganglion receives input only from its sucker rim. The brachial ganglia, $G_{b,n}$ receive input from the immediate vicinity but may also receive direct sensory input from adjacent areas. The values of the connection strengths, **a** and **b** reflect the idea

Table 5.2 The connections in the Figure 5.4 for W_{sg} in matrix form

	G_S (n–1)	G_S (n)	G_S (n+1)	G_B (n–1)	G_B (n)	G_B (n+1)
S_S (n–1)	*a*	0	0	0	0	0
S_S (n)	0	*a*	0	0	0	0
S_S (n+1)	0	0	*a*	0	0	0
S_a (n–1)	0	0	0	*b*	*h*	0
S_a (n)	0	0	0	*h*	*b*	*h*
S_a (n+1)	0	0	0	0	*h*	*b*

that all sensory inputs from one modality would be equal but that those from different modalities need not be.

Returning to the Figure 5.4, there is a large set of interpool connections corresponding to the brachial ganglia neuropil, W_{gg} below W_{sg}, is also set against a gray background. This **g**anglion-to-**g**anglion connectivity matrix shows the connections between the ganglia. Finally, the sensory motor loop is completed with connections in a third neuropil to the motor neurons of the sucker and arm.[5]

The key feature of this analysis is the recurrent or looped feedback connections between the ganglia. The three sucker ganglia are placed slightly higher in the figure and in darker gray than the brachial ganglia to aid in tracing their connectivity. Note that on the input lines of the sucker ganglia there are just three connections, one on each sucker ganglion. This depiction reflects the neuroanatomic fact that each sucker only receives input from its corresponding brachial ganglion. The pattern repeats in the inputs to the brachial ganglia units. Again corresponding to the anatomy, each brachial ganglion receives input from only one sucker ganglion. The upper right corner of this matrix is the most interesting. It shows the connections between the brachial ganglia. The brachial ganglion in the middle, N, receives inputs from itself and the other two units. The proximal brachial ganglion receives inputs from itself and the central brachial ganglion and the same is true of the distal brachial ganglion (i.e. from itself and the central one). This imposes the orderly linear array of brachial ganglia connectivity. If $G_{b,n–1}$ and $G_{b,n+1}$ had been connected, the topology of the network would have been a ring and not a linear array as occurs in the octopus arm.

Table 5.3 presents these interganglionic connections as the matrix W_{gg}.

In Table 5.3, note that the matrix row and column labels are the same. This means that a non-zero connection along the left diagonal (*c, c, c, f, f, f*) in this matrix represents a connection between a unit and itself. So in the upper-left corner of the matrix we see the connection between sucker ganglia n–1 ($G_{s,n–1}$) and itself has a value of "*c*." This feedback means that an input to this ganglion, say from the sucker rim, will persist after the stimulus has disappeared from the receptor and the sensor is inactive. This is

---

[5] Speaking strictly anatomically this "third neuropil" might appropriately have its connections included in the W_{gg} neuropil because some of the connections are located in the brachial ganglion. However, others are found in the eccentric neuropils and this presentation format helps emphasize the functional properties of the brachial ganglia that are central to this paper.

Table 5.3 The interganglionic connections in Figure 5.4 for W_{gg} in a matrix form

	G_S (n−1)	G_S (n)	G_S (n+1)	G_B (n−1)	G_B (n)	G_B (n+1)
G_S (n−1)	*c*	0	0	*k*	0	0
G_S (n)	0	*c*	0	0	*k*	0
G_S (n+1)	0	0	*c*	0	0	*k*
G_B (n−1)	*l*	0	0	*f*	*m*	0
G_B (n)	0	*l*	0	*m*	*f*	*m*
G_B (n+1)	0	0	*l*	0	*m*	*f*

one of the requirements of a representation in the cognitive sense. How long it persists depends on the value of *c*. If the value is 1.0, then a perfect copy of the activation will be continuously supplied to the input of $G_{s,n-1}$. The input will be "remembered" indefinitely. On the other hand if *c* has a value less than 1.0, then the memory of the input in that ganglion will decay with time and be "forgotten." This is the basis by which recurrent networks produce short-term memory, and it is consistent with the existence of the neuropil in the sucker ganglia that reverberate input signals for some time depending on the strength of the connections within the neuropil. We see from Table 5.3 that the self-connections between the brachial ganglia have a value of *f*. If *f* is greater than *c* then the brachial ganglia will "remember" input patterns of equal intensity longer than the sucker ganglia will and vice versa.

The connections between the ganglia, those entries valued *g* in Table 5.3, are another form of memory. If ganglion G_{bn} is activated by the stimulation of the receptors in its LBM it will after some delay pass on that activation to its neighboring ganglia, N−1 and N+1. This just follows from the neuroanatomy which indicates that adjacent brachial ganglia are interconnected. However, because all the brachial ganglia are reciprocally connected, that delayed copy of the activation of G_{bn} will, following another delay, find its way back to G_{bn}. It should be clear that this connectivity pattern means that this reverberation can continue forever through this loop.

How long will this "memory" last? Again, that depends, as it did for *a*, *b*, *c* and *f*, on the value of *g*. These concepts can be summarized in the matrix equations that describe this model.[6]

$$g(t) = s(t - \Delta t)W_{sg} + g(t - \Delta t)W_{gg} \tag{5.1}$$

$$m(t) = g(t - \Delta t)W_{gm} \tag{5.2}$$

Equation 5.1 states that the state of the ganglia at any time step depends on the recent inputs from the primary receptors $[s(t - \Delta t)W_{sg}]$ and the previous state of the system

---

[6] These equations are included as formal specifications for those familiar with matrix mathematics and can be skipped without loss of understanding the important points of this section. These equations follow traditional matrix mathematical forms with capital letters representing matrices and lower case letters representing vectors. Matrix multiplication operators are implied here. Naturally, these equations may be applied to larger matrices representing more spatially realistic models of the CNS components of the octopus arm.

$[g(t - \Delta t)W_{gg}]$, makes this by definition an *adaptive* system. Equation 5.2 closes the sensory-motor arch expressing the motor output of the system (the behavior of the arm and sucker muscles) as the result of the states of the ganglia. The memory built into this system through recurrent loops ensures that the behavior will not be determined by a given stimulus input pattern. Rather it is a product of the current input and the history of the system's state. The behavior of the system is adaptive.

However, because there is now a network of interconnected ganglia we can ask a second question: how *far* will a given stimulus activation travel through the network? Remember that in this toy example we just used three LBMs. If the matrix were sized to represent the 300 of a single arm or the 2400 of all eight arms the input to a single sucker might spread quite far. The answer, again, is determined by the value of g. A larger g will spread 50% of the activation level farther down the chain of brachial ganglia than a smaller one.

There is more to this spatial aspect of the network. The stimulation of two different suckers, adjacent or distant, will lead to a superposition of their activation patterns in the entire network. For a simple example consider two inputs of equal intensity. The stimulation of two nearby suckers will produce a mutually reinforcing activation pattern in both of them that will be spatially localized and longer persisting. Two more distant suckers will produce a mutually reinforcing activation between them that will persist longer than a single activation. Two activations presented to the network at short delays relative to the "forgetting" rate will produce asymmetrical mutually reinforcing signals. And this principle can be extended to numbers of units that are greater than two. This makes evident that in a network of ganglia with recurrent connections, such as the octopus LBMs, *patterns* of activation can be stored and remembered hierarchically *across the network of ganglia*. And these patterns have an ordered spatial arrangement that reflects the attitude of the animal's body and the state of the external world as sensed by contact with surfaces. This exercise demonstrates that such a process is possible within the octopus CNS given what we know of its connectivity.

Figure 5.5 shows a somewhat contrived graphical illustration of this concept. I made it using a photograph of one of our laboratory's favorite octopuses, taken as he was attached to the flat surface of a tank glass. If the words of the text in the lower left had been painted in shrimp extract (a chemical cocktail octopuses detect) on the glass beneath the octopus, the pattern in the lower right panel would be transmitted by the chemo-receptors on the sucker rims into the octopus's CNS. Bear in mind that this is just a single frame and that the network of ganglia in the arms would remember this input for some time. Should the animal move to arrange its suckers with care the entire text might be surveyed, the gaps filled in and been stored in the octopus memory for some time afterwards.[7]

---

[7] I do not mean to imply that an octopus could "read" this text. A problem with this example, and what makes it somewhat contrived, is that the positions of the sucker needs to be known in order to decode the information in this text. It is not clear, and the available evidence makes it seem unlikely, that the Cartesian positions of the pixels in this image would be available from proprioceptive inputs for the octopus to reconstruct between moves. Yet, according to the analysis presented here the information of activated suckers would certainly pass and persist in the network of brachial ganglia.

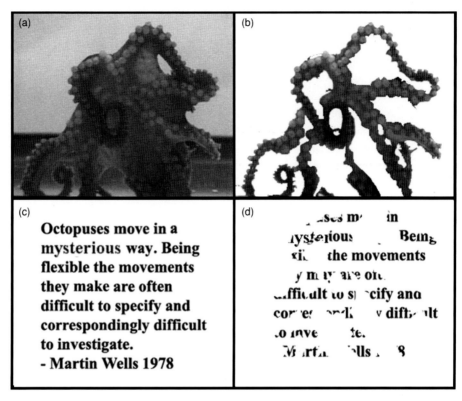

Figure 5.5 Illustration of the chemo-tactile sensory surface of the arms of octopus. Panel (a) shows an image of an *Octopus rubescens* "Benji" attached by his suckers to the glass surface of his tank. Panel (b) shows the same image edited to just the sucker rims which contain the chemical and tactile receptors. Panel (c) shows some sample text. Panel (d) shows the portions of that text that would be transmitted through the collected sensory surface of the suckers visible in this image. Note that much of the text is preserved and would be transmitted to Benji's central nervous system for processing.

A typical metaphor for recurrent networks of this type is of a pool of water. A disturbance, such as a stone thrown into the pool, causes ripples throughout the entire network that can be used at a later time to reconstruct the features of the original stimulus. Multiple stones will cause intersecting patterns of ripples that can be similarly interpreted. In this case the metaphor is of eight canals of water linked at a single pool. And the brain of the octopus sits at the intersection of these canals, in a position to interpret the ripple patterns arriving from the canals.

5.6.2   Tuning the ganglia network

Section 5.4.2 made clear that the brachial ganglia are multitasking entities. It posed the question of how much cognitive load could the network support and answered that there were a lot of neurons available to do a lot of computations. This leads to two possibilities that, if true, have different implications for the evolution of the nervous system.

One possibility is that the information content extracted by and stored by the ganglia network (as illustrated in section 5.6.1) is a by-product of tuning up the network to do well enough in meeting the multiple constraints posed by the different functions that were described in section 5.5. The network does not need to be optimized for the information content or memory function on its own. In the analysis above (Equation 5.2) the observable behavior, (i.e. motor output) occurs on its own regardless of whether or not the reverberating activation patterns in the brachial ganglia are used as a memory mechanism. If the determination of the connectivity strength in the brachial ganglia neuropil (the entries in the W_{gg} matrix of the analysis) were aimed the achieving suitable performance of reaching and grasping and other behaviors the properties described in section 5.5 would emerge to some extent as long as the connection strengths were not zero.

If, on the other hand, there were sufficient neural resources and there was a sufficient evolutionary advantage, then the connectivity of a ganglionic network could have been optimized to some extent for its information content. Octopuses are known to make both chemical and tactile discriminations using their sucker rim inputs (see chapter 7, this volume). The analysis above is at a general and abstracted level. It does not, for example, deal explicitly with the nature of the chemicals that are sensed, nor the mechanical qualities encoded in the receptor neurons. If there are suitable neural resources amongst the 10^5 neurons of each LBM, then separate channels for different chemical qualities, spatial localization on the sucker rim, and intensity of chemical and mechanical stimulation could be encoded across the brachial ganglia network. The same principles could be applied to single modality channels or their combinations.

5.7 Relationships between a network of local brachial modules and the cerebral ganglia

5.7.1 The absence of somatotopic maps

Section 5.4.1 reviewed the literature which expressed the surprising failure to discover somatotopic maps in a brain as complex and large (in numbers of cells) as that of the octopus. Section 5.6.1 has demonstrated that the connectivity of the octopus brachial ganglia could be an implementation of a memory system capable of encoding spatial information about surfaces with which the octopus is in contact. It appears that the absence of somatotopic representations in the cerebral ganglia might find explanation in the LBM network.

Somatotopic maps and spatial maps in general are ubiquitous features of the brain architectures of vertebrates. But it should not be surprising that there should be a different representational strategy in octopuses with soft bodies and different life styles. Perhaps it would be more surprising to find a somatotopic representation of the body of an octopus which lacks rigid physical links of an endoskeleton. The retinotopic representation of the octopus optic lobes makes sense for an invariant physical structure like the retina and, indeed, we see this in a manner similar to that observed in arthropods.

Zullo and Hochner (2011) have suggested that the lack of a central somatotopic representation might reflect the concept of embodiment in neuromechanical systems. The analysis above advances a mechanism that is such an embodiment approach. It begs the question, however, of how the cerebral ganglia might use this representation. We know that the cerebral ganglia are profoundly interconnected with the brachial ganglia so the access to the information contained in the brachial ganglia is not an issue. And, one of the hallmarks of the supraesophageal lobes of the cerebral ganglia is their capacity for learning. Persistence of the pattern of activation and temporal progression of that pattern across the brachial ganglia would provide a trace that could be used to apply trial-and-error learning on the descending inputs to the arm. Why make a copy when you can work with the real thing?

The reciprocal information flow between the arms and cerebral ganglia could be quite informationally impoverished (in the Shannon sense, a few bits) but rich in meaning (in the Bayesian statistical sense). An ordered array of outputs from the individual LBMs to the brain could provide considerable information about the state of the external world in a relatively small number of bits. There is ample evidence that the rich local circuitry of the arm and LBMs support motor programs of their own for local and distributed control. The learned responses to the input patterns might be equally sparse in information, relying on the fixed behavioral repertoires stored in the circuitry of the brachial ganglia.

The reverberant circuits, like the one described in section 5.6.1, produce relatively short-lived traces, minutes or perhaps an hour at the longest, certainly long enough to support the learning of behavioral sequences by the cerebral ganglia but not long enough to make local changes in behavior on a longer time scale. There is no evidence for LTP in the arm and no evidence yet against it. LTP at appropriate synapses would be one way to lengthen the duration of the memory and tune the character of motor responses and information content on a more or less permanent basis. On the other hand, perhaps the predictability of fixed but dynamically complex performance characteristics in the brachial network combined with a plastic brain for long-term changes is a better computational solution than tasking the cerebral ganglia to learn what the brachial ganglia has learned.

5.7.2   The "two brains" of the octopus

I chose the illustrations in Figure 5.1 for two reasons: the first was to illustrate the conventions in representing recurrent neural networks. The second reason was to underscore the idea that a network that connects sensors in the world to effectors in the world is capable of producing behavior. The architecture of the LBM makes clear that the individual LBM is capable of producing autonomous behavior by closing the sensory motor loop in the control of sucker movements. The inputs from other LBMs do not over-ride that autonomy so much as influence the ongoing behavior to support inter-sucker coordination and coordination with the movements of the arm muscles which form a continuum. Thus, the ganglionic network I've proposed here operates rather like a distributed control network. It may not match the neuroanatomical definition of a brain (a collection of *specialized*, interconnected ganglia) but the diversity of behaviors demonstrated by "decerebrate" octopuses indicates that we are not far off from the truth if we were to conceptualize it as one.

There is a parallel example in the nervous system of the starfish. Starfish engage in coherent whole-organism behaviors like chemotactic foraging (Dale, 1999) and dexterous manipulation in the opening of the shells of bivalve mollusks like clams and oysters (Dyal, Owen & Willows, 1973). Yet these animals are without a central structure that could even loosely be considered a brain. Instead the five arms (or more depending on the species) contain a nerve cord organized, among other things, around the control of the hundreds of tube feet that occupy the starfish's oral surface. These nerve cords are connected by a nerve ring that encircles the center of the animal and that is devoid of neurons itself. The choice of direction of walking in a starfish is determined by a democratic "vote" of the neural control units of all the tube feet which is decided by a winner-take-all mechanism.[8] Jellyfish form an even more extreme example of a distributed nervous system, producing coherent behaviors of reproduction, feeding and swimming without even ganglia (Prescott, 2007). They have a diffuse reticulum or diffuse nerve net spread around their bodies to connect patterns of sensory input to muscle commands.

If the starfish, without a central brain, can forage for distant food items, find mates and mate and manipulate objects using dexterous (if stereotyped) methods involving the coordination of arms, why not an octopus with many orders of magnitude more neural hardware in its brachial network alone? In this view the cerebral ganglia simply influence but do not specify the details of ongoing sucker and arm behavior. It is also possible and likely that the cerebral ganglia, as Zullo and Hochner (2011) assert, serve a "gating" function on the ongoing autonomous behavior produced by the brachial ganglia network.

The above demonstrates that computational architecture of a single LBM processes a diversity of sensory modalities and motor outputs, and has a capacity for memory. Many of these powerful LBM information-processing units interconnected with such a large number of central interneurons will be a font of emergent functional properties in the sense described since the early days of connectionism (McCelland & Rumelhart, 1986). One key aspect of that conception of cognitive information processing (the "microstructure of cognition") is that while each unit possesses (in this case large amounts of) local information the properties of the entire network emerge from the interactions of its parts. The network of LBMs in the octopus arm is, from its connectivity and sheer size, a complex distributed information processing structure. Its observable behavior results not from the sum of its parts but from the interactions of its parts (in space and with intrinsic "memory" capacity in time), which is an exponentially larger set of functions than the number of parts.

There is limited evidence from physiological recordings, but what there is suggests that the information from individual sensory modalities is both preserved and propagated

---

[8] It is reported that if this nerve ring is cut in two places to separate two legs from the other three the action of the desynchronized (and strong) tube feet will eventually tear the two arms apart from the other three. I've found this in the literature but not been able to find the original research report. Whether or not this story is apocryphal its point about the distribution of competent autonomous behavior processes is useful here.

between neighboring LBMs. This means that the types of memory and distributed information systems described in the analysis above are likely maintained as parallel systems (e.g. different chemical qualities, mechanical properties, proprioception) up and down a given arm and between arms. It is possible that these modalities also mix in channels of their own ("interaction channels") and that there are also efference copy channels for motor signals that are propagated through the distributed network. In short, the connectivity of the brachial plexus supports its operating as a distributed multimodal representation of sensory and motor states across the arms with memory of past events, which also has the ability to produce action on its own. Even more briefly it is a cognitive behavioral control system.

5.7.3 Communication between cerebral and brachial ganglia

It should be clear now that the conception of the brachial ganglia as an autonomous or semiautonomous behavior-generating explains several odd aspects of octopus dexterous manipulation compared to rigid-bodied animals'. But it does beg the question: how do the brachial ganglia communicate the state of the world in the absence of somatotopic or other forms of maps?

Having raised the question, I will offer the following speculation as a possible answer. Figure 5.6 shows two alternative communication schemes. Figure 5.6a shows how a somatotopic map might be formed by the arm. With direct connectivity between the LBMs and corresponding units in the brain, a literal copy of the orderly sequence from proximal to distal would appear in the brain as a virtual progression from proximal to distal through the brain tissue as, for example, a representation of the body surface does across the sensory cortex (SI) of mammals. For simplicity I show just five LBM units in a single arm, but there is no reason the principles not be extended to all the LBMs of all eight arms. In that case one would expect to find an "Octo-munculus" in the brain of an octopus as Wilder Penfield famously found the "Homunculus" in the brains of his human patients.

Figure 5.6b assigns the cerebral ganglia (lobe deliberately not specified) the role of a decoder of temporal rather than spatial patterns. In the upper left corner of the figure is the chain of LBMs in the arm. Remember that these are interconnected recurrently and, therefore, possessed of "memory" properties of their own to store past patterns. The information in the most proximal node, N_0 would contain information about its state at the present time, the state of N_1 with some delay in the past, N_2 with some greater delay and so on in the distal direction down the arm. The output from N_0 contains therefore the information of the state of the arm at each instant. (If the information carried in this line included both primary sensory and motor state information it might be more useful and certainly more compact than reconstituting the sensory state in the arm in the brain.) A continuous time series of these values contains information about the progression of arm states. The several units in the cerebral ganglia network (N_a, N_b, N_c ...) all receive the identical state-series input. The activation of one could signal the occurrence of a state in the arm that was of behavioral importance. In this architecture the tuning of a particular unit to encode a particular state is accomplished by differential connection strengths

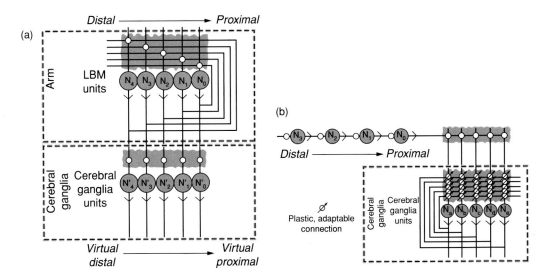

Figure 5.6 An illustration of two network connectivity arrangements. Panel (a) shows one which supports the formation of somatotopic maps. The progression of local brachial modules (LBM) units (N_1, $N_2 \ldots N_n$) from the distal to the proximal ends of a given arm maps in an orderly progression that parallels the distal to proximal sequence of units in the cerebral ganglia (N'_1, $N'_2 \ldots N'_n$) because they are connected that way. Panel (b) shows a connectivity that supports a temporal rather than a spatial encoding approach. Each of the internally recurrent LBM units in one arm progressively pass their activity in a distal to proximal direction. The arm's input to the cerebral ganglia is passed from the most proximal LBM as the accumulated activity of all the LBMs. The delay in propagation between the LBMs produces a temporal code of the arm's state. The cerebral ganglia units encode the patterns (N_a, N_b, $N_c \ldots$) not locations in arm space. The recurrent arrangement of the cerebral network here endows this network with "memory" that permits the units to follow the time course of the input stream. Given that all cerebral ganglia units receive the same input, the discrimination of patterns arm state is acquired through Hebbian learning of the different time encoded sequences at plastic input connections.

on the feedback connections within the cerebral ganglia neuropil. In most animals the acquisition of connectivity, such as that in the feedback matrix here, is as a combination of inherited connections, those acquired during development or those learned through experience. This network architecture supports all three modes but I've drawn them with adaptable connections as a tip-of-the hat to the fact that LTP and Hebbian forms of learning are known to exist in the cerebral ganglia. Neural network methods for learning the connection strengths to store time series like this exist (Williams & Zipser, 1989; Mak, Lu & Ku, 1995; Anastasio, 2010), but it should be remembered that it is the connections in this matrix that make the discrimination possible.

With an architecture like that in Figure 5.6b, which classifies the arm states, the representation in the cerebral ganglia is encoded as a time-series (stream) of events. The cerebral ganglia could combine this compact summary with other information at its disposal and decide which biasing signals to send to the arms to modulate (or gate) the ongoing behavior.

Concluding an alternative encoding scheme from the absence of evidence of this "Octo-munculus" is faulty logic – like *concluding* the null hypothesis when an experiment fails to reject it. The discovery tomorrow of an "Octo-munculus" will invalidate the event-encoding theory that excludes the existence of an "Octo-munculus." Consequently, I tender the conception in Figure 5.6 not as a conclusion but as an example of a mechanism that fits the available evidence. There are many variations on this mechanism and indeed alternative theories (e.g. Hopfield nets [Hopfield, 1982]) that could offer explanations for encoding and representation of arm states in the octopus. Regardless of the algorithm that is used, the theory (in David Marr's sense) that the communication between the brachial ganglia and the cerebral ganglia is a representation of sensory-motor events, offers several advantages in explaining and new opportunities to study cognition in octopuses and, perhaps, cephalopods generally.

Cognitive psychology and cognitive science has made heavy use of reaction time to find quantitative evidence of the levels of cognitive load associated with specific tasks, and to infer various capacities and the nature and number of processing steps involved in the processing of those tasks. Underpinning this approach is the idea that longer processing time reflects the investment of brain resources in the task. The processes described in this chapter rest heavily on the temporal aspects of neural processing and could be used to make specific predictions about performance of tasks by cephalopods that if falsified or supported would reflect the underlying organization of brain processes.

5.8   The octopus with two brains

The two brains of the octopus I alluded to in the title of this chapter are the cerebral ganglia and the ensemble of brachial ganglia (or brachial plexus), and by this point in the chapter we have discussed them from a variety of perspectives. The cerebral ganglia of the octopus are the part of the CNS that most researchers refer to as the "brain" and for good reason – it has all the key features of a brain. The brachial plexus, on the other hand, has some of the features of a brain, namely an aggregation of ganglia and a capacity for the autonomous performance of behavior. I have endeavored to demonstrate that the term "cognitive" could be used to characterize the brachial plexus in that the information processing performed there meets the definition of being adaptive. And yet, constituted as a homogenous chain of ganglia as it is, it does not meet the requirement of specialized ganglia that distinguish a brain. So it is properly referred to as a plexus. So, we can say that, as we use the word, the octopus does not have two brains.

Yet, there is an issue here beyond semantics, beyond the definition of the word "brain." If the conception of the octopus brain (cerebral ganglia) as an agent that biases or gates in the ongoing behavioral processes mediated by the brachial ganglia is true, then the ensemble of brachial ganglia that exist in octopuses is something remarkable: a cognitive information-processing organ for which the term plexus does not seem quite an appropriate name and perhaps not even a proper conception.

We could hedge our bets and, following J. Z. Young's example, (and as I did in the introduction of this chapter) refer to the brachial and cerebral ganglia as "the central nervous system." It makes good sense to consider the brachial plexus and brain as one system for producing the dexterous manipulation behaviors of the octopus. But to think that we understand the processing by claiming the CNS works as a whole is a tautology that obscures the important distinction between the processing modes of the brain and brachial plexus and the important issue of how the two parts of the CNS communicate to produce coherent behavior. Even if the brachial plexus is not an equal partner with the brain, underestimating its degree of autonomy obscures its important cognitive role in the behavior of the octopus. Its size and complexity, a collection of about 2400 ganglia (each composed of about 100 000 interneurons) interacting to produce coherent behavior in eight non-rigid arms and about 2000 moveable suckers makes it a truly remarkable computational instrument rivaling or exceeding the abilities of most whole organisms we know. Perhaps it is the more intriguing and mysterious part than the part of the CNS to which the generic name of plexus does not do appropriate descriptive justice and perhaps one that in its novelty has more to teach us about nervous system function, control systems and the evolution of nervous systems than its better-publicized partner.

I suspect that a vertebrate-centric bias lies behind the neglect of the remarkable brachial plexus. The word "brain" draws on our intuitions about our own brains and how they work. We draw our metaphors often from vertebrate brains because they have been so much more extensively studied. The influence of funding agencies' frequent anthropocentric stance that research should provide discoveries that are useful for human health perpetuates this vertebrate bias. Scientifically, the contrast between vertebrates and cephalopods invites discovery through similarities and differences that are all remarkable because the octopus's body is so novel compared to our own. The counterpoint to the novelty of cephalopod mechanisms is convergent evolution; the idea that animals of different lineages converge from different starting places on the same basic design principles because of the universal utility of those principles (e.g. the wings of bats and birds have shapes that utilize aerodynamic lift). These confirmations of the general utility of a given mechanism give us a sense of their greater explanatory power as theories. It seems likely to me that the brachial ganglia network is an example of convergent evolution that parallels the starfish ring ganglia. The utility of the nerve ring for coordinating many ganglia is a more likely explanation of octopus brain evolution than octopus converged on the solution of somatotopic maps that evolved in vertebrate brains. The question is an interesting one and is at the heart of the comparative method in biology and neuroscience. We should remember the novel solutions to problems that cephalopods can teach us about are true discoveries rather than confirmation of the general utility of the vertebrate approach, and may be of greater value to future human generations than those discoveries that hold a mirror up to ourselves.

Computationally, the LBM network promises to be one of these opportunities for discovering new mechanisms in three ways: first, in an understanding of how to control and coordinate eight (or more, or fewer) soft appendages capable of dexterous manipulation; second, in discovering the emergent properties of computational systems composed of large numbers of very complex homogeneous units; and, third, by studying the nature of the communication between the cerebral ganglia and LBMs we may learn about the control of massive, complex systems with various degrees of distributed autonomy.

One novel idea that I see the brachial plexus as illustrating is its mode of control. One useful engineering definition of a control system is one that is capable of bringing a controlled system, such as the octopus arms and suckers, from its current state to another arbitrary state with a known degree of precision and a finite amount of time. A simple and common instance in octopus behavior might be releasing the 27th sucker on arm R3, moving it 2 cm to the right and reattaching it. Treating the whole CNS as a control system, then *perhaps* the brain and brachial plexus together meet the engineering definition of a control system and together they are able to implement this for any of the ~2400 suckers. It seems more likely that the brain does not know anywhere near this degree of detail and that the truly distributed processes of the brachial plexus serve to give the octopus something *just close enough* to this degree of control using the distributed computational method illustrated in the analysis above.

The communication between the brain and brachial plexus is another novel mechanism that the octopus can teach us. The octopus, like the human species, is profoundly visual in its behaviors. The most prominent externally visible structure in the octopus brain is its paired, enormous, cytoarchitectonically complex visual lobes. The representations in the brain of the octopus, which support processes like visual attention, are intrinsically spatial in the information they encode. They are also, therefore, fundamentally different from the distributed representations in the brachial plexus, which I have argued for here. Young and others have argued similarly for the functional division of the octopus brain into visual and chemotactile division in the organization of the brain, though theirs was a far more centralized, descending control scheme (Young, 1964; Wells, 1978). Those distributed representations, including "memory," are an adaptation to the soft nature of the tissues in the arms and the consequent intedeterminant nature of the sensing and motor control soft tissues. The transformation of the distributed encoding and representation in the arms to something the brain can use and vice versa is a fundamentally novel transformation between a localized representation to a distributed one. The analysis above is one way that this may be achieved, there may be several awaiting discovery in the parallel sensory modalities and levels of motor control in the octopus.

The octopus has a plethora of massively parallel neural control systems: the chromatophore and mantle control systems are two other prominent examples. The non-rigid form of the octopus' body and the evolutionary demands for a complex behavioral repertoire have probably shaped several of these massively parallel and distributed control systems in the coleoid cephalopods. There are undoubtedly variations on the central theme of distributed control amongst them. Cephalopods may be specialists in distributed control systems. However, the behavioral and sensory-motor demands made by the coordinated control of the arms and suckers in the octopus have made the brachial plexus a uniquely cognitive organ, and one with much to teach us about architectures for distributed control and computation.

Aristotle can be forgiven for his claims of octopus stupidity. He did not have access to the abundant behavioral evidence for advanced cognition in cephalopods reviewed in this volume. The octopus may or may not have two kinds of brains in one body. The answer to that question will be resolved by understanding the content and modes of communication between the arms and the brain. Pursuit of that mechanistic understanding will take us a long way towards learning how cognition works in these creatures; and may either define it specifically as a cephalopod innovation that is very different from vertebrate cognition or provide a perspective on a monolithic form of cognition that transcends the details of neural architecture.

Acknowledgements

I thank Dr. Michael Kuba for his assistance with the design and construction of the Octopus Y-maze and Professor Jennifer Basil for helpful discussions of some of the concepts in this manuscript. I am grateful to my home institution, Brooklyn College, CUNY for the wise level of sabbatical year support that facilitated the writing of this chapter.

References

Altmann, J. S. (1971). Control of accept and reject reflexes in the octopus. *Nature*, **229**: 203–207.

Anastasio, T. J. (2010). *Tutorial on neural systems modeling*, Sunderland, MA, Sinauer Associates Inc.

Anderson, R. C. and Mather, J. A. (2007). The packaging problem: bivalve prey selection and prey entry techniques of the octopus *Enteroctopus dofleini. Journal of Comparative Psychology*, **121**: 300–305.

Aristotle, *The history of animals*, Book IX, translated by D'Arcy Wentworth Thompson (2013). ebooks@Adelaide, The University of Adelaide. Available at http://ebooks.adelaide.edu.au/a/aristotle/history/

Braitenberg, V. (1984). *Vehicles: experiments in synthetic psychology*, Cambridge, MA, Bradford Books, MIT Press.

Dale, J. (1999). Coordination of chemosensory orientation in the starfish *Asterias forbesi. Marine and Freshwater Behaviour and Physiology*, **32**: 57–71.

Dyal, J. A., Owen, A. and Willows, D. (1973). Invertebrate learning: cephalopods and echinoderms. In Corning, W. C., Dyal, J. A. and Willows, A. O. D. (eds.) *Invertebrate learning: cephalopods and echinoderms*, New York, NY, Plenum Press.

Edelman, D. B. and Seth, A. K. (2009). Animal consciousness: a synthetic approach. *Trends in Neuroscience*, **32**: 476–484.

Finlay, B. L., Darlington, R. B. and Nicastro, N. (2001). Developmental structure in brain evolution. *Behavioral and Brain Sciences*, **24**: 263–308.

Fiorito, G., Agnisola, C., D'Addio, M., Valanzano, A. and Calamandrei, G. (1998). Scopolamine impairs memory recall in *Octopus vulgaris. Neuroscience*, **253**: 87–90.

Fiorito, G. and Gherardi, F. (1999). Prey-handling behaviour of *Octopus vulgaris* (Mollusca, Cephalopoda) on bivalve preys. *Behavioural Processes*, **46**: 75–88.

Fiorito, G. and Scotto, P. (1992). Observational learning in *Octopus vulgaris. Science*, **256**: 545–547.

Fiorito, G., Von Planta, C. and Scotto, P. (1990). Problem solving ability of *Octopus vulgaris* Lamarck (Mollusca, Cephalopoda). *Behavioral and Neural Biology*, **53**: 217–230.

Grasso, F. W. (2008). Octopus sucker–arm coordination in grasping and manipulation. *American Malacological Bulletin*, **24**: 13–23.

Grasso, F. W. and Basil, J. (2009). The evolution of flexible behavioral repertoires in cephalopod mollusks. *Brain, Behavior and Evolution*, **74**: 231–245.

Graziadei, P. (1965). Muscle receptors in cephalopods. *Proceedings of the Royal Society. B: Biological Sciences*, **161**: 392–402.

Graziadei, P. P. C. (1971). The nervous system of the arms. In Young, J. Z. (ed.) *The anatomy of the nervous system of Octopus vulgaris,* Oxford, UK, Clarendon Press.

Graziadei, P. P. C. and Gagne, H. T. (1976). Sensory innervation of the rim of the octopus sucker. *Journal of Morphology*, **150**: 639–680.

Gutfreund, Y., Flash, T., Fiorito, G. and Hochner, B. (1998). Patterns of arm muscle activation involved in octopus reaching movements. *Journal of Neuroscience*, **18**: 5976–5987.

Gutnick, T., Byrne, R. A., Hochner, B. and Kuba, M. (2011). *Octopus vulgaris* uses visual information to determine the location of its arm. *Current Biology*, **21**: 460–462.

Hanlon, R. T. and Messenger, J. B. (1996). *Cephalopod behaviour*, Cambridge, UK, Cambridge University Press.

Herculano-Houzel, S., Collins, C. E., Wong, P. and Kaas, J. H. (2007). Cellular scaling rules for primate brains. *Proceedings of the National Academy of Sciences*, **104**: 3562–3567.

Hochner, B., Shomrat, T. and Fiorito, G. (2006). The octopus: a model for a comparative analysis of the evolution of learning and memory mechanisms. *The Biological Bulletin*, **210**: 308–317.

Hopfield, J. J. (1982). Neural networks and physical systems with emergent collective computational abilities. *Proceedings of the National Academy of Sciences*, **79**: 2554–2558.

Kier, W. M. (1982). The functional morphology of the musculature of squid (loliginidae) arms and tentacles. *Morphology*, **172**: 179–192.

Mackintosh, N. J. (1965). Discrimination learning in the octopus. *Animal Behaviour suppl*, **1**: 129–134.

Mackintosh, N. J. and Mackintosh, J. (1963). Reversal learning in *Octopus vulgaris* Lamarck with and without irrelevant cues. *Quarterly Journal of Experimental Psychology*, **15**: 236–242.

Mak, M. W., Lu, Y. L. and Ku, K. W. (1995). Improved real time recurrent learning algorithms: a review and some new approaches. *Neurocomputing*, **24**: 13–36.

Marr, D. (1982). *Vision*, New York, NY, W. H. Freeman and Co.

Mather, J. A. (1998). How do octopuses use their arms? *Journal of Comparative Psychology*, **112**: 306–316.

McCelland, J. L. and Rumelhart, D. E. (1986). *Parallel distributed processing: explorations in the microstructure of cognition. Psychological and biological models*, Cambridge, MA, MIT Press.

Packard, A. (1961). Sucker display of octopus. *Nature*, **190**: 736–737.

Prescott, T. J. (2007). Forced moves or good tricks in design space? Landmarks in the evolution of neural mechanisms for action selection. *Journal of Adaptive Behavior*, **15**: 9–31.

Rowell, C. F. H. (1963). Excitatory and inhibitory pathways in the arm of *Octopus*. *Journal of Experimental Biology*, **40**: 257–270.

Rowell, C. F. H. (1966). Activity of interneurons in the arm of Octopus in response to tactile stimulation. *Journal of Experimental Biology*, **44**: 589–605.

Shomrat, T., Graindorge, N., Bellanger, C., Fiorito, G., Loewenstein, Y. and Hochner, B. (2011). Alternative sites of synaptic plasticity in two homologous "Fan-out Fan-in" learning and memory networks. *Current Biology*, **21**: 1773–1782.

Shomrat, T., Zarrella, I., Fiorito, G. and Hochner, B. (2008). The octopus vertical lobe modulates short-term learning rate and uses LTP to acquire long-term memory. *Current Biology*, **18**: 337–342.

Sumbre, G., Fiorito, G., Flash, T. and Hochner, B. (2006). Octopuses use a human-like strategy to control precise point-to-point arm movements. *Current Biology*, **16**: 767–772.

Sumbre, G., Gutfreund, Y., Fiorito, G., Flash, T. and Hochner, B. (2001). Control of octopus arm extension by a peripheral motor program. *Science*, **293**: 1845–1848.

Walløe, S., Nissen, U. V., Berg, R. W., Hounsgaard, J. and Pakkenberg, B. (2011). Stereological estimate of the total number of neurons in spinal segment D9 of the Red Eared turtle. *Journal of Neuroscience*, **31**: 2431–2435.

Wells, M. J. (1964). Tactile discrimination of surface curvature and shape by the octopus. *Journal of Experimental Biology*, **41**: 433–445.

Wells, M. J. (1978). *Octopus: physiology and behaviour of an advanced invertebrate*, Chichester, Sussex, UK, John Wiley and Sons.

Wells, M. J. and Wells, J. (1957a). The function of the brain of *Octopus* in tactile discrimination. *Journal of Experimental Biology*, **34**: 131–142.

Wells, M. J. and Wells, J. (1957b). Repeated presentation experiments and the function of the vertical lobe. *Journal of Experimental Biology*, **34**: 469–477.

Williams, R. J. and Zipser, D. (1989). A learning algorithm for continually running fully recurrent neural networks. *Journal of Neural Computation*, **1**: 270–280.

Young, J. Z. (1964). *A model of the brain*, Oxford, UK, Clarendon Press.

Young, J. Z. (1971). *The anatomy of the nervous system of Octopus vulgaris*, Oxford, UK, Clarendon Press.

Young, J. Z. (1991). Computation in the learning system of cephalopods. *The Biological Bulletin*, **180**: 200 208.

Zullo, L. and Hochner, B. (2011). A new perspective on the organization of an invertebrate brain. *Communicative and Integrative Biology*, **4**: 26–29.

Zullo, L., Sumbre, G., Agnisola, C., Flash, T. and Hochner, B. (2009). Nonsomatotopic organization of the higher motor centers in octopus. *Current Biology*, **19**: 1632–1636.

Part II

Cognition and the environment

6 Foraging and cognitive competence in octopuses

Jennifer A. Mather, Tatiana S. Leite, Roland C. Anderson and James B. Wood

6.1   Introduction

Octopuses and other cephalopods are widely acknowledged to have cognitive ability, where cognition is defined as "All the processes by which the sensory input is transformed, reduced, elaborated, stored, recovered and used" (Neisser, 1976, see Mather, 1995). Over decades, researchers at the Stazione Zoologica in Naples have evaluated both octopuses' visual concept formation and the brain control of their learning (Wells, 1978; Borrelli & Fiorito, 2008). Octopuses play, have personalities and solve problems, capacities which have led to a suggestion that they have a simple form of consciousness (Mather, 2008). Recent research has begun to explore the neurobiology of these processes (Hochner, Shomrat & Fiorito, 2006; Hochner, 2010) and the neural networks underlying them (Williamson & Chrachri, 2004). Yet all these investigations of octopus ability are laboratory-based, and there is a lack of information about how octopuses might process such information in the field, in their daily lives. What is needed to fill this gap is an assessment of the daily activities such as foraging, but in terms of their underlying cognitive processes. The link may not be easy to make as field studies are generally uncontrolled, but it is worth exploring as a foundation for laboratory studies.

High intelligence and complex cognitive processing are theorized to have developed in mammals that live in close social groups for the understanding of cues about conspecifics (Humphrey, 1976; Jolly, 1966). One important aspect of the lives of octopuses is that, in contrast to these mammals, they are generally solitary (Boal, 2006, though see Huffard, Caldwell & Boneka, 2010). Why would a non-social animal need acute sensory processing and quick decision making? The most obvious area in which such solitary animals would use their abilities is in foraging strategies and food selection, which occurs while avoiding predation (Lima & Dill, 1990; Brown & Kotler, 2007) especially given the complex near-shore environment in which many octopus species live.

Classic assessment of animal foraging has been based on the simplistic evaluation of the relative amount of energy expended in finding food versus that produced by its consumption (Stephens & Krebs, 1986), which does not take other variables into account. Such simple analysis is not always adequate. For example, in *Octopus rubescens*

Cephalopod Cognition, eds A.-S. Darmaillacq, L. Dickel and J. Mather. Published by Cambridge University Press. © Cambridge 2014.

(Onthank & Cowles, 2011), energetics does not drive prey choices between crab and clam prey; the animals preferred the crabs but got more nutrition from and had less handling time of the clam. The authors theorized that a difference in digestibility of prey lipids might have driven the choice, although the octopod preference for crabs is a general one (Hanlon & Messenger, 1996). In addition to taking little account of predator risk, the simple energetic model has left little room for other lifestyle influences. However, a recent updating of the area of foraging (Stephens, Brown & Ydenberg, 2007) has begun to point out the role of many aspects of life, including the threat of predation (Bednekoff, 2007) and cognition (Adams-Hunt & Jacobs, 2007), in foraging. The present chapter discusses the potential usefulness of the cognitive skills, some of which have been tested in the laboratory, for the job of finding prey while evading capture.

This cognitive linkage has not been made in octopuses because they have been assumed to be generalist foragers (see O'Brien, Browman & Evans, 1990; Cooper, 2005) and use cruise searching (although pure cruise searching is probably rare). This means that they would range widely across the substrate, unselectively capturing whatever prey they encountered. However, a more detailed assessment of octopus foraging reveals: (1) that individuals are not generalists (see Anderson, Wood & Mather, 2008); (2) they are not cruise searchers but employ the saltatory search described by O'Brien, Browman and Evans (1990) (see Mather, 1991a; Forsythe & Hanlon, 1997; Leite, Haimovici & Mather, 2009), although the secondary search is tactile. Their foraging behavior differs considerably across time and space; and (3) they forage under considerable risk of predation (Bednekoff, 2007, see Mather & O'Dor, 1991; Hanlon, Forsythe & Joneschild, 1999). All these conditions of foraging must be met by the exertion of considerable cognitive ability, evidenced particularly in prey selection, spatial memory and antipredator tactics.

6.2   Octopuses as generalist foragers

The first caveat about octopuses as unselective generalist foragers is that they are usually not. Researchers in this area are fortunate, as octopuses consume the soft parts of prey and discard the skeletal and shell remains near where they have been eating (Mather, 1991a). Although assessment of remains over-represents the proportion of molluscs and under-represents that of crustaceans in the diet (Smith, 2003), it is probably more accurate when sampling is done daily (see Mather, 1991a, for retention of different types of prey remains). But investigators have sometimes been misled by the array of remains of different prey species left in their middens. There were many species: Anderson, Sinn and Mather (2008) found remains of 75 species from *Octopus vulgaris*, Leite, Haimovici and Mather (2009) documented 55 for *Octopus insularis*, Ambrose (1984) found 59 for *Octopus bimaculatus* and Vincent, Scheel and Hough (1998) found 32 for *Enteroctopus dofleini*. Mather (1991a), sampling in one small bay in the isolated islands of Bermuda over a few weeks, found 28. But this array of species remains, taken in some cases from dens of many individuals over a wide area or over several years, is misleading. The aggregate list of prey species hides individual selectivity that is obvious with a further assessment (Anderson, Sinn & Mather, 2008; Mather, Leite & Batista, 2012; Scheel & Anderson, 2012). Such selectivity may be the result of the considerable differences in octopus personality (Mather & Anderson, 1993), leading them to different microhabitats and, thus, influencing their prey choices. Learning can change small individual differences into much larger prey choice ones in silver perch (Warburton, 2003). Kestrels are also generalists, yet the array of prey remains near their nests show that even near-neighbors are selecting different prey species on which to specialize (Costantini, Casagrande, Di Lieto, Fanfani & Dell'Omo, 2005), though the cause is unknown. A shy octopus, avoidant in the face of predation risk (Brown & Kotler, 2007) might forage in short trips to areas well known to contain easy prey such as *Lima (Ctenoides)* bivalves hidden under rocks in Bermuda (Mather 1991a). An active one might explore new habitat areas and find unusual prey, such as clams that have to be dug out of sand at Vancouver Island (Hartwick, Thorarinsson & Tulloch, 1978). Octopuses also opportunistically capture unusual prey such as birds and hatchling turtles on oceanic islands (Leite, Haimovici & Mather, 2009).

The majority of prey remains found in octopus middens comes from just a few, often crustacean, species. *Octopus teheulechus* selected hermit crabs in the laboratory (Iribarne, Fernandez & Zucchini, 1991) and *Octopus cyanea* consumed a small array of four crustacean species in Hawaii in the field (Van Heukelem, 1966; Mather, 2011). Even the octopus species mentioned in the last paragraph were selective of prey species. Two species of crab constituted 51% of the prey remains of *O. insularis* (Leite, Haimovici & Mather, 2009), the snail *Tegula aureocincta* comprised 37% of the diet of *O. bimaculatus* (Ambrose, 1984), and four crustacean species made up 71% of the diet of *E. dofleini (*Vincent, Scheel & Hough, 1998) in Alaska. But variation amongst individuals is high (Mather, Leite & Batista, 2012; Scheel & Anderson, 2012). To know whether this differential consumption represents decision making and preference or simply availability, researchers can use two different approaches. They can contrast preferences in the laboratory with consumption in the field, or consumption in the field against availability of potential prey species (a difficult and time consuming evaluation).

Two studies compared laboratory preferences and prey remains in the field. Ambrose's (1984) thorough evaluation of *Octopus bimaculoides* showed an intersection of preference and availability. In the laboratory, the octopuses much preferred crustaceans as prey, and had a low preference particularly for the snail *Tegula eiseni*, though the species *T. aureocincta* was moderately preferred. In the field crustaceans were rare, gastropods common, with *T. eiseni* the most abundant. The species that constituted 37% of the diet was not this most common one but was *T. aureotincta*, which combined fairly wide availability and reasonable preference. As Ambrose (1984) commented, cruise-searching predators should be opportunistic feeders that attack all encountered prey, and this is clearly not the case for *O. bimaculoides*. With much less data, Mather (1991a) reported preference for *Pachygrapsus* crabs and *Lima* bivalves in the laboratory over *Fissurella* limpets and chitons. In the field, selection was clearly for *Lima* and the crustaceans *Pachygrapsus* and *Mithrax*. Chitons, while very common, were seldom consumed. Informal observation showed that chitons were abundant in the intertidal area where octopuses foraged, despite this lack of consumption. While chitons have a strong hold on the rocky substrate, octopuses are known for their formidable arm strength (Dilly, Nixon & Packard, 1964) and also can drill a hole in one of the chiton valves (J. A. Mather, personal observation) so they can inject a poison that weakens the muscle. They routinely take *Astrea* sp. gastropods in Trindade Island, Brazil, which have a strong shell and also an operculum (T. S. Leite, personal observation). In this case, the laboratory preference reflected the selection in the field, but was likely not the result of encounter rates.

A thorough evaluation of consumption versus prey availability in the field has been carried out for *E. dofleini* (Vincent, Scheel & Hough, 1998; Scheel, Lauster & Vincent, 2007). Again, at the population level octopuses were generalist, with a wide range of prey chosen. However, preferences did not always match availability. Most shell remains (75%) were of decapod crustaceans, and the percentages and abundance of remains in den litter were not significantly different for the top five prey species consumed. The crustacean *Hapalogaster mertensii,* while fairly common, was significantly avoided by the octopuses. More striking, chitons represented a majority of the live suitable prey in the area but were only found as 16 of the 295 prey remains. In further investigation, Scheel, Lauster and Vincent (2007) found that energy content (a factor assumed to dictate prey choice, see Stephens & Krebs, 1986) of the common prey species was not different. As well, variations in density of these crustacean prey across several sampling years did not affect the proportion of their remains in octopus middens. The octopus was a generalist on the surface, but fairly selective (Scheel & Anderson, 2012), perhaps from learning which prey are available or hunting selectivity in specific microhabitats to find them, when preferences and availability were assessed in depth. Cognitive processing of sensory information about places or identity of encountered prey may underlie this selection.

Two pieces of information may reconcile the wide range of prey sampled with the underlying selectivity of the octopuses themselves. First, Leite, Haimovici and Mather (2009) reported a chance visual encounter between a foraging octopus and a gobiid fish leading to its capture, and J. A. Mather (personal observation) saw a similar capture and several visually guided attempts in Bermuda. Such opportunistic visual triggering of attack indicated that chemotactile search (Mather, 1991a) could be modified with a secondary strategy of using visual information either to locate moving prey or to pursue prey that had evaded a first capture. Documenting the use of the Passing Cloud skin display, in which a pale "Blotch" is passed along the skin surface from posterior to anterior, Mather and Mather (2004) found that *O. cyanea* used such a secondary strategy after an unsuccessful attempted capture of crab prey. This display, which is seen in similar circumstances in cuttlefish (Adamo, Ehgoetz, Sangster & Whitehorne, 2006), presumably startled the crab into movement, at which point it would be more easily seen by the octopus and could be captured by a spread-arms Web Over action. An octopus would have to process its capture failure and the likely location of the crab before programming the skin display system to produce the Web Over, while also alerting to future movement of the prey. The control of skin patterns is not well understood, but this was not an automatic "flush" reaction of chromatophore expansion (which is under

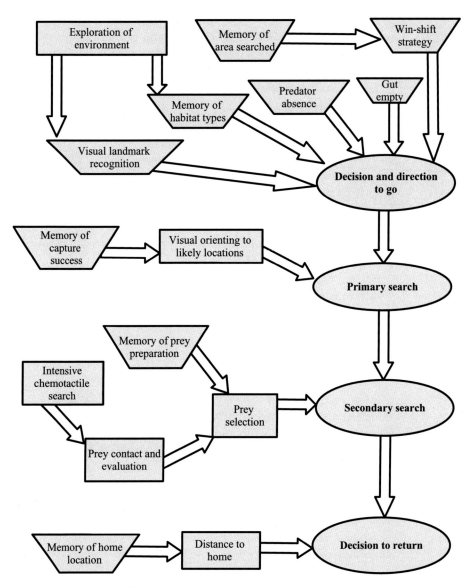

Figure 6.1 A flow chart of the decisions made by octopuses during foraging.

nervous control, see Messenger, 2001), but a forward-directed apparent movement, due to differential chromatophore expansion across the skin surface. Both of these types of evidence show that the octopus can react to changing information and vary strategies and form actions that increase the likelihood of prey capture. In fact, general assessment of detailed hunting behavior sequences (Mather, 1991a; Leite, Haimovici & Mather, 2009) showed variable opportunistic and not fixed sequences.

Second, in a more general approach to prey selection, Anderson, Sinn and Mather (2008) documented the fact that the population of *O. vulgaris* on the island of Bonaire in the Caribbean was a den-specific generalist in prey selection, but that individuals were often specialists; a Cardona niche breadth index of 0.08 confirmed this. As the octopus dens at which prey remains were found lay within a small area of mixed sand/mud, rock and rubble habitat, individuals were not constrained by hunting effort within homogeneous local microhabitats to a restricted choice of prey. It is far more likely that individuals used experience to select particular microhabitats for their foraging or locations where particular types of prey were found, or whose techniques for prey handling they had mastered (see Anderson & Mather, 2007), and in areas of high density they might be influenced by competition. For instance, one of these octopuses selected juvenile *Strombus* conch snails, who were handled by drilling through the shell to poison and weaken the adductor muscle (Wodinsky, 1973), a time-consuming process (Anderson & Mather, 2007; Steer & Semmens, 2003). The "decision" to select this prey, normally found in seagrass beds distant from the octopus dens, and use of this penetration technique would have meant greater energy expenditure but would have gained the octopus a large volume of food.

Another way to look at prey selectivity is to ask whether foraging strategies guide selectivity of prey size, or if octopuses take all sizes of prey encountered. Larger prey, available to larger octopuses, should result in a bigger energy intake, and thus fulfill the selectivity in terms of energetics postulated by Stephens and Krebs (1986). Scheel, Lauster and Vincent (2007) found that the amount of consumable flesh increased exponentially with the size of individuals of common crab prey species of *E. dofleini*, and size of prey remains in middens was shifted upwards, so mean prey size was larger than the mean size found in live crustacean samples from the same area. Thus, logically for energetics but not logically for an unselective predator, octopuses were not taking a representative sample of the prey population but the larger and more energetically rewarding items, though we do not know if they refused small ones or sought areas where larger ones were available. Scheel, Lauster and Vincent (2007) suggested that the octopuses were rate-maximizing foragers. However, this type of selectivity is not always found for octopuses. In *O. insularis* the prey size did not significantly increase with octopus size (Leite, Haimovici & Mather, 2009) and most prey individuals were quite small, suggesting that the animals were time minimizing their duration of foraging under the risk of predation (also see Mather & O'Dor, 1991, for *O. vulgaris*). This lack of size selectivity was also found in the laboratory for *Octopus dierythraeus* (Steer & Semmens, 2003). In both cases the expenditure of energy involved in prey penetration of larger prey items (Steer & Semmens, 2003; Anderson & Mather, 2007) might also have been taken into consideration by the octopus.

6.3   Foraging as cognitively demanding

Classical foraging theory models (Stephens & Krebs, 1986) of decision making were so simple that they were widely criticized, even initially (e.g. see Pierce and Ollason, 1987). Foraging theorists have begun to take note of the complexity of animals' lives, realizing that environments are neither static nor homogeneous (Stephens, Brown &

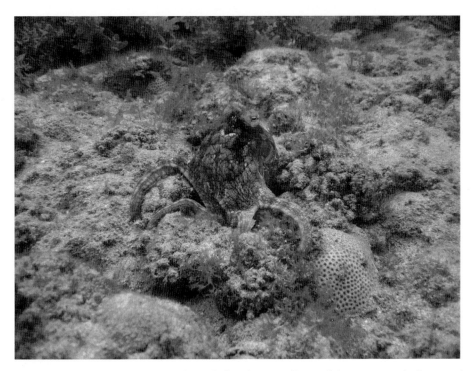

Figure 6.2 An octopus (*Octopus insularis*) during chemotactile search by many arms in the second phase of foraging. (Photograph courtesy of T. S. Leite.) See plate section for color version.

Ydenberg, 2007; Dunlap & Stephens, 2012) and require a foraging animal such as an octopus to spend time and effort acquiring information about them. One way in which such information can be gained proactively is by exploration, and octopuses are highly exploratory animals (Mather & Anderson, 1999; Boal, Dunham, Williams & Hanlon, 2000; Kuba, Byrne, Meisel, Greibel & Mather, 2006). Adams-Hunt and Jacobs (2007) comment that cognitive aspects of foraging include perception and the formation of a search image, conditioning affecting future prey choice, spatial cognition for where to hunt, and acquisition of prey-handling techniques. All of these are relevant to octopus foraging.

Another simplistic model needs to be modified to understand the role of planning and learning in octopus foraging. Theorists originally divided foraging strategies into ambush, when the prey comes to a predator, and cruise searching, when the forager goes to find prey (O'Brien, Browman & Evans, 1990). Either of the choices, which actually belong on the ends of a search-pause ratio continuum, can have a low cognitive demand and may be suitable in a homogeneous habitat and for animals with limited cognitive ability. But O'Brien, Browman and Evans (1990) description of saltatory search based on the pattern of foraging fish and birds (see also Anderson, Stephens & Dunbar, 1997; Cooper, 2005), provides a stop-and-go pattern that fits more closely with octopus foraging movements (Mather 1991a; Leite, Haimovici & Mather, 2009). This pattern of stopping to search for prey, then using results of the search (usually visual) to evaluate whether to continue in the same location or move on (Hill, Burrows & Hughes, 2003) demands information assessment about habitat and decision making on when to leave a patch (O'Brien, Browman & Evans, 1990).

6.3.1   Foraging and search images

When some areas are more suitable for search than others, foraging animals must locate these areas, assess their resources, find and consume prey and then move on. Yet they must also store information about where they have moved and where shelter is, how they have depleted the patch and where similar patches might be found. Hill, Burrows and Hughes (2003) modeled the search of plaice fish and found that a saltatory stop-and-go pattern was most effective, especially with patchy prey distribution. This localized intensive search activity is assisted by the formation of a search image, a pattern of sensory input indicating acceptable prey and focusing attention on important characteristics about it (see Adams-Hunt & Jacobs, 2007; Shettleworth, 2010). Such search images are often visual, and the sophistication of visual search has been studied in depth, often in birds. Search selectivity is controlled by factors such as prey size, microhabitat type, prey crypsis and environmental complexity (O'Brien, Browman & Evans, 1990) and cannot be automatic.

Despite many years of concentration of studies of learning on visual figures in the laboratory (Wells, 1978), saltatory search of octopuses is only visual in the primary stage, but search images of likely habitat must be formed nevertheless. Mather (1991a), continuously observing foraging of *O. vulgaris* in Bermuda, noted that search strategy encompassed two phases. The first phase was visual scan (often before leaving the sheltering home) and location of patch areas in which search could be concentrated – under rocks, in crevices, within algae clusters and in pockets of sand. Location of likely habitat must have been learned and T. S. Leite (personal observation) notes that young *O. insularis* are much less selective of microhabitats for intensive search than adults. In the second phase of search, octopuses employed the focal search strategy in specific locations that was first recorded by Yarnall (1969) for *O. cyanea*. Octopuses extended the flexible arms into these areas, picking up chemical and tactile cues and grasping prey with the many suckers on the arms. The details of foraging behavior varied with habitat to suit its physical constraints (also see Mather, 1991a; Forsythe & Hanlon, 1997; Leite, Haimovici & Mather, 2009). For instance, octopuses approaching a rock extended the arms around and below it, stretching the web between them in the bag-like Web Over posture, enclosing the rock and feeling with arm tips for prey within this balloon-like structure. This is an excellent example of processing learned information for use, Neisser's (1976) final cognitive step. At some giving-up time, the octopus must have chosen to search in another patch or look for a different type of habitat (see Brown & Kotler, 2007), but the rules for and constraints on this switch are unknown.

In the laboratory, Sutherland's (1963) quest for visual shape discrimination "rules" showed how octopus visual search images could be formed. Animals learned to discriminate between two visual shapes based on their horizontal and vertical extents. But they could also encode differences in edge/area ratio, smoothness of margins (square vs. circle), size and other characteristics. Muntz (1970) constructed figures that octopuses could discriminate that did not include any of Sutherland's (1963) cues, and he concluded that the octopuses were "learning how to learn" the important cues for this particular experiment; in other words, forming a search image (see Shettleworth, 2010). If an octopus was given an orientation discrimination that was too subtle to detect at first, further training with closer and closer approximations could allow it to do so (Wells, 1978), thus sharpening this search image. How might octopuses use such information? An octopus in Bonaire that dug into sand to acquire *Pinna* bivalves likely narrowed its search down to sandy patches in order to find this prey species. Hartwick, Breen and Tulloch (1978) commented that *E. dofleini* consumed clams that must have come from scattered sandy patches distant from their sheltering rock homes and likely remembered their location through a series of visits.

As octopuses search for prey in two stages, it is impossible to say at which stage of search and which type of images are formed and used. Still, the rejection by octopuses of nutritious potential prey such as chitons (Mather 1991a; Vincent, Scheel & Hough, 1998) suggests selectivity at both phases. Foraging *O. vulgaris* followed landscape contours (Mather, 1991a) and hunted along these likely areas in which prey might be concealed, ignoring flat open areas with few crevices or little attached algae. Chitons were easily visible in shaded subtidal rocky microhabitats to which octopuses might simply not have oriented, though they sometimes foraged in these areas. But this prey might also have been rejected at touch due to surface chemical cues. The rejection of the crab *H. mertensii* by *E. dofleini* in Alaska (Vincent, Scheel & Hough, 1998) could easily have been at the second stage, in chemotactile search. Its common name is the hairy crab, and a variegated hairy surface makes grasping by the multiple suckers more difficult, a factor used when strips of artificial turf prevent large octopuses from escaping from their tanks in captivity (Wood & Anderson, 2004).

A stronger argument for selection of prey by search image is the extent to which individual octopuses select a much narrower range of prey than the population to which they belong. Mather (1991a) saw that individual *O. vulgaris* in Bermuda concentrated on a few species such as the fragile-shelled *Lima* bivalve, which hides under rocks and in crevices; it is not clear whether this was a prey preference or a microhabitat selection. These individual differences were even stronger in *O. vulgaris* in Bonaire (Anderson, Sinn & Mather, 2008), where Cardona's niche breadth index indicated that, despite the varied habitat and wide total prey choice, individual octopuses were specialists on a few prey species. This selectivity is also true for *E. dofleini* across its range (Scheel & Anderson, 2012). Dukas and Kamil (2000) describe the processing stage of attention underlying such selectivity in blue jay birds, and Dunlap and Stephens (2012) found that birds exposed to a frequent change of environment sampled more often and learned more quickly. See Adams-Hunt and Jacobs (2007) in general and chapter 7, this volume, by Jozet-Alves et al., for cephalopods, but much remains to be assessed about octopuses' ability in this area.

6.3.2   Spatial memory and prey selection

To find and return to productive sites of prey concentration, octopuses and other searching predators use spatial memory (Mather, 1994). Much laboratory testing of animal learning which used food as a reward has focused on "win-stay" strategies, testing an animal's return to rewarded locations or choices (though see the radial maze, Roberts, 1991). Octopuses learned these choices in the laboratory quickly (Wells, 1978). Sometimes, however, they seemed to learn incompletely and did not concentrate on one or a few rewarded stimuli. For instance, Papini and Bitterman (1991) found that *O. cyanea's* ratio of choices of the continually rewarded stimulus of a pair asymptoted at 7/10, as the animals maintained a low rate of checking the unrewarded location.

   This should be a reminder that the shape of learning may vary, and West-Eberhard (2003) reminds us that forgetting is also part of the learning process, especially in a varied environment (Kerr & Feldman, 2003), making way for new information to be stored. What looks like a failure to learn in the laboratory situation may also be the result of a win-switch rather than a win-stay foraging strategy in the field, assisted by learning where one has been and resulting in avoiding returns to a depleted foraging location (Shettleworth, 2010). Radial mazes (Roberts, 1991) reward this approach, as they supply food reward at the end of each arm and the animal must learn and remember which locations are depleted of prey so as not return to them. Continuous observation of areas chosen for intense search by *O. vulgaris* in Bermuda (Mather 1991a, see Figure 6.1) showed that, in a similar pattern, patches recently visited were avoided over the next few days, fulfilling all of Neisser's (1976) cognitive steps. If a crab was taken from under a rock, a snail picked off algae or a clam dug from a pocket of sand, another would not likely reappear, at least for a few days. Such a win-switch strategy, learned before their capture, would not be so adaptive when octopuses were brought into the laboratory and continually rewarded for choice of the same location.

   One aspect of cognitive processing that is poorly understood is exploration to acquire information. Octopuses are highly exploratory animals in the laboratory (Mather & Anderson, 1999; Boal, Dunham, Williams & Hanlon, 2000; Kuba, Byrne, Meisel, Griebel & Mather, 2006). Such behavior (though exploration is poorly understood, see Renner, 1990) is a technique for long-term acquisition of the information about one's environment, which is necessary to make choices such as where to forage intensively or where to find emergency shelter. This type of information gathering may be particularly important for animals in complex environments (see Godfrey-Smith, 2002), such as the rain forest and the tropical nearshore, but is difficult to evaluate by learning studies in the laboratory.

   While we know much about octopuses' visual object perception and memory in the laboratory, how do we know they use memory to control spacing of foraging in the field? Mather's (1991b) continuous tracking of foraging paths gave some clues. The juvenile octopuses (a few hundred grams in weight) that she observed made half of their foraging trips over a long time and distance, nearly an hour and 9 m, so that memory of location in space was involved (Mather, 1991b). The angle of return to the sheltering home compared to the outgoing path was 30 degrees, the percentage of approximate trail overlap was

32% (Mather, 1991b, see Figure 6.1). These returns from far away were jet-propelled and the octopuses lifted off the sea bottom. This is important because gastropod snails also return to a central "home," but they use simple chemical trail following, which can be seen by their trail overlap and minimal angle of deviation (Chelazzi, Innocenti & Della Santina, 1983). The possibility that octopuses form a spatial map of their home ranges (see Shettleworth, 2010) was enhanced by Mather's (1991b) observation of 11 instances of displacement of octopuses from their foraging path, mostly by fish attack, from which all the animals returned directly home, usually orienting by local landmarks that were apparent to the human observers. Such calculation of a novel route home after displacement suggests a cognitive map (Shettleworth, 2010).

Laboratory information about this use of spatial memory is slowly being gathered. Initially, Wells (1964) believed that octopuses could not use a detour to catch a crab that they could see through a window, but they may have been misled by the use of glass for viewing. They were able to move along a corridor if they kept one side continuously in the view of the same eye, perhaps because information was not yet available to the other side of the brain (see Wells, 1978). Mather (1991b) reported fragmentary observations of *O. rubescens* learning to orient to a beacon. Boal, Dunham, Williams and Hanlon (2000) developed a paradigm where octopuses learn the location of deep "wells" in a tank, escaping to one of them as a refuge when the water level in the tank was lowered. A series of papers on this capacity in *Sepia officinalis* cuttlefish showed that they have two memory strategies (Alves, Chichery, Boal & Dickel, 2006), remembering their turns or memorizing landmarks, varying with maturity and sex. Brain lesion studies revealed that the ventral area of the vertical lobe was involved in this memory (Graindorge et al., 2006). Such studies will offer insight into an adaptive use of a type of learning that has already been investigated in arthropods and vertebrates (Shettleworth, 2010). A comparison of cognitive processes and strategies used by animals from three different phyla on the same memory task would be an exciting one, allowing us to isolate whether these are analogous or homologous abilities. Adams-Hunt and Jacobs (2007) already have suggested a cross-phylum bee–gerbil contrast for this ability.

6.3.3   Learned prey handling

When a prey animal is captured, there may be several steps in the consumption process that may influence prey choice. For instance, *O. vulgaris* in Bermuda were timed in handling of the fragile *Lima* bivalves, at 5 minutes between capture and discarding of the shell at the end of consumption, a factor that might have influenced their choice of this species (Mather, 1991a). Larger prey, whose selection was seen by Scheel, Lauster and Vincent (2007), present characteristics that prevent such easy consumption. A predator–prey arms race has evolved over the millennia, with bivalves becoming stronger and stronger resistors as their predators become more able to use a variety of strategies to penetrate them (Vermeij, 1995).

Octopuses can adapt their tactics, probably due to experience, when preying upon difficult-to-access prey like bivalves. When clams resist opening, octopuses have very strong arms to pull the valves apart, a parrot-like beak to chip at the shell, a salivary papilla to drill holes and a posterior salivary gland toxin that immobilizes prey at injection (Hanlon & Messenger, 1996). Steer and Semmens (2003) found that, faced with clam prey, an *O. dierythraeus* first attempted to pull the valves apart. If this procedure failed, it used the more time-consuming technique of drilling a hole in the shell and injecting the paralytic neurotoxin. Anderson and Mather (2007) extended this work with *E. dofleini* and found octopuses had three penetration techniques: they could pull, chip on the valve edge or drill through the shell. Locations of chip and drill holes were not random but near adductor muscles or over the heart, as the vulnerable areas of the clam only occupy some of the area within the shell (also see Hartwick, Breen & Tulloch, 1978; Ambrose & Nelson, 1983; Nixon & Maconnachie, 1988; Cortez, Castro & Guerra, 1998). This drilling location is somewhat dependent on the octopus species and age, and is probably learned after early failures (Anderson, Sinn & Mather, 2008). When the preferred procedure of pulling apart was thwarted by wires holding *Venerupis* clam valves together, *E. dofleini* switched from pulling to drilling and chipping (Anderson & Mather, 2007). Here there is no fixed procedure, but action, evaluation of results and choice of another action.

When *Strombus* snails spires, the preferred drilling location near the adductor muscle insertion, were covered by a metal coating, *O. vulgaris* drilled as close as possible, right at the metal's edge (Wodinsky, 1973). Indicative of the octopod flexibility in solving problems, they pulled more malleable coatings off the shell, but when senescence meant that brooding females had no digestive gland secretion, they simply pulled the snails out of the shell (Wodinsky, 1978). Specific penetration techniques were used, their success stored, and they were then retrieved as guides in preparation of prey for consumption (see the cognitive steps of Neisser, 1976). This process influenced choice of prey species in the laboratory. Octopuses' choice amongst three bivalve species was different when they were opened and offered "on the half shell" compared to those of intact animals (Anderson & Mather, 2007). *Mytilus* valves were easily broken apart and this species was often chosen from intact prey, whereas strong *Protothaca* had to be drilled or chipped and many more were eaten when they had already been opened. The octopuses apparently had taken effort and/or processing time into consideration.

Octopuses may offer a simpler model for the decision-making involved in foraging. Unlike many vertebrates whose foraging is influenced by conspecifics (see Waite & Field, 2007), they are solitary for much of their lifespan and not reproductively active until the end, with a semelparous reproductive strategy. Thus social influences are postponed (see Huffard, Caldwell & Boneka, 2010; T. S. Leite & J. A. Mather, unpublished data). Foraging subadult octopuses in Bermuda did not defend territories and although they noticed conspecifics, they did not fight them and passively avoided contact (Mather & O'Dor, 1991). Their home ranges were fairly small; under 120 m square for an animal of 200 g weight. Octopuses remained in these small areas for a short period, under 2 weeks for juvenile *O. vulgaris* (Mather & O'Dor, 1991) and a month for the much larger *E. dofleini* (Hartwick, Ambrose & Robinson, 1984). Such an occupancy pattern would demand speedy acquisition of information about the environment and equally speedy forgetting (West-Eberhard, 2003), a win-switch foraging strategy, and a relatively quick assessment of prey density and predator risk to decide when to move on. In this

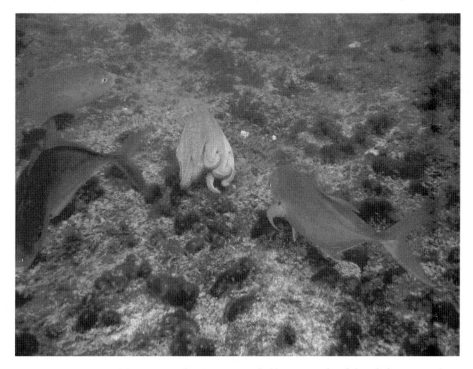

Figure 6.3 An octopus (*Octopus insularis*) accompanied by scavenging fish as it forages on the rocky ground. See plate section for color version.

situation, the number of variables influencing foraging and food intake might be small. A limited test of departure time from these home ranges against food consumption and weight gain for *O. vulgaris* did not produce a significant correlation (Mather & O'Dor, 1991). Instead it suggested another variable for consideration of influences on foraging, time minimizing under the threat of predation (see also Ambrose, 1988, for *O. bimaculatus*).

6.4   Predation avoidance and learning

Modern foraging theory has begun to acknowledge that animal foraging is often carried on under the threat of predation (Lima & Dill, 1990; Bednekoff, 2007; Brown & Kotler, 2007). Octopuses have abandoned the protective molluscan shell and, probably in competition with the bony fishes (Packard, 1972), they have evolved an array of defenses including stunning camouflage (Messenger, 2001), deimatic behavior (Hanlon & Messenger, 1996), inking (Wood et al., 2010) and the cognitive ability to manipulate them. Many animals avoid predation by hiding in shelter (Cooper, 2005) and trading off the risk of emerging with the necessity to forage. Some octopuses are time minimizers who shelter for much of the day, and *O. vulgaris* in Bermuda only hunted for 12% of the daytime (Mather, 1988) and sheltered in homes at night. Provisioned animals or those in areas of abundant prey often minimize their time at risk out foraging (see Shaffery, Ball & Amlaner, 1985, for gulls).

If shelters are so important to the avoidance of predation, have octopuses used cognitive ability to select them? Field studies (Hartwick, Breen & Tulloch, 1978; Mather, 1994; Katsanevakis & Verriopoulos, 2004) demonstrated that octopuses usually shelter in niches, under rocks and in holes in rubble. As they tend to be non-social, octopuses are often primarily constrained in their distribution by the presence of such shelter. *Octopus joubini* in northern Florida was confined mainly to seagrass beds where discarded molluscan shells were available for shelter, and aggregated to a high density when artificial provisioning with gastropod shells was carried out (Mather, 1982a). The low availability of rocky crevice shelter can limit the density of octopuses, as Hartwick, Breen and Tulloch (1978) found for *E. dofleini* on Vancouver Island. Shelter can even allow them to inhabit areas where they would not otherwise be found. Discarded beer bottles allowed *O. rubescens* near Seattle to live in sandy areas that they would otherwise have been eliminated from (Anderson, Hughes, Mather & Steele, 1999).

Little research has been carried out to discover if octopuses have specific sensory preferences for particular shelter dimensions. *O. joubini* preferred shelters of about the same volume as themselves and also ones that had a small aperture (Mather, 1982b), as with their lack of fixed skeletons, octopuses could squeeze through holes that would block out crustacean or fish rivals. Ideal homes do not appear in the natural environment, however, and octopuses appeared instead to select likely shelters and adapt them closer to some desired dimensions (Mather, 1994). They pushed out small rocks with their arms, blew sand with jets of water from the funnel and pulled algae from the top of crevices. More interesting, if an aperture was "too big," an octopus brought small rocks or molluscan shells to block the aperture; the correlation of aperture size with number of rocks was statistically significant, $r = 0.69$. This is a clear example of tool use by Beck's (1980) definition and suggests a proactive strategy of assessment of area and gathering of items to change it – though the cognitive background of tool use is not known. Such a strategy was also observed in Indo-east Pacific octopuses on the sand-mud bottom, who cleaned out a coconut shell and carried it with them for later use as a shelter (Finn, Tregenza & Norman, 2009), a clear proactive strategy of retaining the shell for future use.

Probably depending on predation success, octopuses have many short hunting trips spaced irregularly during the day (Mather, 1988; Scheel & Bisson, 2012) or at night (Meisel, Byrne, Kuba & Mather, 2011), during which they adopt camouflage skin patterns (Packard & Sanders, 1971; Mather 1991a; Forsythe & Hanlon, 2007; Leite et al., 2009). Animals at risk of predation during foraging may adjust the timing and spacing of their hunts (Bednekoff, 2007). For instance, squirrels balance off the risk of eating out of the home with the energy expenditure of returning to it (Lima, Valone & Caraco, 1985) and they compromise by eating small food items outside and large ones in shelter. *O. vulgaris* showed a different compromise. Perhaps because of the small home ranges, 70% of prey were transported home to consume. Prey size did not correlate with transport home, possibly because most prey items were small (Mather, 1991a). Instead, octopuses chose to transport items to a home if it was nearby and eat them outside, though in suboptimal shelter, if home was far away. This tradeoff argues again for the storage, evaluation and use of a spatial memory of the area in which the octopuses hunted.

How important is learning about the presence of predators and adjusting behavior to them? Both the Caribbean reef squid (Mather, 2010) and cuttlefish (Langridge, Broom & Osorio, 2007) carefully adjust their reactions, from camouflage and visual displays to jet-propelled escape, depending on predator species, distance, speed and fish species. But they do not have the shelter opportunities of octopuses. Many animals that come out of shelter to hunt can vary either the amount of this activity or its timing. Nocturnal rodents suppressed activity on moonlit nights when they were more visible to predators (Daly, Behrends, Wilson & Jacobs, 1992) and whiptailed lizards similarly changed their hunting time and pattern in the presence of a predatory lizard (Eifler, Eifler & Harris, 2008). *O. vulgaris* is well known for the flexibility of timing of its activity (Wells, O'Dor, Mangold & Wells, 1983). This activity was influenced particularly in the laboratory by the timing of food provisioning, a kind of temporal learning common in many animals (Shettleworth, 2010). Nevertheless, the daytime cycle of activity of this species in Bermuda was not matched to time of day, height of tides or current in the channel in which the octopuses lived (Mather, 1988), although intertidal animals must be affected by the tidal cycles.

The possibility that octopuses might learn to change their activity to avoid potential predators was explored in a laboratory study by Meisel, Kuba, Byrne, and Mather (2013). Octopuses shared a tank with one of two fish species, separated by a diagonal clear barrier. They shifted activity timing to more nocturnal in the presence of the diurnal *Balistes* trigger fish, a facultative but not major octopod predator. In the presence of a nocturnal moray eel, a well-known predator of octopuses (see Randall, 1967), they did not become more diurnally active. But since the moray hunted by snaking through rocks and rubble, a longer duration of sheltering would not avoid this predator. In fact, the octopuses avoided this potential predator by spending more time out of shelter, suggesting a sophisticated avoidance based on the hunting style of the specific predator.

Animals at risk of predation often have a complex set of avoidance strategies (see Kelley & Magurran, 2011, for fishes) and this is true of octopuses (see Figure 6.2). When they emerge to hunt, their primary antipredator strategy is to avoid being detected. Cephalopods including octopuses have variable camouflage (see Cott, 1940) used in avoidance of detection by vertebrates. Packard (1972) called fish "the designers of octopus skin" and octopuses' appearance is matched to vertebrates' sensory perception. For instance, they are color blind yet produce careful color matches to the substrate on which they move. Many cephalopod species can vary the colors and patterns on the skin surface within 30 ms or less, change their apparent texture by formation of raised papillae on the skin (Allen, Mäthger, Barbosa & Hanlon, 2009), and even alter their posture, including positions of the flexible octopus arms (Packard & Sanders, 1971; Hanlon & Messenger, 1988; Mather, 2004). When out of shelter, they can even change the pattern of movement across the substrate (Huffard, 2006), being bunched up and swaying on two arms and looking like a ball of algae, rather than walking normally

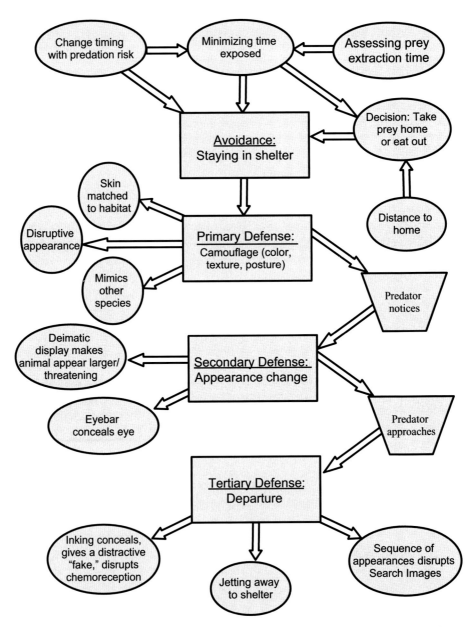

Figure 6.4 A flowchart of the decisions made by an octopus avoiding predation during foraging.

with the eight arms. Without knowing the transformation of sensory input to motor output to the chromatophore muscles, cognitive control of the process is difficult to prove.

There has been some debate as to whether octopuses use a kind of search image to adapt their skin patterns to match the substrate over which they move when foraging, and their repertoire of appearances is so large that this is difficult to determine. Hanlon, Forsythe and Joneschild (1999) did not find that the large *O. cyanea* out foraging used background matching camouflage. However, Leite and Mather (2008) determined a pattern repertoire for the smaller *O. insularis* and evaluated whether this species could vary the set of patterns, dependent on the substrate over which they hunted (Leite, Haimovici & Mather, 2009). Body pattern varied with depth (predicting amount of ambient light), presence of sand or rubble and foraging behavior. Interestingly, larger octopuses (>500 g) used less of the camouflaging Mottle pattern and more of the Disruptive Blotch, almost as if large size (*O. cyanea* is one of the largest octopuses, Hanlon, Forsythe & Joneschild, 1999) meant that camouflage was less vital to predator avoidance. While walking, octopuses used background matching, and swimming octopuses moving from patch to patch adopted countershading camouflage. This automatic reaction to light intensity differences prevents easy detection from above and below and is commonly used by their cuttlefish relatives (Ferguson, Messenger & Budelmann, 1994). Even over a short-distance swim, *O. vulgaris* in Bermuda changed from bottom-matching camouflage to mud-brown and then adopted brown and white stripes (Mather & Mather, 1994). Because of the nervous control of chromatophore muscles, pattern changes can be accomplished in 30 ms and could pinpoint an area as small as 1 mm^2, although regularities of "patch" and "groove" (Packard, 1995) produce overriding patterns.

Changes in skin appearance have led observers to speculate that octopuses in the Indo-east Pacific were mimicking the appearance of common or distasteful prey items, such as lionfish and poisonous snakes or common fish (see Hanlon, Watson & Barbosa, 2010 for a detailed study). One of the problems with assessment of this behavior is that pattern mimicry, such as that of palatable insect mimics for aposematic (warningly colored) models, is generally static and no cognition by mimics is involved (Shettleworth, 2010). Research has instead investigated the role of learning in the behavior of the potential predator (Adams-Hunt & Jacobs, 2007), which would be fish in this case. Mimicking the appearance of distasteful fish would involve octopus assessment of models' patterns, processing of the frequency of different species' appearance, and programming of a specific pattern output during an encounter with a potential visual predator. This is quite a complex set of behaviors, though compatible with Neisser's (1976) cognitive steps of transforming, reducing and elaborating the input, storing the information and recovering and using it. Octopuses might instead carry out the unpredictable sequence of changes in a repertoire of patterns noted above, which Hanlon, Forsythe and Joneschild (1999) documented in *O. cyanea* when threatened by a diver's chase. Hanlon, Watson and Barbosa (2010) delineated a series of appearance changes in *Macrotritopus defilippi*. One of these posture/pattern combinations, which is postulated to be mimicry of flounders (who are not poisonous or aversive) was a dorsoventrally flattened posture also useful for head-first jet propulsion during search over the sandy bottom. More research must be done to sort out the possible causes of these appearance changes. It is possible that octopuses are simply "running through" preset sequences of patterns and not using learning to match the appearance of other species.

The unit of production of skin patterns is smaller on the head and around the eyes (Leite & Mather, 2008), perhaps because these areas are more obvious when the octopus has emerged from hiding. Changes in these areas include production of "eyebars," which extend the horizontal pupil along the skin anterior and posterior to the eye to conceal it (Mather, Anderson & Leite, 2009); an eye is an important search image for a visual predator, indicating the presence of an animal (Coss & Goldthwaite, 1995). This pattern was produced during learned annoyance to keepers in the laboratory (Anderson, Mather, Monette & Zimsen, 2010) and is probably a proactive response to a low level threat of predation, making oneself look less like an animal. Similarly, paired obvious white dots on the dorsal surface of the arms may distract the fish observer from the outline of the octopus behind them (Packard & Sanders, 1971). Again, the control of their production is unknown.

The control of camouflage production is better known in the related cuttlefish. This species has a dazzling pattern repertoire (Hanlon & Messenger, 1988) and its background matching of different patterns is particularly responsive to evaluation of contrast and edges (Zylinski, Osorio & Shohet, 2009; see also chapter 9, this volume, by Zylinski & Osorio). The texture variation of cuttlefish skin by papillae is also the result of matching to the visual appearance (and not due to tactile information) of the substrate below (Allen, Mäthger, Barbosa & Hanlon, 2009). Such matching may be the result of a transformation of the visual image into a "2½ dimension" visual template of the background appearance – Marr's (1983) first step in human cognitive evaluation of visual pattern. Cuttlefish can, however, be foiled in their background matching by color variation, as the cephalopods are color blind (Messenger, 2001). In addition, cuttlefish both change displays and interrupt hunting of shrimp prey when a model bird is "flown" overhead (Adamo, Ehgoetz, Sangster & Whitehorne, 2006).

Detection by a predator despite camouflage does not mean capture, and octopuses and other cephalopods can avoid capture by breaking a potential predator's search image during pursuit, as in the Hanlon, Forsythe and Joneschild (1999) study of unpredictable pattern changes, stop-and-go movement and concealment within a cloud of dark ink for *O. cyanea* pursued by a diver. This is a general secondary antipredatory response of cephalopods, as Anderson and Mather (1996) noted camouflage matched to different backgrounds, jet escape, inking and digging into the sand substrate in small *Euprynna scolopes* sepiolid squid. Cephalopod ink can also hold together in a "blob" and these animals can darken, squirt out an ink blob, pale and then jet away, leaving the predator attacking the blob that still matches its search image (Hanlon & Messenger, 1996). The selection and use of these common secondary tactics, which also have physiological costs, have been little studied across the cephalopods, though see Hanlon and Messenger (1996) for discussion.

Cephalopods that are threatened can change their appearance to look more menacing. Moynihan (1975) speculated that the dymantic (deimatic) visual skin display of squid, cuttlefish and octopuses showed a production parallel across the cephalopods. The purpose is likely the same but the displays are different. Both cuttlefish (Langridge, Broom & Osorio, 2007; Langridge, 2009) in the laboratory and squid (Mather, 2010) in the sea produce eye spots on the dorsal surface. The cognitive control of this pattern was demonstrated by their directional production towards the threatening fish and selection towards visual predators and at lesser threat. Octopuses spread the web between the arms, darken the area around the eyes and the edges of the web, orienting this spread dorsal surface towards the potential threat (Packard & Sanders, 1971). However, no evaluation of the circumstances of the production of this display has been carried out in octopuses. Differential use of varied antipredator responses is widely documented across the animal

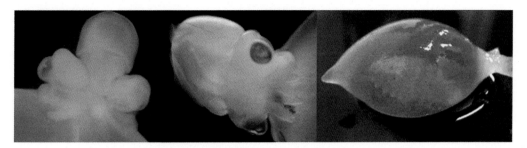

Figure 1.1 *Sepia officinalis* embryonic stages according to Lemaire (1970) from left to right: (A) stage 23, (B) stage 25 and (C) stage 30 (copyright L. Bonnaud and A.-S. Darmaillacq).

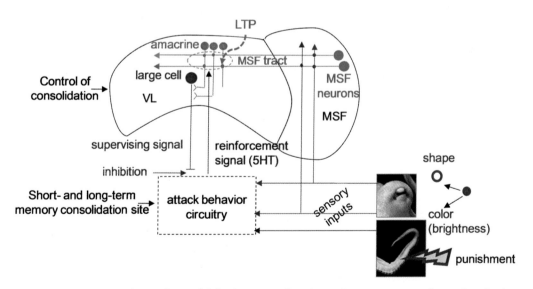

Figure 4.12 A tentative model for the octopus learning and memory system. See explanation in text.

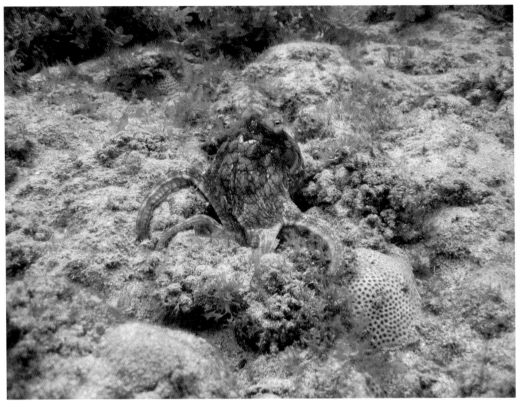

Figure 6.2 An octopus (*Octopus insularis*) during chemotactile search by many arms in the second phase of foraging (Photograph courtesy of T. S. Leite.)

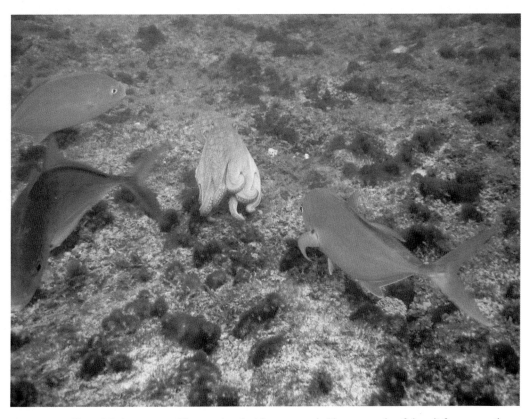

Figure 6.3 An octopus (*Octopus insularis*) accompanied by scavenging fish as it forages on the rocky ground.

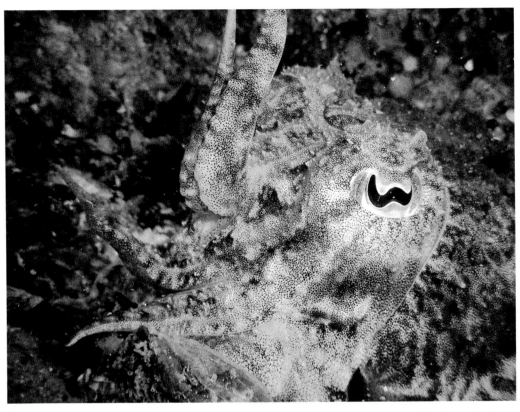

Figure 7.1 Cuttlefish *Sepia officinalis*. The picture has been taken in the English Channel off Granville (Manche, France). The ocular globe is particularly voluminous. The eye is characterized by the w-shaped papillae. (Copyright, F. Sichel).

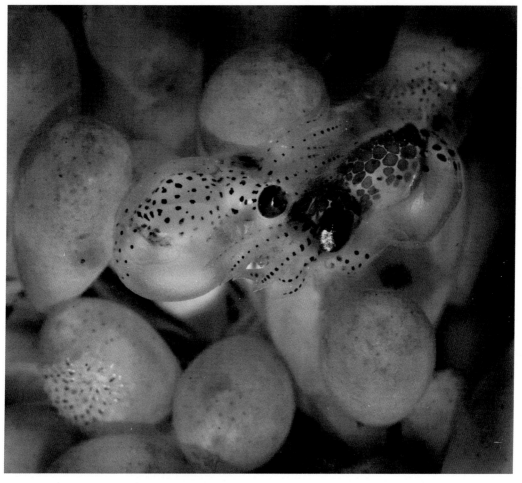

Figure 7.2 Giant Pacific Octopus, *Enteroctopus dofleini*, paralarvae. They do not have the same way of life as adults, which are generally benthic. Photo courtesy of J. Kocian.

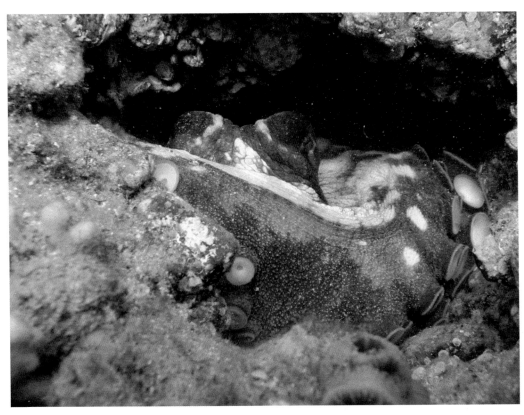

Figure 7.3 *Octopus cyanea* in its den. Note the stones surrounding the den entrance. (Copyright, A.-S. Darmaillacq).

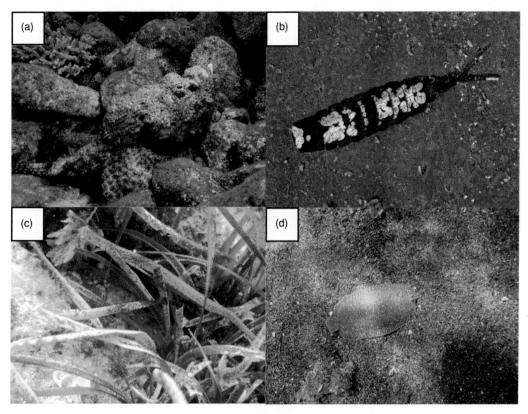

Figure 8.1 Camouflage examples in marine animals. (a) A stone fish, *Synanceia verrucosa* choosing a place to settle which matches its body pattern. (b) An isopod: displaying disruptive coloration. (c) A Posidonia pipefish, *Syngnathus* sp. using object resemblance in hiding between seagrass leafs. (d) A Moses sole, *Pardachirus mormoratus* showing a static Mottle pattern; note partial missmatch with such a static camouflage.

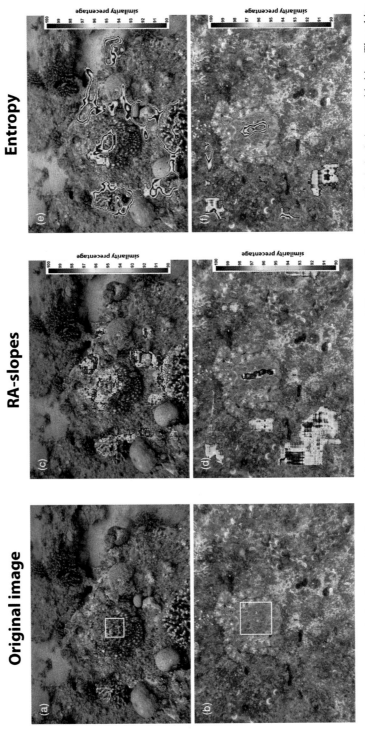

Figure 8.5 Image analysis of camouflaged octopuses. (a,b) Cryptic *Octopus cyanea* and *Octopus vulgaris* respectively in their natural habitat. The white square marks the sampled mantle for similarity comparison. (c,d) Computer-generated similarity map of the RA-slopes descriptor. For clarity reasons only 90% similarity or higher is presented. (e,f) Computer-generated similarity map of the entropy descriptor.

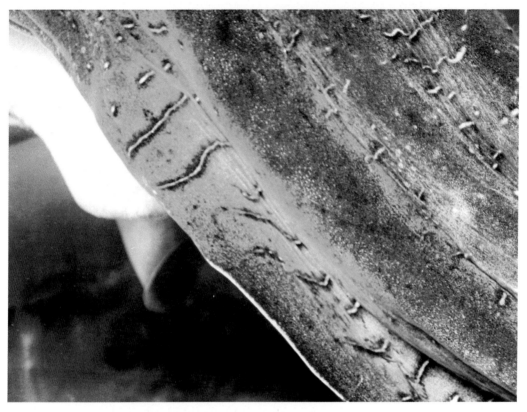
Figure 9.2 The bright blues and greens in the mating displays of the Australian giant cuttlefish *Sepia apama* are primarily due to wavelength specific reflectors. The animals themselves are most likely colour-blind.

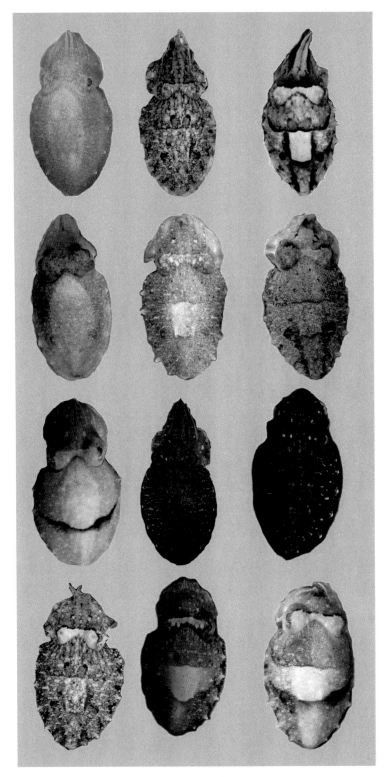

Figure 9.3 Demonstration of just some of the body pattern variation *Sepia officinalis* uses in camouflage body pattern responses to the visual environment. The top row shows the primary characteristics of the main three *classes* of body pattern referred to in the text: Uniform (left), Mottle (centre) and Disruptive (right). The remaining images show how individual chromatic components patterns can be varied in their expression, along with the overall contrast of the body pattern, to give a wide range of body patterns that cannot always be readily identified as Uniform, Mottle or Disruptive.

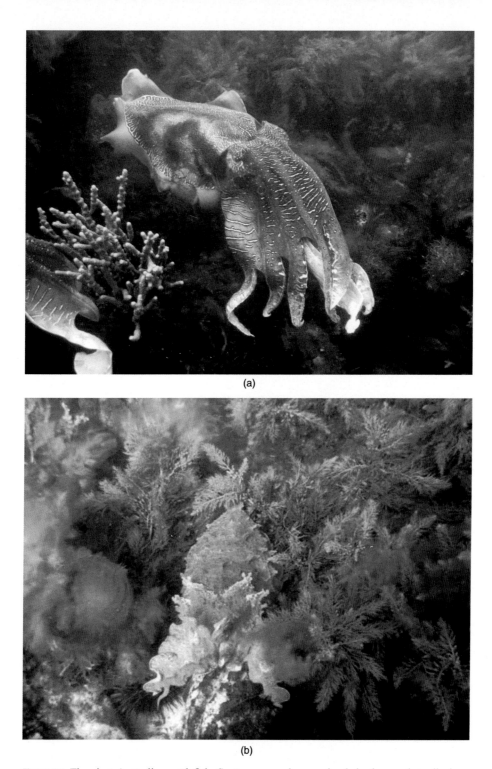

(a)

(b)

Figure 9.7 The giant Australian cuttlefish, *Sepia apama*, chooses simple backgrounds to display against, which probably acts to increase signal efficacy, and more complex backgrounds to camouflage against making visual search more difficult for potential predators. (a) A male engaged in an agonistic display to another male. (b) A camouflaging individual uses chromatic and textural components. Adapted from Zylinski, How, Osorio, Hanlon and Marshall (2011).

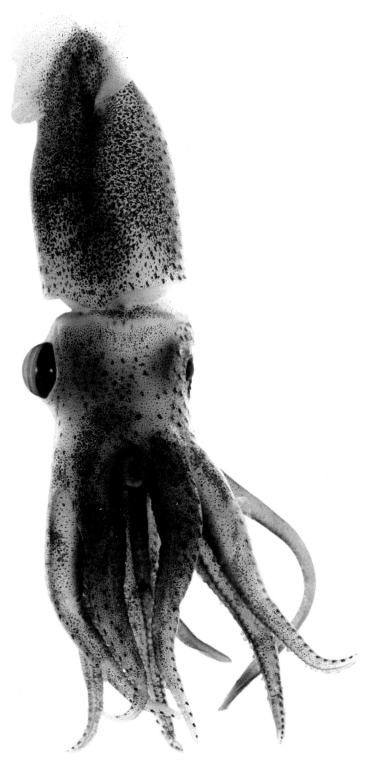

Figure 10.2 The lower-mesopelagic squid *Histeoteuthis* has asymmetrical eyes and optic lobes, with a large left eye for looking up for passing silhouettes of potential prey against the weak downwelling light, and a small right eye orientated downwards, probably specialized for detecting point-source bioluminescence.

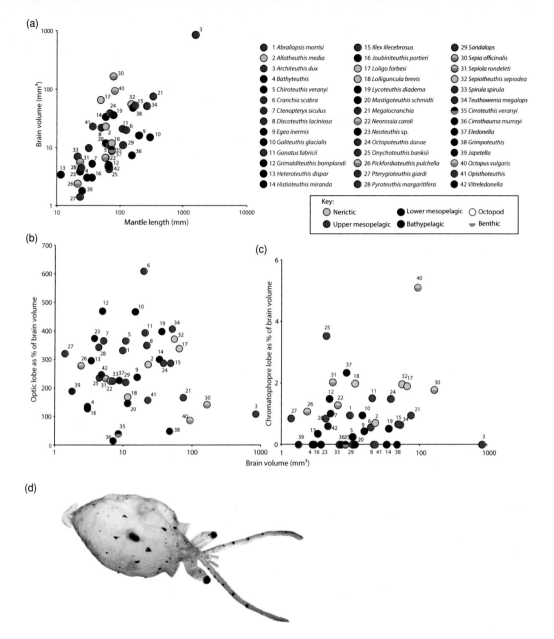

Figure 10.3 Brain size and brain regions in a range of cephalopods from different habitats (data taken from Maddock & Young, 1987). The 34 species of decapods plotted on each graph are listed on the right in alphabetical order. A further eight species of octopods are then listed in alphabetical order and are distinguished by a red marker ring. Numbers relate to the placement on the plot. The colour of marker represents a common habitat type (or usual collection depth range) for adults during daylight hours (the depth occurrence of many species changes with size and life-stage, and many of the species listed undergo vertical migration so will be found in shallower waters at night), as given in the key. (a) Absolute brain volume plotted against mantle length, showing a positive correlation between brain volume and body length, although there is a tendency for shallow-water benthic taxa (namely *Loligo*, *Sepia* and *Octopus*) to fall above the trend, and bathypelagic/bathybenthic species to fall below the trend, be they octopod or decapod (note log scales). (b) Plotting optic lobe volume (given as a percentage of brain volume, measured separately because of location and large size (d)) against absolute brain volume shows that optic lobe volume varies greatly and is not correlated with overall brain volume. Interestingly, many pelagic and mesopelagic species have comparatively larger optic lobes than neritic/benthic species that are considered highly visual. (c) Plotting the chromatophore lobe volume against brain volume shows chromatophore lobe volume varies greatly between species. There is a trend for shallow-water species to have relatively larger chromatophore lobes, with notable exceptions (e.g. the deep-water pelagic octopod *Eledonella*). Many deep-sea species had no chromatophore lobes or lobes too small to be measured. (d) An oegopsid squid paralarva showing eye stalks with the large optic lobe located behind the eye on the stalk and separate from the brain.

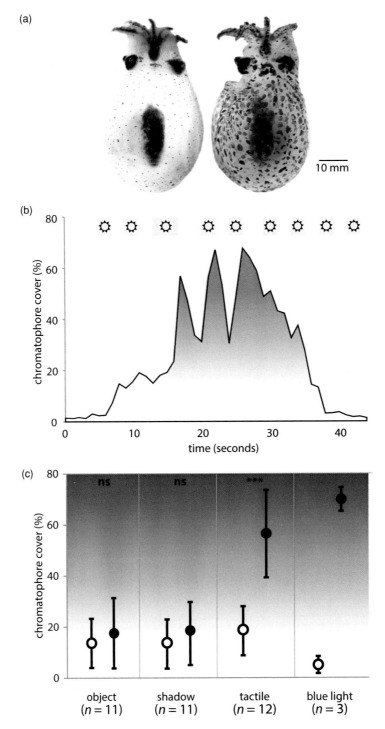

Figure 10.4 (a) The same individual *Japetella heathi* octopus in transparent mode (left) and pigmented mode (right). (b) Responses of a single *J. heathi* to directed blue light. Yellow boxes and icon indicate onset and cessation of individual lighting 'bouts', consisting of a flashing blue light at one flash per second. Most bouts lasted for 3 seconds and, therefore, subjected the animal to three flashes. Chromatophores can be seen to expand seconds after initial exposure. After continued exposure the animal ceased reacting to the light with chromatophore responses, and instead displayed evasive behaviour such as swimming away from the light-source and retraction of the head into the mantle. (c) Responses of *J. heathi* to four different stimuli. Objects passed in front of the animals, and shadows passed overhead, failed to evoke a significant increase in chromatophore expression. A tactile stimulus (touching the arms with a blunt needle) resulted in the rapid expansion of chromatophores. By comparison, directed blue light resulted in a rapid and strong expression of chromatophores. White circles = pre-stimulus, black circles = post-stimulus. Error bars show standard deviation from mean. From Zylinski & Johnson 2011.

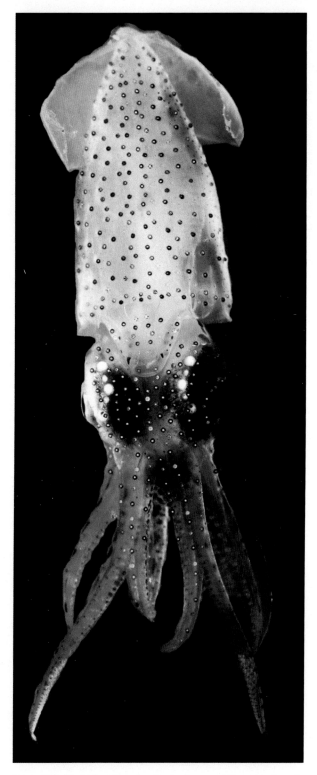

Figure 10.5 Ventral and ocular photophores on the ventral surface of an *Abraliopsis* squid.

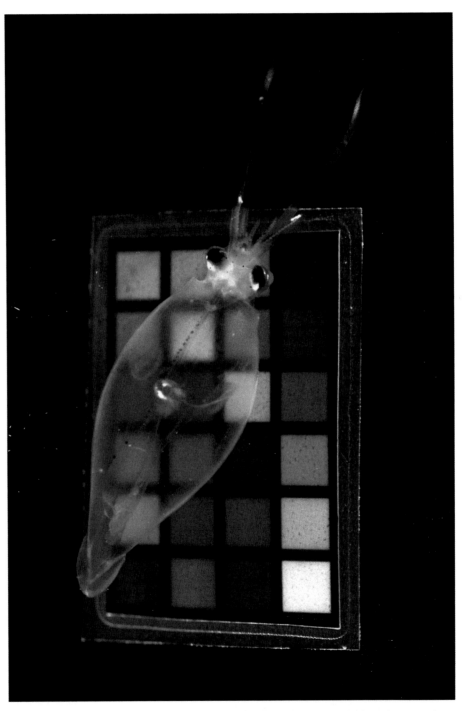

Figure 10.7 Transparency is a common form of camouflage in the mesopelagic realm. Here the transparency of a chranchiid squid is demonstrated as it rests over a colour standard.

kingdom (Owings, Hennessy, Leger & Gladney, 1986; Owings & Morton, 1998), and such selection of responses must come after sensory information storage, risk evaluation and then action selection.

Little is known about the selection, learning or brain control of appearance in these antipredator responses. The optic lobe of the brain contains the circuits controlling pattern production (Williamson & Chrachri, 2004) and the suboesophageal lobe has an output-controlling chromatophoric lobe. The octopuses may use open-loop production of these camouflage patterns and not monitor their own output. Still, cephalopods certainly utilize the visual cues about background, which Sutherland (1963) proved long ago in the laboratory, that they can recognize, to form the behavioral sequence. As Hanlon, Forsythe and Joneschild (1999) pointed out, this sequence of responses to predator threat must include pattern and/or movement production, assessment of predator response, selection of a new response and a movement option, a clear cognitive accomplishment in the sequence proposed by Neisser (1976).

6.5   Conclusion

The results of this closer look at foraging of octopuses is both a realization of the complexity of their behavior and a better understanding of the pressures that likely caused the cognitive ability that we see demonstrated in laboratory situations. Prey selectivity, saltatory search and spatial memory, as well as predator avoidance, tap the considerable information processing capacity of the octopus (see Mather, 2008) and demonstrate its cognitive ability.

Many of these field studies could form the basis for extensive laboratory research. Foraging of octopuses under predatory threat, as Adamo, Ehgoetz, Sangster and White-horne (2006) have done for cuttlefish, would be revealing. It would be possible to study octopuses' Search Images for prey, perhaps using a Y-maze to evaluate chemical cues. More research needs to be carried out on prey choice, taking into account the variables of search, penetration ability and handling time, as well as energetic costs and food value. As octopuses live in a changing environment, laboratory studies could evaluate their responses to frequent changes in prey cues (see Dunlap & Stephens, 2012). Developmental studies could evaluate acquisition of foraging competence. The link between personality, learning and foraging competence could be established (see Warburton, 2003). A wonderful opportunity exists for a cross-phyla comparison for spatial memory (Alves, Chichery, Boal & Dickel, 2006). And, of course, laboratory studies should begin to evaluate the nervous system control of these behaviors (see chapter 5, this volume, by Grasso).

Acknowledgements

The first and second authors would like to thank the Brazilian science funding agency, CNPq, for a grant that allowed J. M. to travel to Brazil so the two could work on the manuscript together. The authors would like to dedicate this chapter to Roland Anderson, in memory of his many contributions to cephalopod biology.

References

Adamo, S. A., Ehgoetz, K., Sangster, C. and Whitehorne, I. (2006). Signaling to the enemy? Body pattern expression and its response to external cues during hunting in the cuttlefish *Sepia officinalis* (Cephalopoda). *The Biological Bulletin*, **210**: 192–200.

Adams-Hunt, M. M. and Jacobs, L. F. (2007). In *Foraging: behavior and ecology*. Chicago, IL: University of Chicago Press, pp. 105–138.

Allen, J. J., Mäthger, L. M., Barbosa, A. and Hanlon, R. T. (2009). Cuttlefish use visual cues to control three-dimensional skin papillae for camouflage. *Journal of Comparative Physiology*, **195**: 547–555.

Alves, C., Chichery, R., Boal, J. G. and Dickel, L. (2006). Orientation in the cuttlefish *Sepia officinalis*, response versus place learning. *Animal Cognition*, **10**: 29–36.

Ambrose, R. F. (1984). Food preferences, prey availability, and the diet of *Octopus bimaculatus* Verrill. *Journal of Experimental Marine Biology and Ecology*, **77**: 29–44.

Ambrose, R. F. (1988). Population dynamics of *Octopus bimaculatus*: influence of life history patterns, synchronous reproduction and recruitment. *Malacologia*, **29**: 23–39.

Ambrose, R. F. and Nelson, B. V. (1983). Predation by *Octopus vulgaris* in the Mediterranean. *PSZN Marine Ecology*, **4**: 251–261.

Anderson, J. P., Stephens, D. W. and Dunbar, S. R. (1997). Saltatory search: a theoretical analysis. *Behavioral Ecology*, **8**: 307–317.

Anderson, R. C., Hughes, P. D., Mather, J. A. and Steele, C. W. (1999). Determination of the diet of *Octopus rubescens* Berry, 1953 (Cephalopoda: Octopodidae) through examination of its beer bottle dens in Puget Sound. *Malacologia*, **41**: 455–460.

Anderson, R. C. and Mather, J. A. (1996). Escape responses of *Euprymna scolopes* Berry, 1911 (Cephalopoda: Sepiolidae). *Journal of Molluscan Studies*, **62**: 543–545.

Anderson, R. C. and Mather, J. A. (2007). The packaging problem: bivalve prey selection and prey entry techniques of the octopus *Enteroctopus dofleini*. *Journal of Comparative Psychology*, **121**: 300–305.

Anderson, R. C., Mather, J. A., Monette, M. Q. and Zimsen, S. R. M. (2010). Octopuses (*Enteroctopus dofleini*) recognize individual humans. *Journal of Applied Animal Welfare Science*, **13**: 261–272.

Anderson, R. C, Sinn, D. L. and Mather, J. A. (2008). Drilling localization on bivalve prey by *Octopus rubescens* (Cephalopoda: Octopodidae). *The Veliger*, **50**: 326–328.

Anderson, R. C., Wood, J. B. and Mather, J. A. (2008). *Octopus vulgaris* in the Caribbean is a specializing generalist. *Marine Ecology Progress Series*, **371**: 199–202.

Beck, B. B. (1980). *Animal tool behavior: the use and manufacture of tools by animals*. New York, NY: Garland Publishing.

Bednekoff, P. A. (2007). Foraging in the face of danger. In *Foraging: behavior and ecology*. Chicago, IL: University of Chicago Press, pp. 305–330.

Boal, J. G. (2006). Social recognition: a top-down view of cephalopod behavior. *Vie et Milieu*, **56**: 69–79.

Boal, J. G., Dunham, A. W., Williams, K. T. and Hanlon, R. T. (2000). Experimental evidence for spatial learning in octopuses (*Octopus bimaculoides*). *Journal of Comparative Psychology*, **114**: 246–252.

Borrelli, L. and Fiorito, G. (2008). Behavioral analysis of learning and memory in cephalopods. In *Learning and memory: a comprehensive reference*. London, UK: Elsevier, pp. 605–627.

Brown, J. S. and Kotler, B. P. (2007). The ecology of fear. In *Foraging: behavior and ecology*. Chicago, IL: University of Chicago Press, pp. 437–480.

Chelazzi, G., Innocenti, R. and Della Santina, P. (1983). Zonal migration and trail following of an intertidal gastropod analyzed by LED tracking in the field. *Marine Behaviour and Physiology*, **10**: 121–136.

Cooper, W. E., Jr. (2005). The foraging mode controversy and foraging space. *Journal of Zoology*, **267**: 179–190.

Cortez, T., Castro, B. G. and Guerra, A. (1998). Drilling behaviour of *Octopus mimus* Gould. *Journal of Experimental Marine Biology and Ecology*, **224**: 193–203.

Coss, R. G. and Goldthwaite, R. O. (1995). The persistence of old designs for perception. In *Perspectives in ethology, II*. New York, NY: Plenum Press, pp. 83–148.

Costantini, D., Casagrande, S., Di Lieto, G., Fanfani, A. and Dell'Omo, G. (2005). Consistent differences in feeding habits between neighbouring breeding kestrels. *Behaviour*, **142**: 1409–1421.

Cott, H. B. (1940). *Adaptive coloration in animals*. London, UK: Methuen Publishing.

Daly, M., Behrends, P. R., Wilson, M. I. and Jacobs, L. F. (1992). Behavioral modulation of predation risk: moonlight avoidance and crepuscular compensation in a nocturnal desert rodent, *Dipodomys merriami*. *Animal Behaviour*, **44**: 1–9.

Dilly, P. N., Nixon, M. and Packard, A. (1964). Forces exerted by *Octopus vulgaris*. *Pubblicazioni della Stazione Zoologica di Napoli*, **34**: 86–97.

Dukas, R. and Kamil, A. (2000). The cost of limited attention in blue jays. *Behavioral Ecology*, **11**: 502–506.

Dunlap, A. S. and Stephens, D. W. (2012). Tracking a changing environment: optimal sampling, adaptive memory and overnight effects. *Behavioral Processes*, **89**: 86–94.

Eifler D. A, Eifler, M. A. and Harris, B. R. (2008). Foraging under the risk of predation in desert grassland whiptail lizards (*Aspidoscelis uniparens*). *Journal of Ethology*, **26**: 219–223.

Ferguson, G. P., Messenger, J. B. and Budelmann, B. U. (1994). Gravity and light influence the countershading reflexes of the cuttlefish *Sepia officinalis*. *Journal of Experimental Biology*, **191**: 247–256.

Finn, J. T., Tregenza, T. and Norman, M. D. (2009). Defensive tool use in a coconut-carrying octopus. *Current Biology*, **19**: 1069–1070.

Forsythe, J. W. and Hanlon, R. T. (1997). Foraging and associated behavior by *Octopus cyanea* Gray, 1849 on a coral atoll, French Polynesia. *Journal of Experimental Marine Biology and Ecology*, **209**: 15–31.

Godfrey-Smith, R. (2002). Environmental complexity and the evolution of cognition. In *The evolution of intelligence*. Mahwah, NJ: Lawrence Erlbaum Associates, pp. 223–250.

Graindorge, N., Alves, C., Darmaillacq, A. S., Chichery, R., Dickel, L. and Bellanger, C. (2006). Effects of dorsal and ventral electrolytic lesions of the vertical lobe on spatial learning and locomotor activity in *Sepia*. *Behavioral Neurosciences*, **120**: 1151–1158.

Hanlon R. T., Forsythe J. W. and Joneschild, D. E. (1999). Crypsis, conspicuousness, mimicry and polyphenism as antipredator defences of foraging octopuses on Indo-Pacific coral reefs, with a method of quantifying crypsis from video tapes. *Biological Journal of the Linnean Society*, **66**: 1–22.

Hanlon, R. T. and Messenger, J. B. (1988). Adaptive coloration in young cuttlefish (*Sepia officinalis* L.): the morphology and development of body patterns and their relation to behaviour. *Philosophical Transactions of the Royal Society of London. Series B*, **320**: 437–487.

Hanlon, R. T. and Messenger, J. B. (1996). *Cephalopod behaviour*. New York, NY: Cambridge University Press.

Hanlon, R. T., Watson, A. C. and Barbosa, A. (2010). A "mimic octopus" in the Atlantic: flatfish mimicry and camouflage by *Macrotritopus defilippi*. *The Biological Bulletin*, **218**: 15–24.

Hartwick, E. B., Ambrose, R. F. and Robinson, S. M. C. (1984). Den utilization and the movements of tagged *Octopus dofleini*. *Marine Behaviour and Physiology*, **11**: 95–110.

Hartwick, E. B., Breen, P. A. and Tulloch, L. (1978). A removal experiment with *Octopus dofleini* (Wülker). *Journal of the Fisheries Research Board of Canada*, **35**: 1492–1495.

Hartwick, E. B., Thorarinsson, G. and Tulloch, L. (1978). Methods of attack by *Octopus dofleini* (Wülker) on captured bivalve and gastropod prey. *Marine Behaviour and Physiology*, **5**: 193–200.

Hill, S. L., Burrows, M. T. and Hughes, R. N. (2003). The efficiency of adaptive search tactics for different prey distribution patterns: a simulation model based on the behavior of juvenile plaice. *Journal of Fish Biology*, **63** (Supplement A): 117–130.

Hochner, B. (2010). Functional and comparative assessments of the octopus learning and memory system. *Frontiers in Bioscience*, **2**: 764–771.

Hochner, B., Shomrat, T. and Fiorito, G. (2006). The octopus: a model for comparative analysis of the evolution of learning and memory. *The Biological Bulletin*, **210**: 308–317.

Huffard, C. L. (2006). Locomotion by *Abdopus aculeatus* (Cephalopoda: Octopodidae): walking the line between primary and secondary defenses. *Journal of Experimental Biology*, **209**: 3697–3707.

Huffard, C. L., Caldwell, R. L. and Boneka, F. (2010). Male–male and male–female aggression may influence mating associations in wild octopuses (*Abdopus aculeatus*). *Journal of Comparative Psychology*, **124**: 38–46.

Humphrey, N. K. (1976). The social function of intellect. In *Growing points in ethology*. Cambridge, UK: Cambridge University Press, pp. 303–317.

Iribarne, O. O., Fernandez, M. E. and Zucchini, H. (1991). Prey selection by the small Patagonian octopus *Octopus tehuelchus* d'Orbigny. *Journal of Experimental Marine Biology and Ecology*, **148**: 271–281.

Jolly, A. (1966). Lemur social behavior and primate intelligence. *Science*, **139**: 764–766.

Katsanevakis, S. and Verriopoulos, G. (2004). Den ecology of *Octopus vulgaris* Cuvier, 1797, on soft sediment: availability and types of shelters. *Scientia Marina*, **68**: 147–157.

Kelley, J. L. and Magurran, A. E. (2011). Learned defences and counterdefences in predator-prey interactions. In *Fish cognition and behavior*. Chichester, UK: Wiley-Blackwell, pp. 36–58.

Kerr, B. and Feldman, M. W. (2003). Carving the cognitive niche: optimal learning strategies in homogeneous and heterogeneous environments. *Journal of Theoretical Biology*, **220**: 169–188.

Kuba, M., Byrne, R. A., Meisel, D. V., Griebel, U. and Mather, J. A. (2006). When do octopuses play? Effects of repeated testing, object type, age, and food deprivation on object play in *Octopus vulgaris*. *Journal of Comparative Psychology*, **120**: 184–190.

Langridge, K. V. (2009). Cuttlefish use startle displays, but not against large predators. *Animal Behaviour*, **77**: 847–856.

Langridge, K. V., Broom, M. and Osorio, D. (2007). Selective signaling by cuttlefish to predators. *Current Biology*, **17**: 1044–1045.

Leite, T. S., Haimovici, M. and Mather, J. A. (2009). *Octopus insularis* (Octopodidae): evidences of a specialized predator and a time-minimizing forager. *Marine Biology*, **156**: 2355–2367.

Leite, T. S. and Mather, J. A. (2008). A new approach to octopuses' body pattern analysis: a framework for taxonomy and behavioral studies. *American Malacological Bulletin*, **24**: 31–41.

Lima, S. L. and Dill, L. M. (1990). Behavioural decisions made under the risk of predation: a review and prospectus. *Canadian Journal of Zoology*, **68**: 619–640.

Lima, S. L., Valone, T. J. and Caraco, T. (1985). Foraging efficiency-predation risk trade-off in the grey squirrel. *Animal Behaviour*, **33**: 155–165.

Marr, D. (1983). *Vision: a computational investigation into the human representation and processing visual information*. San Francisco, CA: W. H. Freeman and Co.

Mather, J. A. (1982a). Factors affecting the spatial distribution of natural populations of *Octopus joubini* Robson. *Animal Behaviour*, **30**: 1166–1170.

Mather, J. A. (1982b). Choice and competition: their effects on occupancy of shell homes by *Octopus joubini*. *Marine Behaviour and Physiology*, **8**: 285–293.

Mather, J. A. (1988). Daytime activity of juvenile *Octopus vulgaris* in Bermuda. *Malacologia*, **29**: 69–76.

Mather, J. A. (1991a). Foraging, feeding and prey remains in middens of juvenile *Octopus vulgaris* (Mollusca: Cephalopoda). *Journal of Zoology, London*, **224**: 27–39.

Mather, J. A. (1991b). Navigation by spatial memory and use of visual landmarks in octopuses. *Journal of Comparative Physiology*, **168**: 491–497.

Mather, J. A. (1994). "Home" choice and modification by juvenile *Octopus vulgaris* (Mollusca: Cephalopoda): specialized intelligence and tool use? *Journal of Zoology, London*, **233**: 359–368.

Mather, J. A. (1995). Cognition in cephalopods. *Advances in the Study of Behavior*, **24**: 316–353.

Mather, J. A. (2004). Cephalopod displays: from concealment to communication. In *Evolution of communication systems*. Cambridge, MA: MIT Press, pp. 193–213.

Mather, J. A. (2008). Cephalopod consciousness: behavioral evidence. *Consciousness and Cognition*, **17**: 37–48.

Mather, J. A. (2010). Vigilance and antipredator responses of Caribbean reef squid. *Marine and Freshwater Behaviour and Physiology*, **43**: 357–370.

Mather, J. A. (2011). Why is *Octopus cyanea* Gray in Hawaii specializing in crab prey? *Vie et Milieu*, **61**: 181–184.

Mather, J. A. and Anderson, R. C. (1993). Personalities of octopuses (*Octopus rubescens*). *Journal of Comparative Psychology*, **107**: 336–340.

Mather, J. A. and Anderson, R. C. (1999). Exploration, play and habituation in octopuses (*Octopus dofleini*). *Journal of Comparative Psychology*. **113**: 333–338.

Mather, J. A., Anderson, R. C. and Leite, T. S. (2009). "The octopus eyebar: anatomy of a skin display." Presented at the meeting of the Animal Behavior Society, Pirenopolis, Brazil, June, 2009.

Mather, J. A., Leite, T. S. and Batista, A. T. (2012). Individual prey choices of octopuses: are they generalist or specialist? *Current Zoology*, **58**: 596–602.

Mather, J. A. and Mather, D. L. (1994). Skin colours and patterns of juvenile *Octopus vulgaris* (Mollusca, Cephalopoda) in Bermuda. *Vie et Milieu*, **44**: 267–272.

Mather, J. A. and Mather, D. L. (2004). Apparent movement in a visual display: the passing cloud in *Octopus cyanea*. *Journal of Zoology, London*, **263**: 89–94.

Mather, J. A. and O'Dor, R. K. (1991). Foraging strategies and predation risk shape the natural history of juvenile *Octopus vulgaris*. *Bulletin of Marine Science*, **49**: 256–269.

Meisel, D. V., Byrne, R. A., Kuba, M. and Mather, J. A. (2011). Behavioural sleep in *Octopus vulgaris*. *Vie et Mileu*, **61**: 185–190.

Meisel, D. V., Kuba, M., Byrne, R. A. and Mather, J. Λ. (2013). The effect of predatory presence on the temporal organization of activity in *Octopus vulgaris*. *Journal of Experimental Marine Biology and Ecology*, **447**: 75–79.

Messenger, J. B. (2001). Cephalopod chromatophores: neurobiology and natural history. *Biological Reviews*, **76**: 473–528.

Moynihan, M. (1975). Conservatism of displays and comparable stereotyped patterns among cephalopods. *Function and evolution in behavior: essays in honor of Professor Niko Tinbergen, F.R.S.* Oxford, UK: Oxford University Press, pp. 276–291.

Muntz, W. R. A. (1970). An experiment in shape discrimination and signal detection in *Octopus*. *Quarterly Journal of Experimental Psychology*, **22**: 82–90.

Neisser, U. (1976). *Cognition and reality*. San Francisco, CA: W. H. Freeman and Co.

Nixon, M. and Maconnachie, E. (1988). Drilling by *Octopus vulgaris* (Mollusca: Cephalopoda) in the Mediterranean. *Journal of Zoology, London*, **216**: 687–716.

O'Brien, W. J., Browman, H. I. and Evans, B. I. (1990). Search strategies of foraging animals. *American Scientist*, **78**: 152–160.

Onthank, K. L. and Cowles, D. L. (2011). Prey selection in *Octopus rubescens*: Possible roles of energy budgeting and prey nutritional composition. *Marine Biology*, **158**: 2795–2804.

Owings, D. H., Hennessy, D. F., Leger, D. W. and Gladney, A. B. (1986). Different functions of "alarm" calling for different time scales: a preliminary report on ground squirrels. *Behaviour*, **99**: 101–116.

Owings, D. H. and Morton, E. (1998). *Animal vocal communication: a new approach*. Cambridge, UK: Cambridge University Press.

Packard, A. (1972). Cephalopods and fish: the limits of convergence. *Biological Reviews*, **47**: 241–307.

Packard, A. (1995). Organization of cephalopod chromatophore systems: a neuromuscular image generator. In *Cephalopod neurobiology*. Oxford, UK: Oxford University Press. pp. 331–367.

Packard, A. and Sanders, G. D. (1971). Body patterns of *Octopus vulgaris* and maturation of the response to disturbance. *Animal Behaviour*, **19**: 780–790.

Papini, M. R. and Bitterman, M. E. (1991). Appetitive conditioning in *Octopus cyanea*. *Journal of Comparative Psychology*, **105**: 107–113.

Pierce, G. J. and Ollason, J. G. (1987). Eight reasons why optimal foraging theory is a complete waste of time. *Oikos*, **49**: 111–118.

Randall, J. E. (1967). Food habits of reef fishes of the West Indies. *Studies in Tropical Oceanography*, **5**: 665–847.

Renner, M. J. (1990). Neglected aspects of exploratory and investigatory behavior. *Psychobiology*, **18**: 16–22.

Roberts, W. A. (1991). Testing optimal foraging theory on the radial maze. *Animal Learning and Behavior*, **19**: 305–316.

Scheel, D. and Anderson, R. C. (2012). Variability in the diet specialization of *Enteroctopus dofleini* in the eastern Pacific examined from midden contents. *American Malacological Bulletin*, **30**: 1–13.

Scheel, D and Bisson, L. (2012). Movement patterns of giant Pacific octopuses, *Enteroctopus dofleini* (Wülker, 1910). *Journal of Experimental Marine Biology and Ecology*, **416**–417: 21–31.

Scheel, D., Lauster, A. and Vincent, T. L. S. (2007). Habitat ecology of *Enteroctopus dofleini* from middens and live prey surveys in Prince William Sound, Alaska. In *Cephalopods present and past: new insights and fresh perspectives*. New York, NY: Springer, pp. 434–458.

Shaffery, J. P., Ball, N. J. and Amlaner, C. J. (1985). Manipulating daytime sleep in herring gulls (*Larus argentatus*). *Animal Behaviour*, **33**: 566–572.

Shettleworth, S. J. (2010). *Cognition, evolution, and behavior*, 2nd edn. New York, NY: Oxford University Press.

Smith, C. D. (2003). Diet of *Octopus vulgaris* in False Bay in South Africa. *Marine Biology*, **143**: 1127–1133.

Steer, M. A. and Semmens, J. M. (2003). Pulling and drilling, does size or species matter? An experimental study of prey handling in *Octopus dierythraeus* (Norman, 1992). *Journal of Experimental Marine Biology and Ecology*, **290**: 165–178.

Stephens, D. W., Brown, J. S. and Ydenberg, R. C. (Eds.) (2007). *Foraging: behavior and ecology*. Chicago, IL: University of Chicago Press.

Stephens, D. W. and Krebs, J. R. (1986). *Foraging Theory*. Princeton, NJ: Princeton University Press.

Sutherland, N. S. (1963). Shape discrimination and receptive fields. *Nature*, **197**: 118–122.

Van Heukelem, W. F. (1966). Some aspects of the ecology and ethology of *Octopus cyanea* Gray. Unpublished MSc. Thesis, University of Hawaii.

Vermeij, G. J. (1995). *A natural history of shells*. Princeton, NJ: Princeton University Press.

Vincent, T. L. S., Scheel, D. and Hough, K. R. (1998). Some aspects of diet and foraging behavior of *Octopus dofleini* (Wülker, 1910) in its northernmost range. *Marine Ecology*, **19**: 13–29.

Waite, T. A. and Field, K. L. (2007). Foraging with others: games social foragers play. In *Foraging: behavior and ecology*. Chicago, IL: University of Chicago Press, pp. 331–362.

Warburton, K. (2003). Learning of foraging skills by fish. *Fish and Fisheries*, **4**: 203–215.

Wells, M. J. (1964). Detour experiments with octopus. *Journal of Experimental Biology*, **41**: 621–642.

Wells, M. J. (1978). *Octopus: physiology and behaviour of an advanced invertebrate*. London, UK: Chapman and Hall.

Wells, M. J., O'Dor, R. K., Mangold, K. and Wells, M. J. (1983). Diurnal changes in activity and metabolic rate in *Octopus vulgaris*. *Marine Behaviour and Physiology*, **9**: 275–287.

West-Eberhard, M. J. (2003). *Developmental plasticity and evolution*. Oxford, UK: Oxford University Press.

Williamson, R. and Chrachri, A. (2004). Cephalopod neural networks. *Neurosignal*, **13**: 87–98.

Wodinsky, J. (1973). Mechanism of hole boring in *Octopus vulgaris*. *Journal of General Psychology*, **88**: 179–183.

Wodinsky, J. (1978). Feeding behavior of broody *Octopus vulgaris*. *Animal Behaviour*, **26**: 803–813.

Wood, J. B. and Anderson, R. C. (2004). Interspecific evaluation of octopus escape behavior. *Journal of Applied Animal Welfare Science*, **7**: 96–106.

Wood, J. B., Maynard, A. E., Lawlor, A. G., Sawyer, E. K., Simmons, D. M., Pennoyer, K. E. and Derby, C. E. (2010). Caribbean reef squid, *Sepioteuthis sepioidea*, use ink as a defense against predatory French grunts, *Haemulon flavolineatum*. *Journal of Experimental Marine Biology and Ecology*, **388**: 20–27.

Yarnall, J. L. (1969). Aspects of the behaviour of *Octopus cyanea* Gray. *Animal Behaviour*, **17**: 747–75.

Zylinski, S., Osorio, D. and Shohet, A. J. (2009). Edge detection and texture classification by cuttlefish. *Journal of Vision*, **9**: 1–10.

7 Navigation in cephalopods

Christelle Jozet-Alves, Anne-Sophie Darmaillacq and Jean G. Boal

7.1 Introduction

The coleoid cephalopods exhibit three classes of natural movement patterns: dispersal, local movements and migrations. How are these movements accomplished? The coleoid cephalopods (octopuses, cuttlefishes and squids) have complex nervous systems and multiple types of sensory information at their disposal, including vision (contrast, polarization), chemoreception (contact, distance) and mechanoreception (touch, vibration). Based on information gleaned from field and laboratory studies, what can we infer about cephalopod orientation and navigation?

Multiple words are in use to describe the movement patterns of organisms in space. *Orientation* is a term used for directional movements, such as phototaxis or rheotaxis, orientation with respect to light or water currents, respectively (Dunn, 1990). Complex cognition is not necessary for orientation behavior. The term *navigation* is used for the process of determining and maintaining a course or trajectory to a goal location (Franz & Mallot, 2000). Navigation requires at least some cognition (attention, memory, learning): learning particular landmarks, travel routes, associations between particular environmental features, or some combination of these. If an animal uses the configuration of several landmarks to localize the goal; this behavior is called *piloting* (Gallistel, 1993).

In this chapter, we first describe the sensory systems of coleoid cephalopods (octopuses, cuttlefishes and squids) that enable them to collect spatial information and then explore current field and laboratory evidence for short- and long-distance navigation. Throughout the chapter, we will discuss possible mechanisms to support such navigation. For a discussion of orientation and navigation in *Nautilus*, see chapter 2, this volume, by Basil & Crook; for excellent overviews of spatial orientation in animals, see Wehner et al. (1996), Healy (1998), Golledge (1999), Brown and Cook (2006) and Dolins and Mitchell (2010).

7.2 Sensory systems

Navigation requires complex sense organs to collect information, a sophisticated central nervous system to process the information and make decisions and efficient effectors

Cephalopod Cognition, eds A.-S. Darmaillacq, L. Dickel and J. Mather. Published by Cambridge University Press. © Cambridge 2014.

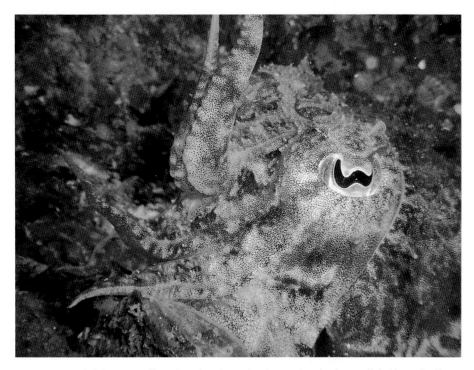

Figure 7.1 Cuttlefish *Sepia officinalis*. The picture has been taken in the English Channel off Granville (Manche, France). The ocular globe is particularly voluminous. The eye is characterized by the w-shaped papillae. (Copyright, F. Sichel.) See plate section for color version.

to carry out the behavioral response. Cephalopods possess all of these (for reviews, Budelmann, 1995; Hanlon & Messenger, 1996). Their prodigious capabilities for complex cognition are covered elsewhere (for a review, Mather, 1995), including within this volume; here we assess the types of sensory information available to support cephalopod navigation.

7.2.1   Vision

Eyes are one of the most conspicuous features of cephalopods (Figure 7.1). Cephalopod eyes are structurally very similar to those of vertebrates (for reviews, Messenger, 1991; Budelmann, 1994; Gleadall & Shashar, 2004). The visual information from the eyes is considerable and the brain has large visual areas. The size of the optic lobes represents 85% of the whole central nervous system in *Octopus vulgaris*, about 140% in *Sepia* sp. and more than 330% in *Loligo* sp. (reviewed in Nixon & Young, 2003). It is interesting to note that the relative size of these lobes increases as the way of life changes from the most benthic individuals (octopuses) to the most pelagic (squids). Cephalopods' excellent visual discrimination abilities are evident from the extensive body of research addressing visual discrimination learning (e.g. in *Sepia:* Karson, 2003; in *Octopus*: Sutherland et al., 1963; Mackintosh & Mackintosh, 1964; for reviews, Mather, 1995; Boal, 1996).

Experimental evidence indicates that cephalopod vision is highly sensitive to brightness contrast. For example, cephalopods show an optomotor or an optokinetic response when placed within a rotating cylinder painted with black and white vertical stripes (in *Sepia*: Messenger, 1970; Groeger et al., 2005). To date, there is no evidence that cephalopods see colors (Marshall & Messenger, 1996; Mäthger et al., 2006). Color vision requires at least two visual pigments (Tansley, 1965) and, except in *Watasenia scintillans*, a deep-sea squid, cephalopod eyes contain only a single visual pigment (Hanlon & Messenger, 1996; Bellingham et al., 1998). Cephalopods do perceive light polarization (Hanlon & Messenger, 1996; Horváth & Varjú, 2004), however, which can be considered as analogous to color vision (Cronin et al., 2003). This polarization sensitivity (PS) arises from the orthogonal positioning of the microvilli of neighboring photoreceptors in the retina. Linear PS can be used to break camouflage by enhancing contrast; for example, when attacking transparent or silvery prey (in *Sepia officinalis*: Shashar et al., 2000). It is also possibly involved in intraspecific communication (Shashar et al., 1996; Boal et al., 2004). Most notably, polarization is used in orientation behavior by many animals (bees: Kraft et al., 2011; fish: Waterman, 2006; see also Shettleworth, 2010 and Marshall & Cronin, 2011); recent laboratory experiments have demonstrated that cephalopods also can use the *e*-vector when orientating (*S. officinalis*; Cartron et al., 2012, see below).

7.2.2   Chemoreception

Detection of chemical cues can be either through contact chemoreception (gustation) or distance chemoreception (olfaction). Contact chemoreception is achieved through chemoreceptors located on the suckers and lips (Budelmann et al., 1997). There are about 10 000 receptors on each sucker in *Octopus* and only about 100 in *Sepia*, illustrating the relative importance of this sense to octopuses (Graziadei, 1964; Graziadei & Gagne, 1976). Chemotactile discrimination learning has been demonstrated in octopuses (Wells, 1978). Distance chemoreception is achieved through olfactory organs located close to the eyes (Budelmann, 1996). Octopuses and cuttlefish are capable of sensing a variety of different chemicals, even at very low concentrations and can orient with respect to these odors (in *Eledone*: Boyle, 1986; in *Octopus*: Lee, 1992; Walderon et al., 2011; in *Sepia*: Boal & Golden, 1999; Boal et al., 2010; in *Loligo*: Cummins et al., 2011; for a review, Hanlon & Messenger, 1996).

As with the optic lobes, the relative size of the brain structures that process chemosensory information depends on the animals' way of life. Octopuses and cuttlefish, which are benthic or necto-benthic, are more likely to use their arms for crawling or manipulating prey than squids, which swim in the open water. This difference is reflected in the organization of the brain where the sub-esophageal mass is much less condensed and the brachio-pedal connectives much longer in squids than in cuttlefish and octopuses.

7.2.3   Mechanoreception

Cephalopods have a complex mechanoreceptive system that comprises the statocysts, the lateral line analogue and touch and pressure receptors (Budelmann, 1996).

The statocysts are the most complex of all invertebrate equilibrium receptor systems (Young, 1960; Dilly et al., 1975). Their level of sophistication rivals that of the vestibular system of vertebrates. There are receptors for the detection of gravity, angular acceleration and linear acceleration; by integrating this information, cephalopods can assess their location and their active and passive movements in the water (Budelmann, 1980). This sophisticated equilibration system may allow cephalopods to move efficiently in a three-dimensional environment.

Like other aquatic species, cephalopods are highly sensitive to local water movements ("sound"). The lateral line analogue (in *Sepia* and *Lolliguncula*: Budelmann & Bleckmann, 1988; Bleckmann et al., 1991) provides cephalopods with the equivalent of "hearing" (Hanlon & Budelmann, 1987). Physiological studies have shown that the hair cells respond to local water movements at 0.5–400 Hz (Bleckmann et al., 1991); behavioral responses have been documented to frequencies from 20 to 600 Hz (in *Sepia*: Komak et al., 2005). Recordings from the statocysts suggest that these receptors also play a role in detecting particle movements (*Loligo*: Mooney et al., 2010). It is possible that this sensory system detects sounds from predators and prey, or the low-frequency environmental sound signatures that may aid navigation.

Cephalopods possess also other mechanoreceptors. Octopuses are particularly sensitive to touch and can learn to discriminate different degrees of roughness (Wells, 1978). Benthic cephalopods could use texture to orient (Hvorecny et al., 2007). Cuttlefish possess mechanoreceptors in the fins; according to Kier et al. (1985), they probably use this peripheral mechanical information during swimming to regulate and control their fin beat.

7.2.4 Geomagnetism perception

The mechanisms underlying the perception of the geomagnetic field are not fully understood; however, this ability is important to the navigation of many birds, fishes and reptiles (Winklhofer, 2009). The mollusk *Tritonia diomedea* appears to use its perception of the geomagnetic field to orient towards the shore (Willows, 1999). No evidence yet exists for whether cephalopod mollusks can detect the geomagnetic field.

7.2.5 Summary

Cephalopods have well-developed sensory systems that could support orientation and navigation in the field. Vision is clearly useful for orienting in shallow, lit waters. Chemoreception could allow cephalopods to locate prey, particular water currents, spawning locations or conspecific aggregations. Mechanoreception could provide orientation cues to support short-distance navigation (e.g. integration of movements in the three-dimensional environment) as well as onshore and offshore seasonal migrations.

7.3 Dispersal

Dispersal refers to moving away from a particular location, often the natal location, that is typically undirected and without a later return. These latter features distinguish dispersal

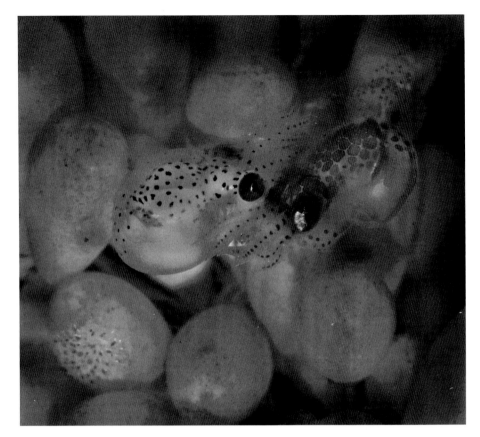

Figure 7.2 Giant Pacific Octopus, *Enteroctopus dofleini*, paralarvae. They do not have the same way of life as adults, which are generally benthic. (Photograph courtesy of J. Kocian.) See plate section for color version.

from migration. Dispersal is often accomplished by passive means, such as drifting with currents (e.g. planktonic larvae, Figure 7.2). Cephalopod hatchlings, whether benthic or planktonic, likely use similar mechanisms to disperse, but further investigation is required (Boletzky, 2003).

7.3.1   Field observations

The lives of cephalopods between hatching and adult recruitment are poorly described, with particular difficulties in both sampling and species identification (Boyle & Rodhouse, 2005). Field samples yield distinct cohorts (Arkhipkin, 1993) with different physiographic distributions (*Octopus*: Faraj & Bez, 2007; *Todarodes*: Kawabata et al., 2006), adding to the confusion.

Cephalopod adults are semelparous and a single species can spawn at different times of the year within the same area (*Loligo*: Ito, 2007). The duration of the hatching period of a single egg mass can range from 2 days (*Octopus laqueus*, Kaneko et al., 2006) to 78 days (*Enteroctopus dofleini*, Gabe, 1975). Hatchlings may be either planktonic or benthic, depending on the species (Boletzky, 2003) and the duration of a planktonic stage can range from 3 weeks (*Octopus joubini*, Forsythe & Toll, 1991) to 6 months (*E. dofleini,* Villanueva & Norman, 2008).

The horizontal distances covered during dispersal may range from several hundreds of meters in small bottom dwelling species without a planktonic phase (e.g. sepiolid squids) to hundreds of kilometers in pelagic species (e.g. teuthid squids and octopods; Boyle & Boletzky, 1996; for a review, see Villanueva & Norman, 2008). Several approaches have been taken to assess dispersal distance. Genetic structuring of the common cuttlefish (*S. officinalis*) in the Atlantic–Mediterranean region was evaluated using cytochrome oxidase mitochondrial DNA (Pérez-Losada et al., 2007) and isolation by distance was shown to be the main factor driving genetic structuring of *Sepia* populations. This result supports the hypothesis of restricted dispersal ability probably due to its nectobenthic way of life along with the absence of any planktonic stage. An analysis of natural elemental signatures in cephalopod statoliths suggested that juvenile squid (*Gonatus fabricii*) inhabit surface waters while larger animals move to colder, deeper waters (Arkhipkin et al., 2004; Zumholz et al., 2007). Few studies to date have specifically examined the potential of mass-marking techniques for the early life-history stages of cephalopods (Pecl et al., 2010; Payne et al., 2011). Such techniques offer considerable potential for understanding juvenile dispersal.

7.3.2   Possible mechanisms

"Paralarvae," planktonic stages that do not undergo metamorphosis before settlement (Young & Harman, 1988), possess considerable potential for dispersal. Hatchlings may disperse actively both in the water column and along the seabed (Boletzky, 2003). Strong positive phototaxis is a common response for hatchlings and some later paralarval (immature; see Young & Harman, 1988) stages, but among benthic species, this response reduces, disappears or reverses after settlement (Villanueva & Norman, 2008). It is not known what factors control settlement of the planktonic paralavae of benthic species (Semmens et al., 2007).

All hatchlings may undergo some passive dispersal due to water movements. Soon after hatching, squid paralarvae are active predators on other zooplankton; although they are active swimmers using jet propulsion during this life stage, their distribution is essentially dependent on oceanic circulation (Moreno et al., 2009). In western Iberia, temperature and upwellings were shown to be the most important variables in modulating seasonality and distribution of the paralarvae of *Loligo vulgaris, O. vulgaris,* sepiolids and ommastrephids (Moreno et al., 2009). The influence of the physical environment is particularly pronounced for the paralarvae of *O. vulgaris,* which follows distinct patterns according to the oceanography of the western Iberia and the Gulf of Cádiz systems (Moreno et al., 2009).

7.3.3   Individual differences

Differences between individual cephalopods could influence individual movement trajectories. Animal personalities (temperaments, behavioral syndromes) are common across taxa and have important evolutionary and ecological implications that have only recently come under close scrutiny (e.g. Reale et al., 2007; Stamps, 2007). Individual differences have been found in exploration, aggressiveness, reactivity and boldness in the dumpling squid (*Euprymna:* Sinn & Moltschaniwskyj, 2005; Sinn et al., 2010) and enduring individual differences in reactions have been documented in octopuses (Mather & Anderson, 1993). Among vertebrates, variations in boldness, sociability or aggressiveness influence dispersal tendency (Cote et al., 2010). This possibility remains to be explored in cephalopods.

7.3.4   Discussion and conclusions

Dispersal is an important component of spatial behavior, yet relatively little is known about the life histories of juvenile cephalopods. Mechanisms for dispersal are unlikely to involve complex cognition, however.

7.4   Migrations

Migration typically refers to long-distance movements, often in connection to seasonal or ontogenetic changes. Often, but not always, migrations are cyclical and involve a return to the original location by either the individuals or the population. Most of what we know about migrations in cephalopods comes from fisheries data, tagging studies (both traditional tag/recapture and electronic tracking), systematic sampling and statolith and other tissue composition analyses (reviewed in Semmens et al., 2007).

7.4.1   Field observations

Cephalopod migrations range from diel vertical migrations of a few hundred meters (e.g. *Dosidicus gigas*, Gilly et al., 2006; multiple species, Watanabe et al., 2006) to annual horizontal movements of hundreds of kilometers (e.g. *Illex argentinus*, Arkhipkin, 1993; see Boyle & Rodhouse, 2005) to the combination of vertical and horizontal components in onshore-offshore migrations (e.g. Villanueva, 1992; Olyott et al., 2007; reviewed in Hanlon & Messenger, 1996). Cephalopod migrations support the combined needs of foraging, avoiding predators, mating and spawning and, in the case of vertical migrations, managing thermal stress (*D. gigas*, Zeidberg & Robison, 2007; reviewed in Olson & Young, 2007). When migrating, some species traverse the same path in both directions, e.g. traveling north as they grow and traveling south along the same route when they return to traditional spawning grounds as mature adults (e.g. Kiyofuji & Saitoh, 2004), but other species traverse different routes (e.g. Choi et al., 2008).

Field observations suggest that the key factors in many cephalopod migrations are ocean productivity and hydrographic/physiographic parameters: temperature, light, salinity, oxygen and water currents (Sims et al., 2001; Wang et al., 2003; Gilly et al., 2006; Stark, 2008; Chen C. S. et al., 2007, Chen X. J., 2007; Ito, 2007; Onitsuka et al., 2010; Rosa & Seibel, 2010; Sakaguchi, 2010; for a review, Pierce et al., 2008).

Consistent with these observations is the apparent shift in migrations and distributions with climate change (Sims et al., 2001; Kidokoro et al., 2010).

Most cephalopods are semelparous, spawning just once before they die, and live only for about a year (Hanlon & Messenger, 1996), providing little opportunity to learn from previous migratory experience. Curiously, although some populations show clear evidence of genetic mixing (e.g. *Loligo opalescens*, Reichow & Smith, 2001; *O. vulgaris*: Oosthuizen et al., 2004), other species show genetically distinct spawning populations (e.g. *S. officinalis*: Pérez-Losada et al., 2002; *Loligo forbesi*: Shaw et al., 1999; *Martialia hyadesi*: Brierley et al., 1993; *Loligo pealeii*: Buresch et al., 2006) suggestive of population-level site fidelity in spawning locations.

7.4.2   Possible mechanisms

The mechanisms underlying long-distance migration, particularly for a first or only transit, are not fully understood for any animal (Wehner et al., 1996). For marine migrants, potential cues for orientation include celestial cues, the geomagnetic field, vibrations and water currents.

Celestial cues can provide directional information for migrating animals. Navigation based on the movements and configurations of the sun and stars has been demonstrated in insects (e.g. Akesson & Wehner, 2002) and birds (e.g. Able & Able, 1996). Navigation based on polarization patterns in the sky has been documented in insects (Marshall & Cronin, 2011). An ability to perceive polarized light could also support underwater navigation, especially under restricted conditions (e.g. turbidity; Lerner et al., 2011). Some squids exhibit spontaneous preferential swimming direction relative to the *e*-vector orientation of polarized light (*Eupryma morsei, Sepioteuthis lessoniana*: Jander et al., 1963). It remains unclear whether this polarization-based body orientation is biologically meaningful in the context of navigation and migration. It could play a role comparable to phototaxis (see Saidel et al., 1983 for further discussion).

The geomagnetic field can provide both directional and map information for migrating animals (e.g. Lohmann et al., 2004). It is not known whether any cephalopods detect the geomagnetic field.

Vibration (e.g. reef sounds, surf) provides directional information that is used for orientation by some marine species (*Pomacentrid* larvae, Tolimieri et al., 2004; decapod crustaceans, Montgomery et al., 2006). Behavioral studies in *S. officinalis* showed that young animals (<4 months post-hatching) responded to low frequencies ranging from 20 to 600 Hz by changing their body patterns, moving and trying to bury (Komak et al., 2005). Vibration cues could be used for orientation in cephalopods, but this possibility has still to be investigated.

Water currents can provide both directional and map information from the speed and direction of the flow, the temperature, salinity and clarity of the water, and the chemicals carried in the current, whether of biologic or geologic origin. Detection of the spatial gradient of chemical cues in water can also be used to orient (Moore et al., 1991). Laboratory experiments have demonstrated that both octopuses and cuttlefishes detect biologically relevant odors (different waters, conspecifics and prey items;

e.g. *S. officinalis*: Boal & Golden, 1999) and can use these odors to orient (*S. officinalis*: Boal et al., 2010; *Octopus bimaculoides*: Walderon et al., 2011); presumably, squids are similarly capable.

It is not currently understood how cephalopods locate traditional, common spawning grounds (e.g. *Sepia apama* in the Spencer Gulf, South Australia: Hall & Hanlon, 2002). Such sites may be consistent from a large scale viewpoint, but the exact locations can vary from year to year (e.g. *Doryteuthis opalescens*: Young et al., 2011). Late arrivers could be guided by odors from conspecifics or conspecific eggs (*S. officinalis*: Boal et al., 2010; *O. bimaculoides*: Walderon et al., 2011) or, at close range, the sight of the eggs, themselves (King et al., 2003). Early learning (imprinting) could account for this location fidelity. Recent research has demonstrated that biologically significant learning occurs at or even before hatching (e.g. *S. officinalis*: Dickel et al., 2000; Darmaillacq et al., 2006, 2008; Guibé et al., 2010) and that adults are capable of oriented movements in response to the odors of conspecifics or conspecific eggs (*S. officinalis*: Boal et al., 2010; *O. bimaculoides*: Walderon et al., 2011). It is possible that young cephalopods could learn the characteristics of the hatching location and then later return to that location to spawn, similar to salmon (Scholz et al., 1976); this hypothesis remains to be explored. Alternatively, developmentally timed responses to physiographic features could allow a return to particular locations via specific water currents.

7.4.3   Discussion and conclusions

Long-distance migrations can be accomplished through sensory and developmentally linked orientation behavior (Shea & Vecchione, 2010) as well as through true navigation. Simple diel vertical movements within the pelagic ocean probably do not involve cognition, for example. Long-distance horizontal migrations could involve cognition if return travel followed outbound travel routes, implicating learning and early learning of the hatching site could facilitate a later return to that location for spawning, suggestive of imprinting. Alternatively, endogenous biologic timing mechanisms coupled with internal biases, attention or preferences for particular physical parameters could facilitate such movement patterns. Such mechanisms, while both complex and fascinating, do not require complex cognition. There is ample room for further investigation of these topics.

7.5   Local movements

Local movements include travels within a home range. Such travels open the possibility of learning local landmarks and the locations of significant resources. Such learning can result in more efficient and potentially purposeful movements in space.

7.5.1   Field observations

At least some cephalopods navigate within a local area. Many octopus species are central place foragers, traveling away from one or more (*O. dofleini*: Mather et al., 1985) home

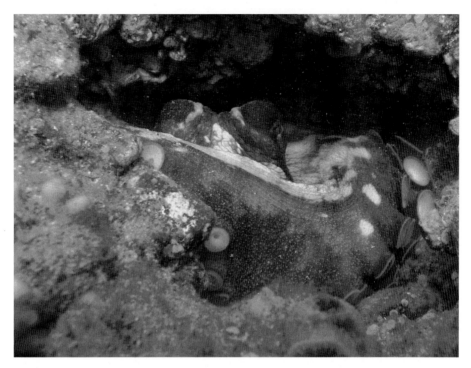

Figure 7.3 *Octopus cyanea* in its den. Note the stones surrounding the den entrance. (Copyright, A.-S. Darmaillacq.) See plate section for color version.

den and then returning to the den repeatedly for shelter (*O. bimaculatus*: Ambrose, 1982; *Octopus briareus*: Aronson, 1986, 1989, 1991; *Octopus cyanea*: Van Heukelem, 1966; Yarnall, 1969; Forsythe & Hanlon, 1997; *O. dofleini*: Hartwick et al., 1978, 1984; Mather et al., 1985; *O. vulgaris*: Altman, 1967; Kayes, 1974; Mather, 1988, 1991a, 1991b; Mather & O'Dor, 1991; for reviews, Boyle, 1983, 1987; Figure 7.3).

The local movements of octopuses are likely supported by sophisticated spatial orientation abilities. At least some octopuses travel considerable distances before returning to their dens (up to 40 m, *O. cyanea,* Forsythe & Hanlon, 1997) and they sometimes remain away for extended periods of time before returning (up to 7 h, *O. dofleini,* Mather et al., 1985). They often jet-swim directly home without contacting the bottom substrate or retracing their outbound routes (*O. vulgaris*, Mather, 1991a; *O. cyanea,* Forsythe & Hanlon, 1997). Individuals avoid recently visited areas on subsequent hunting trips, suggesting that they remember where they foraged previously (*O. vulgaris*: Mather, 1991a; *O. cyanea*: Forsythe & Hanlon, 1997). Octopuses may use a particular den continuously for anywhere from 1 day to as long as 5 months (*O. dofleini,* Hartwick et al., 1984), after which they move to a new location, presumably because of prey depletion. Moving to a new location with new features and spatial relationships is likely to promote flexible and long-term spatial memory.

The natural history of cuttlefish also provides evidence for spatial learning (*S. officinalis*: Boletzky, 1983; Hanlon & Messenger, 1988). In particular, cuttlefish appear to minimize their hunting time and then quickly return to safe places. Recent tagging experiments indicate that *S. apama* forages away from and then returns to specific rocky outcroppings (Aitken et al., 2005). Monitored individuals showed high site fidelity and small home ranges (between 5300 m² and 27 300 m²), suggesting that the cuttlefish confined their foraging to a restricted area. Tagged cuttlefish produced fewer data from movements after several days. They hypothesize that the cuttlefish may have settled into a den (rock crevice, no signal) emitting only brief signals during foraging excursions. *S. apama* rest more than 95% of the time (Aitken et al., 2005), supporting the idea that long rest periods in safety are punctuated by brief foraging bouts in the open, nearby. Regular travels between safe resting places and good hunting grounds would promote spatial learning.

In the field, cuttlefish frequently swim in and around vertical barriers. Spatial learning could aid in negotiating these obstacles (Sanders & Young, 1940). In the old harbor of Cesarea, Israel, a single cuttlefish (*S. officinalis*) was tracked for over 50 m, at water depth of 5–3 m (N. Shashar, personal communication), as it swam in a straight line until it reached a small (2 m tall) underwater wall. There, without touching any surfaces and with great speed, it swam approximately 3 m up an inclined ledge and turned into a small crevice, not much larger than the animal, where it went into hiding. The animal did not seem to hesitate, change speed or collide with obstacles, indicating that it was familiar with the spatial layout of the area. Its behavior suggests the use of three-dimensional navigation to reach a location that was both distant and higher than its original position. Alternatively, it could have used two orthogonal yet flat representations of the environment, one leading to the wall and the other leading up the surface of the wall into the crevice.

Squids are predominantly neritic (e.g. *L. forbesi*) or pelagic (e.g. *D. gigas*) and direct underwater observations are difficult to obtain. Most of the daily activities of squids are known from tracking experiments and results to date vary widely. Individual *L. vulgaris reynaudii* were monitored as they circled egg beds in South Africa (Sauer et al., 1997). Each dawn, the squid moved onshore (several kilometers) to mate in small and well-defined areas near egg beds on the substrate; at dusk, most individuals moved offshore, probably for feeding or resting. In *L. forbesi*, most individuals (except the largest ones) tended to remain in the vicinity of the reef (*L. forbesi*: O'Dor et al., 1994; *Sepioteuthis australis*: O'Dor et al., 2002) and most of the smaller individuals moved very little over periods of up to 19 days. Tracking experiments are more scarce for pelagic species. Individual *D. gigas* spent most daylight hours at depths greater than 250 m and foraged in near-surface waters at night (Yatsu et al., 1999; Gilly et al., 2006). Similar daily vertical migrations have been documented in other squid species (e.g. *Ommastrephes bartramii*: Murata & Nakamura, 1998; Hiroyuki, 2001). Such diel migrations do not require spatial learning.

7.5.2   Laboratory evidence of spatial memory

Octopuses are good candidates to study spatial learning. In the wild, they are central-place foragers that relocate periodically, depending on den size and the presence of preferred prey (Mather, 1994). Spatial memory in octopuses was initially demonstrated by Walker et al. (1970), who trained octopuses (*Octopus maya*) to find a goal location with water in a dry, T-shaped apparatus. The stem of the "T" served as a start box and the two identical arms of the "T" led to the goal compartments situated at either side of the stem. In this experiment, five octopuses learned to enter the goal compartment opposite to their initial side-turning preference to regain access to seawater. After 27 days of training, all octopuses were performing without errors, providing convincing evidence of spatial learning in octopuses.

Exploratory learning is considered a natural manifestation of spatial learning (Gallistel, 1993). According to O'Keefe and Nadel (1978), exploration is necessary for animals to build maps of new environments and to update existing maps. To test the hypothesis that octopuses show exploratory learning, Boal and collaborators performed two separate experiments (*O. bimaculoides,* Boal et al., 2000). To determine if octopuses spontaneously move about, they placed individual octopuses in an unfamiliar environment and recorded the octopuses' behavior. The octopuses gradually decreased their activity over the course of 3 days, consistent with the hypothesis that the octopuses had been exploring. To evaluate whether they actually learned (retained information) about their new environment during their movements, the octopuses were placed in a different aquatic environment with two inset (deeper water) burrow sites, only one of which was open, for a period of 23 h and then removed (Boal et al., 2000). After a 24 h delay, the octopuses were placed back into this same environment, but with much shallower water in the arena. Most octopuses approached the previously open burrow first, demonstrating that they had learned the location of the open burrow, evidence for exploratory learning.

More recently, Hvorecny et al. (2007) demonstrated that octopuses can learn two different spatial problems simultaneously (conditional discrimination). They tested octopuses (*O. bimaculoides*) in two distinct maze apparatuses that differed in the visual and tactile cues provided. As before, each maze was provided with two inset burrows, one open and one closed. The octopuses were placed for 16 h per day in one of the two maze configurations, which were presented alternately throughout training (10 days total, 5 days in each maze). Six out of ten octopuses learned to go directly to the open burrow in both mazes.

Unlike many octopus species, cuttlefishes have not been described as having dens (but see Aitken et al., 2005 in *S. apama*) and are thought to rely primarily on camouflage for defense. This behavior pattern could explain why researchers have started to explore the abilities of cuttlefish to orient and navigate only recently. Preliminary observations showed that cuttlefish (*S. officinalis*) placed in a large artificial pond spontaneously moved around and appeared to learn its features (Karson et al., 2003). This result suggested that cuttlefish, too, explore a new environment. Karson et al. (2003) then designed mazes to assess cuttlefish (*S. officinalis*) spatial learning abilities. Although food reinforcement is used in mazes classically (in rats, birds, fish or even insects), escape was chosen to make the task more comparable to a natural spatial learning problem. The cuttlefish were trained to exit a circular testing arena with two exit holes cut on opposite sides. The exit holes were surrounded by visual cues (striped or spotted panels of fabric), with only one exit hole opened. The cuttlefish demonstrated the ability to solve the task; moreover, cuttlefish improved over serial reversals (once the cuttlefish trained, the open hole was closed and the opposite one was opened), showing that the cuttlefish were able to quickly update their spatial memory with the most recent information. More recently, Hvorecny et al. (2007) tested the cuttlefish *S. officinalis* and *Sepia pharaonis* in modified versions of this same procedure. This time, the presence of a centrally located cue indicated which of the two exit holes was open (striped or spotted; right or left). Cuttlefish learned to select the correct exit hole, even when the learning trials with the two different central cues were intermixed. These experiments clearly demonstrate that complex spatial memory is well within the abilities of cuttlefishes.

7.5.3   Possible mechanisms

There are four systems in which spatial information is represented (Dolins & Mitchell, 2010). In order of cognitive complexity, these systems include: (i) use of a single cue or beacon (self in response to a cue); (ii) use of sequential cues or route following (self in response to individual cues within a sequence); (iii) path integration (self as a cue); and (iv) piloting (relational and simultaneous use of multiple cues). The first three of these are self-referential mechanisms. With (i) single cues or beacons, individuals orient their own position in space according to one or more cues. This form of orientation can take the form of trail following (e.g. gastropod slime trails, Davies & Blackwell, 2007), taxes (i.e. orienting with respect to a sensory gradient, Campan, 1997) or beaconing (i.e. movements directed towards a particular landmark, Cheng & Spetch, 1998). (ii) The use of sequential cues or route following can be accomplished through motor patterns that link sequences of movements or responses into stereotyped series (e.g. arthropods, Bell, 1985). (iii) Path integration, also called "dead reckoning," is a navigational process by which signals generated during locomotion allow the subject to update its position as if it had summed the vectors of its outbound journey. This computation allows the subject to return directly home without tracing the path of its outbound journey. This strategy is found in many species, from arthropods to humans (ants: Müller & Wehner, 1988; Wehner, 2003; crabs: Layne et al., 2003; mammals: Etienne et al., 1996). (iv) Piloting is the most sophisticated navigational mechanism and is not self-referential. Environmental features are combined together with a directional sense to accomplish orientation ("cognitive mapping"; Save et al., 1998). Laboratory experiments with octopuses and cuttlefish have explored the first two of these systems. Unfortunately, no study has yet directly tested either path integration or piloting hypotheses in cephalopods (see Alves et al., 2008, for further discussion about piloting in cephalopods).

Single cues

Many animals return home by secreting a chemical trail on a solid substrate on their outbound route and then retrace that trail when returning. This strategy, called trail following, depends on contact chemoreception (e.g. limpets, Cook, 1971; termites, Kaib et al., 1982). In the field, Mather (1991a) and Forsythe and Hanlon (1997) observed that octopuses (*O. vulgaris* and *O. cyanea*) traveled by jetting through the water when leaving or returning home; consequently, they were not in contact with the substrate. In addition, they returned directly to their den afterwards rather than tracing their outbound route.

As a consequence, it is unlikely that octopuses use contact chemoreception for short-distance navigation. In support of this hypothesis, raking the gravel substrate between trials in a laboratory maze experiment had no effect on the octopuses' orientation behavior (Boal et al., 2000). However, these observations do not exclude the possibility that octopuses are able to use this strategy in particular environmental conditions (low visibility, for example). Neither cuttlefishes nor squids maintain regular, tactile contact with the substrate when they travel, making it unlikely that these species use trail following, either.

For local travel, cephalopods seem more likely to orient using visual landmarks, particularly those with high contrast and distinctive polarization. One possible orienting strategy consists of using landmark guidance or beaconing (Gallistel, 1993; also called stimulus-approach behaviour, Schmajuk & Thieme, 1992). In this case, the animal will learn to go to a particular feature that marks the location of a goal, regardless of the motor behavior involved. In a series of experiments, Mather (1991a) has investigated octopuses' ability to use visual landmarks to orient. These cues can be used in a variety of ways to provide information about the location of a goal. The simplest way of using them is to rely on a single visual cue as a beacon marking a goal: for example, goldfish can learn to use simple objects as beacons to locate food which has been buried under a gravel substrate in a testing tank (Warburton, 1990). Mather (1991a) trained octopuses (*Octopus rubescens*) to go to a piece of plastic tubing (the beacon) to find a food reward located within a featureless circular tank. The octopuses learned to approach the plastic tubing even when it was moved around the tank. This experiment clearly showed octopuses' ability to rely on a single landmark to label the location of a goal.

Some learning experiments are designed to provide very precise information about the features that cephalopods attend to and how they learn to solve spatial problems. These studies used an experimental technique called the transformational approach (Tinbergen, 1972). Animals are trained to solve a spatial task and then their environment is modified in some way (e.g. by displacing landmarks) to determine which strategy the animals were using to solve the task (e.g. using landmarks or a motor sequence). Using this approach, cuttlefish (*S. officinalis*) were tested in a cross-maze apparatus (Alves et al., 2007). The task required animals to locate a goal compartment at the end of one arm of the maze. The reward for solving the task was 15 min in a darkened goal compartment with a sandy bottom into which the cuttlefish could bury. The cuttlefish could either learn a motor sequence (e.g. turn left) or orient using distal visual cues (water-pipes, sets of shelving in the laboratory room). At the end of training, the cuttlefish were placed again in the maze but in the opposite starting arm. Most of the cuttlefish made the formerly rewarded motor sequence (turn right or left), swimming in the opposite direction of the rewarded goal compartment. Interestingly, one out of the ten cuttlefish swam in the correct direction, apparently using the distal visual cues rather than a motor sequence. In a second version of the experiment, the cross-maze was surrounded by black curtains and two proximate visual cues were provided just above the water (striped and spotted PVC panels). When tested in the opposite start arm of this maze configuration, half of the cuttlefish used the proximate visual cues while the other half used a motor sequence. These two experiments demonstrated that cuttlefish can use at

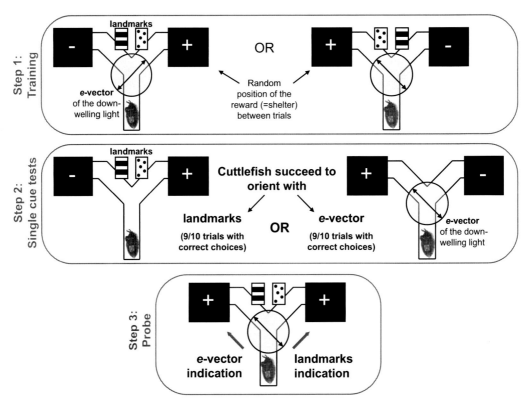

Figure 7.4 Schematic representation of three steps of the learning procedure. See Cartron et al. (2012) for the detailed procedure.

least two different strategies to solve spatial tasks: visual cues and motor sequences. The availability and salience of the visual cues influenced which strategy was used. Similar results have been obtained previously with vertebrates (Restle, 1957; Carman & Mactutus, 2001).

Cartron et al. (2012) trained cuttlefish (*S. officinalis*) in a Y-maze with two kinds of visual cues, the *e*-vector of a polarized light (either perpendicular or parallel) and two PVC panels (one striped and one spotted). Cues were placed just above the water surface (Figure 7.4). During training, both visual cues were available. At the end of training, the experimenters provided just one of the two types of cues (i.e. either the PVC panels or the filter linearly polarizing the light). All cuttlefish tested were able to orient with either one of the visual cues, presented separately. This study also showed for the first time that cuttlefish can orient either parallel or perpendicular to the *e*-vector of a polarized light. The results clearly indicate that cuttlefish, like marine mammals (Gibson & Shettleworth, 2005) and insects (Heinze & Homberg, 2007), acquire redundant information simultaneously.

Sequential cues

Animals can also use a series or chain of landmarks to compose a route when multiple landmarks are available. For example, ants learn and recognize landmarks distributed along a route and they correct their course relative to these landmarks (Collett et al., 1992). In Mather's experiments (1991a; above), when a box and a dish were added in the tank, the octopus (*O. rubescens*) moved first to the larger landmark (the box) and, next, oriented to the plastic tubing associated with food. These results could be interpreted as the use of a chain of landmarks to follow a route leading to the food location.

Accurate assessment of the layout of multiple objects in the immediate environment allows animals to plan routes and to solve spatial problems, such as those posed by obstructions. Detouring around objects can be cognitively challenging, requiring the animal to synthesize spatial memories in potentially new ways. Octopuses, at least, appear to be capable of this type of spatial reasoning. Schiller (1949), Boycott (1954) and Wells (1964) tested the ability of octopuses (*O. vulgaris*) to detour around opaque partitions to reach a prey item (a live crab). The crab was either (a) shown in the corner of an opaque partition and then displaced behind that partition (Boycott 1954) or (b) directly visible but located behind a transparent partition (Schiller, 1949; Boycott, 1954; Wells, 1964). How animals responded to their first trial in these apparatuses was indicative of their spatial representation of the location of the goal. Some, although not all, of the octopuses successfully reached the crab at the first trial (1 in 5 when the crab was displaced behind the partition, Boycott, 1954; 8 in 29 when the crab was visible behind a transparent wall, Wells, 1964). In Schiller (1949) and Wells (1964) experiments, the transparent partition that separated the octopuses from the prey could have been such an unnatural stimulus that the animals failed to perceive it as an obstacle (for further discussion of possible explanations for the behavior of the octopuses that failed this task, see Alves et al., 2008). The authors then attempted to train the octopuses that had failed by providing repeated trials with the same detour problem. The octopuses showed an improvement in performance over time, as measured by a decrease in the time spent pushing and attacking the transparent partition. Performances were erratic, however, and the octopuses never went straight to the edge of the partition (Boycott, 1954). Upon closer analysis, Schiller (1949) and Wells (1964) found that the octopuses needed to remain in tactile contact with the wall separating them from the goal (Schiller, 1949) and if the tactile contact was lost, they needed to maintain a continuous visual fixation on the wall itself (Wells, 1964).

More recently, Moriyama and Gunji (1997) tested octopuses (*O. vulgaris*) in a tank with four partitioning boards, either transparent or opaque. Animals had to learn to detour these obstacles to reach the end of the tank to obtain a food reward. With repeated trials, octopuses reduced the time they spent detouring around the obstacles. By studying swimming actions, the researchers asserted that octopuses "evaluated" their environment and estimated their actions, before proceeding. Octopuses in such situations may be planning their route. Taken together, experiments suggest that octopuses, at least, have the ability to maintain orientation towards a goal while detouring around obstacles.

7.5.4   Individual differences

Spatial learning can vary between individuals, based on differences in age, experience and sex. The range size hypothesis predicts sex dimorphism in spatial learning abilities in species in which range expansion is different between males and females (e.g. sex differences in promiscuous meadow voles) and not in other species (e.g. no sex difference in monogamous voles; Gaulin & FitzGerald, 1986, 1989; reviewed in Jones et al., 2003). Jozet-Alves et al. (2008) assessed spatial learning performances of male and female cuttlefish (*S. officinalis*), either before or after sexual maturation, in a T-maze (procedure described above; Alves et al., 2007). They also determined the spatial strategy preferentially used by each cuttlefish to evaluate whether males and females use different spatial orientation strategies. Although cuttlefish males and females did not differ in the time they took to learn the spatial task in a T-maze, sexually mature males were more likely to attend to the visual cues provided above the apparatus to solve the T-maze task while sexually mature females preferentially relied on a motor sequence (right versus left turn). This difference in strategy did not lead to a sex difference in overall performance. The authors also showed that sexually mature males traveled a longer distance when placed in an open-field compared with female and immature cuttlefish, suggesting a possible greater propensity for exploring new environments by males. This study was the first to demonstrate cognitive differences between sexes in an invertebrate. Moreover, the data conform to the predictions of the range size hypothesis.

7.5.5   Discussion and conclusions

Both field observations and laboratory experiments provide clear evidence that at least some cephalopods navigate within local areas for the purposes of foraging and sheltering. These travels are accomplished by learning the locations of external cues (both single and sequential; see above) and learning and remembering patterns of movements (turning right/left, route following; see above). The more cognitively complex forms of orientation, path integration and piloting (see above), merit further investigation, particularly in light of anecdotal observations indicating complex and purposeful traveling behavior.

7.6   Summary and future directions

Cephalopods show a wide range of orientation behavior in the field, ranging from precise short-distance navigation, particularly in octopuses, to long-distance orientation with respect to physiographic characteristics, particularly in squids. Newer methods, ranging from electronic tags (e.g. Gilly et al., 2006) to molecular analyses (see Semmens et al., 2007) are likely to provide more precise information about particular species' movement patterns in the near future. Data arising from these methods will allow the generation of testable hypotheses for mechanisms underlying cephalopod orientation behavior. In parallel, brain studies (e.g. electrophysiology, pharmacology and immuno-histochemistry) have the potential to uncover how cephalopods represent space and the sensory bases for these representations. Different spatial behavior mechanisms may be supported by different neural representational mechanisms.

A better understanding of cephalopod movements will be of both theoretical and practical value. For evolutionary biologists, results of research with cephalopods in comparison with other lineages will provide clearer understanding of the evolution of spatial orientation. For industrial and artisanal fisheries, such research can provide practical information useful for improving stock assessment and fisheries management (Boyle & Rodhouse, 2005; Faraj & Bez, 2007). The greatest benefit will come from an interdisciplinary approach that integrates population-level analyses obtained from fisheries investigations with individual-level analyses obtained from laboratory and field studies. Such an approach will require greater teamwork between disparate subdisciplines than has been typical in the past.

Acknowledgements

We would like to express our gratitude to the long history of curious and dedicated scientists, both in the field and in laboratories worldwide, who have carefully and painstakingly built our understanding of the natural world.

References

Able, K. P. and Able M. A. (1996). The flexible migratory orientation system of the savannah sparrow (*Passerculus sandwichensis*). *Journal of Experimental Biology*, **199**: 3–8.

Aitken, J. P., O'Dor, R. K. and Jackson, G. D. (2005). The secret life of the giant Australian cuttlefish *Sepia apama* (Cephalopoda): behaviour and energetics in nature revealed through radio acoustic positioning and telemetry (RAPT). *Journal of Experimental Marine Biology and Ecology*, **320**: 77–91.

Akesson, S. and Wehner, R. (2002). Visual navigation in desert ants *Cataglyphis fortis*: are snapshots coupled to a celestial system of reference? *Journal of Experimental Biology*, **205**: 1971–1978.

Altman, J. S. (1967). The behaviour of *Octopus vulgaris* Lam. in its natural habitat: a pilot study. *Underwater Association Reports*, **1966–1967**: 77–83.

Alves, C., Chichery, R., Boal, J. G. and Dickel, L. (2007). Orientation in the cuttlefish *Sepia officinalis*: response versus place learning. *Animal Cognition*, **10**: 29–36.

Alves, C., Boal, J. G. and Dickel, L. (2008). Short-distance navigation in cephalopods: a review and synthesis. *Cognitive Processing*, **9**: 239–247.

Ambrose, R. F. (1982). Shelter utilization by the molluscan cephalopod *Octopus bimaculatus*. *Marine Ecology Progress Series*, **7**: 67–73.

Arkhipkin, A. I. (1993). Age, growth, stock structure and migratory rate of pre-spawning short-finned squid *Illex argentinus* based on statolith ageing investigations. *Fisheries Research*, **16**: 313–338.

Arkhipkin, A. I., Campana, S. E., Fitzgerald, J. and Thorrold, S. R. (2004). Spatial and temporal variation in elemental signatures of statoliths from the Patagonian longfin squid (*Loligo gahi*). *Canadian Journal of Fisheries and Aquatic Sciences*, **61**: 1212–1224.

Aronson, R. B. (1986). Life history and den ecology of *Octopus briareus* Robson in a marine lake. *Journal of Experimental Marine Biology and Ecology*, **95**: 37–56.

Aronson, R. B. (1989). The ecology of *Octopus briareus* Robson in a Bahamian saltwater lake. *American Malacological Bulletin*, **7**: 47–56.

Aronson, R. B. (1991). Ecology, paleobiology and evolutionary constraint in the octopus. *Bulletin of Marine Science*, **49**: 245–255.

Bell, W. J. (1985). Sources of information controlling motor patterns in arthropod local search orientation. *Journal of Insect Physiology*, **31**: 837–847.

Bellingham, J., Morris, A. G. and Hunt, D. M. (1998). The rhodopsin gene of the cuttlefish *Sepia officinalis*: sequence and spectral tuning. *Journal of Experimental Biology*, **201**: 2299–2306.

Bleckmann, H., Budelmann, B. U. and Bullock, T. H. (1991). Peripheral and central nervous responses evoked by small water movements in a cephalopod. *Journal of Comparative Physiology A*, **168**: 247–257.

Boal, J. G. (1996). A review of simultaneous visual discrimination as a method of training octopuses. *Biological Reviews*, **71**: 157–190.

Boal, J. G. and Golden, D. K. (1999). Distance chemoreception in the common cuttlefish, *Sepia officinalis* (Mollusca, Cephalopoda). *Journal of Experimental Marine Biology and Ecology*, **235**: 307–317.

Boal, J. G., Dunham, A. W., Williams, K. T. and Hanlon, R. T. (2000). Experimental evidence for spatial learning in octopuses (*Octopus bimaculoides*). *Journal of Comparative Psychology*, **114**: 246–252.

Boal, J. G., Shashar, N., Grable, M. M., et al. (2004). Behavioral evidence for intraspecific signaling with achromatic and polarized light by cuttlefish (Mollusca: Cephalopoda). *Behaviour*, **141**: 837–861.

Boal, J. G., Prosser, K. N., Holm, J. B., et al. (2010). Sexually mature cuttlefish are attracted to the eggs of conspecifics. *Journal of Chemical Ecology*, **36**: 834–836.

Boletzky, S. v. (1983). *Sepia officinalis*. In *Cephalopod life cycles. Species accounts*, vol. 1. London, Academic Press, pp. 31–52.

Boletzky, S. v. (2003). Biology of early life stages in cephalopod mollusks. *Advances in Marine Biology*, **44**: 143–200.

Boycott, B. B. (1954). Learning in *Octopus vulgaris* and other cephalopods. *Pubblicazioni Della Stazione Zoologica di Napoli*, **25**: 67–93.

Boyle, P. R. (1983). *Cephalopod life cycles. Species accounts*, vol. 1. London, Academic Press.

Boyle, P. R. (1986). Responses to water-borne chemicals by the octopus *Eledone cirrhosa* (Lamarck, 1798). *Journal of Experimental Marine Biology and Ecology*, **104**: 23–30.

Boyle, P. R. (1987). *Cephalopod life cycles. Comparative reviews*, vol. 2. London, Academic Press.

Boyle, P. R. and Boletzky, S. v. (1996). Cephalopod populations: definition and dynamics. *Philosophical Transactions of the Royal Society of London. Series B*, **351**: 985–1002.

Boyle, P. R. and Rodhouse, P. (2005). *Cephalopods: ecology and fisheries*. Oxford, Blackwell.

Brierley, A. S., Rodhouse, P. G., Thorpe, J. P. and Clarke, M. R. (1993). Genetic evidence of population heterogeneity and cryptic speciation in the ommastrephid squid *Martialia hyadesi* from the Patagonian Shelf and Antarctic Polar Frontal Zone. *Marine Biology*, **116**: 593–602.

Brown, M. F. and Cook, R. G. (2006). *Animal spatial cognition: comparative, neural, and computational approaches* [online]. Available from www.pigeon.psy.tufts.edu/asc/

Budelmann, B. U. (1980). Equilibrium and orientation in cephalopods. *Oceanus*, **23**: 34–43.

Budelmann, B. U. (1994). Cephalopod sense organs, nerves and the brain: adaptations for high performance and life style. *Marine and Freshwater Behaviour and Physiology*, **25**: 13–33.

Budelmann, B. U. (1995). The cephalopod nervous system: what evolution has made of the molluscan design. In *The nervous systems of invertebrates: an evolutionary and comparative approach*. Basel, Birkhäuser Verlag, pp. 115–138.

Budelmann, B. U. (1996). Active marine predators: the sensory world of cephalopods. *Marine and Freshwater Behaviour and Physiology*, **27**: 59–75.

Budelmann, B. U. and Bleckmann, H. (1988). A lateral line analogue in cephalopods: water waves generate microphonic potentials in the epidermal head lines of *Sepia* and *Lolliguncula*. *Journal of Comparative Physiology A*, **164**: 1–5.

Budelmann, B. U., Schipp, R. and Boletzky, S. v. (1997). *Cephalopoda*. In *Microscopic anatomy of invertebrates*. New York, Wiley-Liss, pp. 119–414.

Buresch, K. C., Gerlach, G. and Hanlon, R. T. (2006). Multiple genetic stocks of longfin squid *Loligo pealeii* in the NW Atlantic: stocks segregate inshore in summer, but aggregate offshore in winter. *Marine Ecology Progress Series*, **310**: 263–270.

Campan, R. (1997). Tactic components in orientation. In *Orientation and communication in arthropods*. Basel, Birkhäuser Verlag, pp. 1–40.

Carman, H. M. and Mactutus, C. F. (2001). Proximal versus distal cue utilization in spatial navigation: the role of visual acuity? *Neurobiology of Learning and Memory*, **78**: 332–346.

Cartron, L., Darmaillacq, A. S., Jozet-Alves, C., Shashar, N. and Dickel, L. (2012). Cuttlefish rely on both polarized light and landmarks for orientation. *Animal Cognition*, **15**: 591–596.

Chen, C. S., Chiu T. S. and Haung, W. B. (2007). The spatial and temporal distribution patterns of the Argentine short-finned squid, *Illex argentinus*, abundances in the Southwest Atlantic and the effects of environmental influences. *Zoological Studies*, **46**: 111–122.

Chen, X. J., Zhao, X. H. and Chen, Y. (2007). Influence of *El Niño/La Niña* on the western winter–spring cohort of neon flying squid (*Ommastrephes bartramii*) in the northwestern Pacific Ocean. *ICES Journal of Marine Science*, **64**: 1152–1160.

Cheng, K. and Spetch, M. L. (1998). Mechanisms of landmark use in mammals and birds. In *Spatial representation in animals*. Oxford, Oxford University Press, pp. 1–17.

Choi, K., Lee, C. I., Hwang, K., et al. (2008). Distribution and migration of Japanese common squid, *Todarodes pacificus*, in the southwestern part of the East (Japan) Sea. *Fisheries Research*, **91**: 281–290.

Collett, T. S., Dillmann, E., Giger, A. and Wehner, R. (1992). Visual landmarks and route-following in desert ants. *Journal of Comparative Physiology A*, **170**: 435–442.

Cook, S. B. (1971). A study of homing behavior in the limpet *Siphonaria alternata*. *The Biological Bulletin*, **141**: 449–457.

Cote, J., Clobert, J., Brodin, T., Fogarty, S. and Sih, A. (2010). Personality-dependent dispersal: characterization, ontogeny and consequences for spatially structured populations. *Philosophical Transactions of the Royal Society of London. Series B*, **365**: 4065–4076.

Cronin, T. W., Shashar, N., Caldwell, R. L., et al. (2003). Polarization vision and its role in biological signaling. *Integrative and Comparative Biology*, **43**: 549–558.

Cummins, S. F., Boal, J. G., Buresch, K. C., et al. (2011). Extreme aggression in male squid induced by a b-MSP-like pheromone. *Current Biology*, **21**: 322–327.

Darmaillacq, A -S., Chichery, R. and Dickel, L. (2006). Food imprinting, new evidence from the cuttlefish *Sepia officinalis*. *Biology Letters*, **2**: 345–347.

Darmaillacq, A -S., Lesimple, C. and Dickel, L. (2008). Embryonic visual learning in the cuttlefish *Sepia officinalis*. *Animal Behaviour*, **76**: 131–134.

Davies, M. S. and Blackwell, J. (2007). Energy saving through trail following in a marine snail. *Proceedings of the Royal Society. B: Biological Sciences*, **274**: 1233–1236.

Dickel, L., Boal, J. G. and Budelmann, B. U. (2000). The effect of early experience on learning and memory in cuttlefish. *Developmental Psychobiology*, **36**: 101–110.

Dilly, P. N., Stephens, P. R. and Young, J. Z. (1975). Receptors in the statocyst of squids. *Journal of Physiology*, **249**: 59–61.

Dolins, F. L. and Mitchell, R. W. (2010). *Spatial cognition, spatial perception, mapping the self and space*. Cambridge, Cambridge University Press.

Dunn, G. A. (1990). Conceptual problems with kinesis and taxis. In *Biology of the Chemotactic Response*. Cambridge, Cambridge University Press, pp. 1–13.

Etienne, A. S., Maurer, R. and Séguinot, V. (1996). Path integration in mammals and its interaction with visual landmarks. *Journal of Experimental Biology*, **199**: 201–209.

Faraj, A. and Bez, N. (2007). Spatial considerations for the Dakhla stock of *Octopus vulgaris*: indicators, patterns, and fisheries interactions. *ICES Journal of Marine Science*, **64**: 1820–1828.

Forsythe, J. W. and Hanlon, R. T. (1997). Foraging and associated behavior by *Octopus cyanea* Gray, 1849 on a coral atoll, French Polynesia. *Journal of Experimental Marine Biology and Ecology*, **209**: 15–31.

Forsythe, J. W. and Toll, R. B. (1991). Clarification of the Western Atlantic Ocean pigmy octopus complex: the identity and life history of *Octopus joubini* (Cephalopoda: Octopodinae). *Bulletin of Marine Science*, **49**: 88–97.

Franz, M. O. and Mallot, H. A. (2000). Biomimetic robot navigation. *Robotics and Autonomous Systems*, **30**: 133–153.

Gabe, S. H. (1975). Reproduction in the giant octopus of the North Pacific, *Octopus dofleini martini*. *Veliger*, **18**: 146–150.

Gallistel, C. R. (1993). *The organization of learning*. Cambridge, MIT Press.

Gaulin, S. J. C. and FitzGerald, R. W. (1986). Sex differences in spatial ability: an evolutionary hypothesis and test. *The American Naturalist*, **127**: 77–88.

Gaulin, S. J. C. and FitzGerald, R. W. (1989). Sexual selection for spatial-learning ability. *Animal Behaviour*, **37**: 322–331.

Gibson, B. M. and Shettleworth, S. J. (2005). Place versus response learning revisited: tests of blocking on the radial maze. *Behavioral Neuroscience*, **119**: 567–586.

Gilly, W. F., Markaida, U., Baxter, C. H., et al. (2006). Vertical and horizontal migrations by the jumbo squid *Dosidicus gigas* revealed by electronic tagging. *Marine Ecology Progress Series*, **324**: 1–17.

Gleadall, I. G. and Shashar, N. (2004). The octopus's garden: the visual world of cephalopods. In *Complex worlds from simpler nervous systems*. Cambridge, MIT Press, pp. 269–307.

Golledge, R. G. (1999). *Wayfinding behavior: cognitive mapping and other spatial processes*. Baltimore, Johns Hopkins University Press.

Graziadei, P. (1964). Receptors in the sucker of the cuttlefish. *Nature*, **203**: 384–386.

Graziadei, P. P. C. and Gagne, H. T. (1976). Sensory innervation in the rim of the octopus sucker. *Journal of Morphology*, **150**: 639–679.

Groeger, G., Cotton, P. A. and Williamson, R. (2005). Ontogenetic changes in the visual acuity of *Sepia officinalis* measured using the optomotor response. *Canadian Journal of Zoology*, **83**: 274–279.

Guibé, M., Boal, J. G. and Dickel, L. (2010). Early exposure to odors changes late visual preferences in cuttlefish. *Developmental Psychobiology*, **52**: 833–837.

Hall, K. C. and Hanlon, R. T. (2002). Principal features of the mating system of a large spawning aggregation of the giant Australian cuttlefish *Sepia apama* (Mollusca: Cephalopoda). *Marine Biology*, **140**: 533–545.

Hanlon, R. T. and Budelmann, B. U. (1987). Why cephalopods are probably not "deaf." *The American Naturalist*, **129**: 312–317.

Hanlon, R. T. and Messenger, J. B. (1988). Adaptive coloration in young cuttlefish (*Sepia officinalis* L.): the morphology and development of body patterns and their relation to behaviour. *Philosophical Transactions of the Royal Society of London. Series B*, **320**: 437–487.

Hanlon, R. T. and Messenger, J. B. (1996). *Cephalopod behaviour*. Cambridge, Cambridge University Press.

Hartwick, E. B., Breen, P. A. and Tulloch, L. (1978). A removal experiment with *Octopus dofleini* (Wülker). *Journal of the Fisheries Research Board of Canada*, **35**: 1492–1495.

Hartwick, E. B., Ambrose, R. F. and Robinson, S. M. C. (1984). Den utilization and the movements of tagged *Octopus dofleini*. *Marine Behaviour and Physiology*, **11**: 95–110.

Healy, S. D. (1998). *Spatial representation in animals*. Oxford, Oxford University Press.

Heinze, S. and Homberg, U. (2007). Maplike representation of celestial *e*-vector orientations in the brain of an insect. *Science*, **315**: 995–997.

Hiroyuki, T. (2001). Tracking the neon flying squid by the biotelemetry system in the central North Pacific Ocean. *Aquabiology*, **23**: 533–539.

Horváth, G. and Varjú, D. (2004). *Polarized light in animal vision: polarization patterns in nature*. Berlin, Springer.

Hvorecny, L. M., Grudowski, J. L., Blakeslee, C. J., et al. (2007). Octopuses (*Octopus bimaculoides*) and cuttlefishes (*Sepia pharaonis*, *S. officinalis*) can conditionally discriminate. *Animal Cognition*, **10**: 449–459.

Ito, K. (2007). Studies on migration and causes of stock-size fluctuations in the northern Japanese population of spear squid, *Loligo bleekeri*. *Bulletin of Aomori Prefectural Fisheries Research Center*, **5**: 11–75.

Jander, R., Daumer, K. and Waterman, T. H. (1963). Polarized light orientation by two Hawaiian decapod cephalopods. *Zeitschrift für vergleichende Physiologie*, **46**: 383–394.

Jones, C. M., Braithwaite, V. A. and Healy, S. D. (2003). The evolution of sex differences in spatial ability. *Behavioral Neuroscience*, **117**: 403–411.

Jozet-Alves, C., Modéran, J. and Dickel, L. (2008). Sex differences in spatial cognition in an invertebrate: the cuttlefish. *Proceedings of the Royal Society. B: Biological Sciences*, **275**: 2049–2054.

Kaib, M., Bruinsma, O. and Leuthold, R. H. (1982). Trail-following in termites: evidence for a multicomponent system. *Journal of Chemical Ecology*, **8**: 1193–1205.

Kaneko, N., Oshima, Y. and Ikeda, Y. (2006). Egg brooding behavior and embryonic development of *Octopus laqueus* (Cephalopoda: Octopodidae). *Molluscan Research*, **26**: 113–117.

Karson, M. A. (2003). Simultaneous discrimination learning and its neural correlates in the cuttlefish *Sepia officinalis* (Cephalopoda: Mollusca). Doctoral dissertation. East Lansing, Michigan State University.

Karson, M. A., Boal, J. G. and Hanlon, R. T. (2003). Experimental evidence for spatial learning in cuttlefish (*Sepia officinalis*). *Journal of Comparative Psychology*, **117**: 149–155.

Kawabata, A., Yatsu, A., Ueno, Y., Suyama, S. and Kurita, Y. (2006). Spatial distribution of the Japanese common squid, *Todarodes pacificus*, during its northward migration in the western North Pacific Ocean. *Fisheries Oceanography*, **15**: 113–124.

Kayes, R. J. (1974). The daily activity pattern of *Octopus vulgaris* in a natural habitat. *Marine Behaviour and Physiology*, **2**: 337–343.

Kidokoro, H., Goto, T., Nagasawa, T., et al. (2010). Impact of a climate regime shift on the migration of Japanese common squid (*Todarodes pacificus*) in the Sea of Japan. *ICES Journal of Marine Science*, **67**: 1314–1322.

Kier, W. M., Messenger, J. B. and Miyan, J. A. (1985). Mechanoreceptors in the fins of the cuttlefish, *Sepia officinalis*. *Journal of Experimental Biology*, **119**: 369–373.

King, A. J., Adamo, S. A. and Hanlon, R. T. (2003). Squid egg mops provide sensory cues for increased agonistic behaviour between male squid. *Animal Behaviour*, **66**: 49–58.

Kiyofuji, H. and Saitoh, S. -I. (2004). Use of nighttime visible images to detect Japanese common squid *Todarodes pacificus* fishing areas and potential migration routes in the Sea of Japan. *Marine Ecology Progress Series*, **276**: 173–186.

Komak, S., Boal, J. G., Dickel, L. and Budelmann, B. U. (2005). Behavioural responses of juvenile cuttlefish (*Sepia officinalis*) to local water movements. *Marine and Freshwater Behaviour and Physiology*, **38**: 117–125.

Kraft, P., Evangelista, C., Dacke, M., Labhart, T. and Srinivasan, M. V. (2011). Honeybee navigation: following routes using polarized-light cues. *Philosophical Transactions of the Royal Society B*, **366**: 703–708.

Layne, J. E., Barnes, W. J. P. and Duncan, L. M. J. (2003). Mechanisms of homing in the fiddler crab *Uca rapax*. 2. Information sources and frame of reference for a path integration system. *Journal of Experimental Biology*, **206**: 4425–4442.

Lee, P. G. (1992). Chemotaxis by *Octopus maya* Voss et Solis in a Y-maze. *Journal of Experimental Marine Biology and Ecology*, **153**: 53–67.

Lerner, A., Sabbah, S., Erlick, C. and Shashar, N. (2011). Navigation by light polarization in clear and turbid waters. *Philosophical Transactions of the Royal Society of London. Series B*, **366**: 671–679.

Lohmann, K. J., Lohmann, C. M. F., Ehrhart, L.M., Bagley, D.A. and Swing, T. (2004). Animal behaviour: geomagnetic map used in sea-turtle navigation. *Nature*, **428**: 909–910.

Mackintosh, N. J. and Mackintosh, J. (1964). Performance of *Octopus* over a series of reversals of a simultaneous discrimination. *Animal Behaviour*, **12**: 321–324.

Marshall, N. J. and Cronin, T. W. (2011). Polarisation vision. *Current Biology*, **21**: R101–105.

Marshall, N. J. and Messenger, J. B. (1996). Colour-blind camouflage. *Nature*, **382**: 408–409.

Mather, J. A. (1988). Daytime activity of juvenile *Octopus vulgaris* in Bermuda. *Malacologia*, **29**: 69–76.

Mather, J. A. (1991a). Navigation by spatial memory and use of visual landmarks in octopuses. *Journal of Comparative Physiology A*, **168**: 491–497.

Mather, J. A. (1991b). Foraging, feeding and prey remains in middens of juvenile *Octopus vulgaris* (Mollusca: Cephalopoda). *Journal of Zoology*, **224**: 27–39.

Mather, J. A. (1994). "Home" choice and modification by juvenile *Octopus vulgaris* (Mollusca: Cephalopoda): specialized intelligence and tool use? *Journal of Zoology*, **233**: 359–368.

Mather, J. A. (1995). Cognition in cephalopods. *Advances in the Study of Behavior*, **24**: 317–353.

Mather, J. A. and Anderson, R. C. (1993). Personalities of octopuses (*Octopus rubescens*). *Journal of Comparative Psychology*, **107**: 336–340.

Mather, J. A. and O'Dor, R. K. (1991). Foraging strategies and predation risk shape the natural history of juvenile *Octopus vulgaris*. *Bulletin of Marine Science*, **49**: 256–269.

Mather, J. A., Resler, S. and Cosgrove, J. (1985). Activity and movement patterns of *Octopus dofleini*. *Marine Behavior and Physiology*, **11**: 301–314.

Mäthger, L. M., Barbosa, A., Miner, S. and Hanlon, R. T. (2006). Color blindness and contrast perception in cuttlefish (*Sepia officinalis*) determined by a visual sensorimotor assay. *Vision Research*, **46**: 1746–1753.

Messenger, J. B. (1970). Optomotor responses and nystagmus in intact, blinded and statocystless cuttlefish (*Sepia officinalis* L.). *Journal of Experimental Biology*, **53**: 789–796.

Messenger, J. B. (1991). Photoreception and vision in Mollusks. In *Evolution of the eye and visual system*. London, Macmillan, pp. 364–97.

Montgomery, J. C., Jeffs, A., Simpson, S. D., Meekan, M. and Tindle, C. (2006). Sound as an orientation cue for the pelagic larvae of reef fishes and decapod crustaceans. *Advances in Marine Biology*, **51**: 143–196.

Mooney, T. A., Hanlon, R. T., Christensen-Dalsgaard, J., et al. (2010). Sound detection by the longfin squid (*Loligo pealeii*) studied with auditory evoked potentials: sensitivity to low-frequency particle motion and not pressure. *Journal of Experimental Biology*, **213**: 3748–3759.

Moore, P. A., Scholz, N. and Atema, J. (1991). Chemical orientation of lobsters, *Homarus americanus*, in turbulent odor plumes. *Journal of Chemical Ecology*, **17**: 1293–1307.

Moreno, A., Dos Santos, A., Piatkowski, U., Santos, M. P. and Cabral, H. (2009). Distribution of cephalopod paralarvae in relation to the regional oceanography of the western Iberia. *Journal of Plankton Research*, **31**: 73–91.

Moriyama, T. and Gunji, Y. -P. (1997). Autonomous learning in maze solution by *Octopus*. *Ethology*, **103**: 499–513.

Müller, M. and Wehner, R. (1988). Path integration in desert ants, *Cataglyphis fortis*. *Proceedings of the National Academy of Sciences of the United States of America*, **85**: 5287–5290.

Murata, M. and Nakamura, Y. (1998). Seasonal migration and diel vertical migration of the neon flying squid, *Ommastrephes bartramii* in the North Pacific. In *Contributed papers to international symposium on large pelagic squids, July 18–19, 1996, for JAMARC's 25th anniversary of its foundation*. Tokyo, JAMARC, pp. 13–30.

Nixon, M. and Young, J. Z. (2003). *The brains and lives of cephalopods*. Oxford, Oxford University Press.

O'Dor, R. K., Hoar, J. A., Webber, D. M., et al. (1994). Squid (*Loligo forbesi*) performance and metabolic rates in nature. *Marine and Freshwater Behaviour and Physiology*, **25**: 163–177.

O'Dor, R. K., Adamo, S., Aitken, J.P., et al. (2002). Currents as environmental constraints on the behavior, energetics and distribution of squid and cuttlefish. *Bulletin of Marine Science*, **71**: 601–617.

O'Keefe, J. and Nadel, L. (1978). *The hippocampus as a cognitive map*. Oxford, Oxford University Press.

Olson, R. J. and Young, J. W. (Eds.) (2007). *The role of squid in open ocean ecosystems. Report of the GLOBEC-CLIOTOP/PFRP workshop, 16–17 November 2006. GLOBEC Report 24: VI*. Honolulu, Hawaii, GLOBEC.

Olyott, L. J. H., Sauer, W. H. H. and Booth, A. J. (2007). Spatial patterns in the biology of the chokka squid, *Loligo reynaudii* on the Agulhas Bank, South Africa. *Reviews in Fish Biology and Fisheries*, **17**: 159–172.

Onitsuka, G., Hirose, N., Miyahara, K., et al. (2010). Numerical simulation of the migration and distribution of diamond squid (*Thysanoteuthis rhombus*) in the southwest Sea of Japan. *Fisheries Oceanography*, **19**: 63–75.

Oosthuizen, A., Jiwaji, M. and Shaw, P. (2004). Genetic analysis of the *Octopus vulgaris* population on the coast of South Africa. *South African Journal of Science*, **100**: 603–607.

Payne, N. L., Semmens, J. M. and Gillanders, B. M. (2011). Elemental uptake via immersion: a mass-marking technique for the early life-history stages of cephalopods. *Marine Ecology Progress Series*, **436**: 169–176.

Pecl, G. T., Doubleday, Z. A., Danyushevsky, L., Gilbert, S. and Moltschaniwskyj, N. A. (2010). Transgenerational marking of cephalopods with an enriched barium isotope: a promising tool for empirically estimating post-hatching movement and population connectivity. *ICES Journal of Marine Science*, **67**: 1372–1380.

Pérez-Losada, M., Guerra, A., Carvalho, G. R., Sanjuan, A. and Shaw, P. W. (2002). Extensive population subdivision of the cuttlefish *Sepia officinalis* (Mollusca: Cephalopoda) around the Iberian Peninsula indicated by microsatellite DNA variation. *Heredity*, **89**: 417–424.

Pérez-Losada, M., Nolte, M. J., Crandall, K. A. and Shaw, P. W. (2007). Testing hypotheses of population structuring in the Northeast Atlantic Ocean and Mediterranean Sea using the common cuttlefish *Sepia officinalis*. *Molecular Ecology*, **16**: 2667–2679.

Pierce, G. J., Valavanis, V. D., Guerra, A., et al. (2008). A review of cephalopod-environment interactions in European seas. *Hydrobiologia*, **612**: 49–70.

Reale, D., Reader, S. M., Sol, D., McDougall, P. T. and Dingemanse, N. J. (2007). Integrating animal temperament within ecology and evolution. *Biological Reviews*, **82**: 291–318.

Reichow, D. and Smith, M. J. (2001). Microsatellites reveal high levels of gene flow among populations of the California squid *Loligo opalescens*. *Molecular Ecology*, **10**: 1101–1109.

Restle, F. (1957). Discrimination of cues in mazes: a resolution of the "place-vs.-response" question. *Psychological Review*, **64**: 217–228.

Rosa, R. and Seibel, B. A. (2010). Metabolic physiology of the Humboldt squid, *Dosidicus gigas*: implications for vertical migration in a pronounced oxygen minimum zone. *Progress in Oceanography*, **86**: 72–80.

Saidel, W. M., Lettvin, J. Y. and McNichol, E. F. (1983). Processing of polarized light by squid photoreceptors. *Nature*, **304**: 534–536.

Sakaguchi, K. (2010). Migration of tagged Japanese common squid, *Todarodes pacificus*, in waters around Hokkaido [Japan]. *Scientific Reports of Hokkaido Fisheries Experimental Station*, **77**: 45–72.

Sanders F. K. and Young, J. Z. (1940). Learning and other functions of the higher nervous centres of *Sepia*. *Journal of Neurophysiology*, **3**: 501–526.

Sauer, W. H., Roberts, M. J., Lipinski, M. R., et al. (1997). Choreography of the squid's "nuptial dance." *The Biological Bulletin*, **192**: 203–207.

Save, E., Poucet, B. and Thinus-Blanc, C. (1998). Landmark use and the cognitive map in the rat. In *Spatial representation in animals*. Oxford, Oxford University Press, pp. 119–132.

Schiller, P. H. (1949). Delayed detour response in the octopus. *Journal of Comparative and Physiological Psychology*, **42**: 220–225.

Schmajuk, N. A. and Thieme, A. D. (1992). Purposive behavior and cognitive mapping: a neural network model. *Biological Cybernetics*, **67**: 165–174.

Scholz, A. T., Horrall, R. M., Cooper, J. C. and Hasler, A. D. (1976). Imprinting to chemical cues: the basis for home stream selection in salmon. *Science*, **192**: 1247–1249.

Semmens, J. M., Pecl, G. T., Gillanders, B. M., et al. (2007). Approaches to resolving cephalopod movement and migration patterns. *Reviews in Fish Biology and Fisheries*, **17**: 401–423.

Shashar, N., Rutledge, P. S. and Cronin, T. W. (1996). Polarization vision in cuttlefish in a concealed communication channel? *Journal of Experimental Biology*, **199**: 2077–2084.

Shashar, N., Hagan, R., Boal, J. G. and Hanlon, R. T. (2000). Cuttlefish use polarization sensitivity in predation on silvery fish. *Vision Research*, **40**: 71–75.

Shaw, P. W., Pierce, G. J. and Boyle, P. R. (1999). Subtle population structuring within a highly vagile marine invertebrate, the veined squid *Loligo forbesi*, demonstrated with microsatellite DNA markers. *Molecular Ecology*, **8**: 407–417.

Shea, E. K. and Vecchione, M. (2010). Ontogenic changes in diel vertical migration patterns compared with known allometric changes in three mesopelagic squid species suggest an expanded definition of a paralarva. *ICES Journal of Marine Science*, **67**: 1436–1443.

Shettleworth, S. J. (2010). *Cognition, evolution and behavior*, 2nd edn. Oxford, Oxford University Press.

Sims, D. W., Genner, M. J., Southward, A. J. and Hawkins, S. J. (2001). Timing of squid migration reflects North Atlantic climate variability. *Proceedings of the Royal Society. B: Biological Sciences*, **268**: 2607–2611.

Sinn, D. L. and Moltschaniwskyj, N. A. (2005). Personality traits in dumpling squid (*Euprymna tasmanica*): context-specific traits and their correlation with biological characteristics. *Journal of Comparative Physiology*, **119**: 99–110.

Sinn, D. L., Moltschaniwskyj, N. A., Wapstra, E. and Dall, S. R. X. (2010). Are behavioral syndromes invariant? Spatiotemporal variation in shy/bold behavior in squid. *Behavioral Ecology and Sociobiology*, **64**: 693–702.

Stamps, J. A. (2007). Growth-mortality tradeoffs and "personality traits" in animals. *Ecology Letters*, **10**: 355–363.

Stark, K. E. (2008). Ecology of the arrow squid (*Nototodarus gouldi*) in Southeastern Australian waters: a multi-scale investigation of spatial and temporal variability. PhD thesis, Tasmania, University of Tasmania.

Sutherland, N. S., Mackintosh, N. J. and Mackintosh, J. (1963). Simultaneous discrimination training of *Octopus* and transfer of discrimination along a continuum. *Journal of Comparative and Physiological Psychology*, **56**: 150–156.

Tansley, K. (1965). *Vision in vertebrates*. London, Chapman and Hall.

Tinbergen, N. (1972). *The animal in its world*. Cambridge, MA, Harvard University Press.

Tolimieri, N., Haine, O., Jeffs, A., McCauley, R. and Montgomery, J. (2004). Directional orientation of pomacentrid larvae to ambient reef sound. *Coral Reefs*, **23**: 184–191.

Van Heukelem, W. F. (1966). Some aspects of the ecology and ethology of *Octopus cyanea* Gray. MS thesis. Honolulu, University of Hawaii.

Villanueva, R. (1992). Deep-sea cephalopods of the north-western Mediterranean: indications of up-slope ontogenetic migration in two bathybenthic species. *Journal of Zoology*, **227**: 267–276.

Villanueva, R. and Norman, M. D. (2008). Biology of the planktonic stages of benthic octopuses. *Oceanography and Marine Biology*, **46**: 105–202.

Walderon, M. D., Nolt, K. J., Haas, R. E., et al. (2011). Distance chemoreception and the detection of conspecifics in *Octopus bimaculoides*. *Journal of Molluscan Studies*, **77**: 309–311.

Walker, J. J., Longo, N. and Bitterman, M. E. (1970). The octopus in the laboratory. Handling, maintenance, training. *Behavior Research Methods and Instrumentation*, **2**: 15–18.

Wang, J., Pierce, G. J., Boyle, P. R., et al. (2003). Spatial and temporal patterns of cuttlefish (*Sepia officinalis*) abundance and environmental influences – a case study using trawl fishery data in French Atlantic coastal, English Channel, and adjacent waters. *ICES Journal of Marine Science*, **60**: 1149–1158.

Warburton, K. (1990). The use of local landmarks by foraging goldfish. *Animal Behaviour*, **40**: 500–505.

Watanabe, H., Kubodera, T., Moku, M. and Kawaguchi, K. (2006). Diel vertical migration of squid in the warm core ring and cold water masses in the transition region of the western North Pacific. *Marine Ecology Progress Series*, **315**: 187–197.

Waterman, T. H. (2006). Reviving a neglected celestial underwater polarization compass for aquatic animals. *Biological Reviews*, **81**: 111–115.

Wehner, R. (2003). Desert ant navigation: how miniature brains solve complex tasks. *Journal of Comparative Physiology A*, **189**: 579–588.

Wehner, R., Lehrer, M., Harvey, W. R. (1996). Navigation. *Journal of Experimental Biology*, **199**: 1–261.

Wells, M. J. (1964). Detour experiments with octopuses. *Journal of Experimental Biology*, **41**: 621–642.

Wells, M. J. (1978). *Octopus: physiology and behaviour of an advanced invertebrate*. London, Chapman and Hall.

Willows, A. O. D. (1999). Shoreward orientation involving geomagnetic cues in the nudibranch mollusc *Tritonia diomedea*. *Marine and Freshwater Behaviour and Physiology*, **32**: 181–192.

Winklhofer, M. (2009). The physics of geomagnetic-field transduction in animals. *IEEE Transactions on Magnetics*, **45**: 5259–5265.

Yarnall, J. L. (1969). Aspects of the behaviour of *Octopus cyanea* Gray. *Animal Behaviour*, **17**: 747–754.

Yatsu, A., Yamanaka, K.and Yamashiro, C. (1999). Tracking experiments of the jumbo flying squid, *Dosidicus gigas*, with an ultrasonic telemetry system in the Eastern Pacific Ocean. *Bulletin of the National Research Institute of Far Seas Fisheries*, **36**: 55–60.

Young, J. Z. (1960). The statocysts of *Octopus vulgaris*. *Proceedings of the Royal Society. B: Biological Sciences*, **152**: 3–29.

Young, M. A., Kvitek, R. G., Iampietro, P. J., et al. (2011). Seafloor mapping and landscape ecology analyses used to monitor variations in spawning site preference and benthic egg mop abundance for the California market squid (*Doryteuthis opalescens*). *Journal of Experimental Marine Biology and Ecology*, **407**: 226–233.

Young, R. E. and Harman, R. F. (1988). "Larva," "paralarva," and "subadult" in cephalopod terminology. *Malacologia*, **29**: 201–207.

Zeidberg, L. D. and Robison, B. H. (2007). Invasive range expansion by the Humboldt squid, *Dosidicus gigas*, in the eastern North Pacific. *Proceedings of the National Academy of Sciences of the United States of America*, **104**: 12948–12950.

Zumholz, K., Klügel, A., Hansteen, T. and Piatkowski, U. (2007). Statolith microchemistry traces the environmental history of the boreoatlantic armhook squid *Gonatus fabricii*. *Marine Ecology Progress Series*, **333**: 195–204.

8 Camouflage in benthic cephalopods: what does it teach us?

Noam Josef and Nadav Shashar

8.1 Brief historical review

Neither the scientist nor the curious diver can remain impassive after witnessing an octopus camouflaging itself in a reef. Intriguing, beautiful and efficient camouflagers, cephalopods can produce thousands of different patterns (Packard, 1972; Packard & Hochberg, 1977; Hanlon, 1982; Moynihan, 1985; Hanlon & Messenger, 1988, 1996; reviewed in Borrelli, Fiorito & Gherardi, 2006).

Cephalopods are an ancient group dating from the upper Cambrian. Although they are mollusks, coleoid cephalopods present an extraordinary resemblance to teleosts in morphology, physiology, ecology and behavior (Packard, 1972; Hanlon & Messenger, 1996). A variety of physiological structures, crafted by evolution, enables cephalopods to change their body patterning continuously and rapidly, conferring on them the cryptic, communicative and aesthetically appealing characteristics typical of this group. The ability of octopuses, cuttlefish and squid to quickly and dramatically change their appearance has thrilled scientists from antiquity (Aristotle 350 BCE; Darwin, 1870; Parker, 1948). Like many past researchers who witnessed their amazing displays, movements and behaviors, we, too, have been captivated. Throughout this chapter, we use the word "cephalopod" to refer to the benthic coleoid cephalopod taxa. However, the reader should bear in mind that many pelagic coleoids are also capable of remarkable changes in body patterning that may be similarly important in camouflage (e.g. Bush, Robison & Caldwell, 2009; Zylinski & Johnsen, 2011).

8.2 Definitions and nomenclature

Camouflage is the common term describing the capacity of an animal to disguise itself and avoid detection by visual seekers. The term crypsis (Endler, 1981) includes behavioral as well as morphological strategies to prevent detection. Although easy to understand, the concepts of camouflage and concealment are difficult to define and quantify. As many as 15 different mechanisms and definitions can be found in the literature. Some mechanisms operate synergistically and, as such, it is likely that some phenomena would

Cephalopod Cognition, eds A.-S. Darmaillacq, L. Dickel and J. Mather. Published by Cambridge University Press. © Cambridge 2014.

Table 8.1 Commonly used camouflage terminology (modified after Stevens & Merilaita, 2009)

Term	Definition
Camouflage	All concealment strategies, including prevention of detection and recognition
Crypsis	Initially preventing detection
(a) Background matching	Appearance generally matches the color, lightness and pattern of one (specialist) or several (compromise) background types
(b) Self-shadow concealment	Elimination or concealment of shadows that are created by directional light, occasionally achieved by countershading
(c) Obliterate shading	Countershading leads to the obliteration of three-dimensional form
(d) Disruptive coloration	A set of markings that creates the appearance of false edges and boundaries and hinders the detection or recognition of either part or all of an object's true outline or shape
(e) Flicker-fusion camouflage	Markings such as stripes blur during motion to match the color/lightness of the general background, preventing detection of the animal when in motion
(f) Distractive markings	Direct the "attention" or gaze of the receiver from traits that would give away the animal (such as the outline)
Motion camouflage	Movement in a fashion that decreases the probability of movement detection
Motion dazzle	Markings complicate receiver estimation of speed and trajectory
Masquerade	Resemblance to an uninteresting object, such as a leaf or a stick
Countershading (Thayer's Law)	Using dark dorsal coloration or light ventral colors or photophores for concealment by matching overall brightness. When viewed from above, the animal has the backdrop of dark, deep waters; in the opposite perspective, the animal is viewed against brighter downwelling light, which ventral photoluminescent organs can match
Silvering	Common in aquatic environments and where an animal's body is highly reflective making it difficult to detect when light incidence is non-directional (such as due to strong scattering by waterborne particles)
Transparency	Animal's body (or a part of it) is transparent, reducing detection; like a hood

be best described by a combination of several terms. To clarify this somewhat confusing use of terms and guide the reader, Table 8.1 contains the terms and definitions used in this chapter.

With predator avoidance as an evolutionary driving force, camouflage has generated some classic examples of selection (e.g. the peppered moth; Bacot, 1907). Therefore, since predators tend to select conspicuous individuals during their search for prey, good camouflage can be defined as the phenotypic appearance of the survivor. Nonetheless, one should note that animals also use warning colors that are deliberately conspicuous to their predators (e.g. Cronin, 2005).

Existent in amazing variety, camouflage can be found in distant phylogenetic groups, from flatworms and insects to reptiles and mammals. But its manifestation in cephalopods is exceptional not only in the speed with which they can match their visual backgrounds, but also in the diversity of colors and patterns they can express.

8.3   Dynamic versus static camouflage

While most animals exhibit fixed or slowly changing, "static camouflage" patterns (Stevens & Merilaita, 2011), the "dynamic camouflage" of cephalopods describes their ability to rapidly change their patterns, color and even texture to match the background on which they are found.

The avoidance of visual detection by predators or by prey has driven the creation of outstanding adaptations. Examples of amazing camouflage can be found throughout the marine environment, including markings to match color, pattern and brightness of the background (e.g. stonefish, *Synanceia* sp.) and Disruptive coloration that disturbs the visual appearance of the outline of the body (e.g. some marine isopods, Merilaita, 1998) as well as the capacity of some fish to resemble sea-grass leaves and the sand-like skin patterns possessed by others (Figure 8.1a–d). Camouflage achieves even greater efficiency, however, in the dynamic coloration found in some cephalopods (Hanlon & Messenger, 1988) and chameleons (Stuart-Fox & Moussalli, 2008).

Either type of camouflage, dynamic or static, entails a particular set of strategies and behaviors the camouflaged individual uses to decrease detection, including remaining motionless (Eilam, 2005), selecting a suitable body position and changing its orientation according the ambient light conditions (Barbosa, Allen, Mäthger & Hanlon, 2012). What distinguishes dynamic from static camouflage, however, is the ability of animals with the former to match and therefore occupy a wide range of distinct visual environments. For example, imagine a flatfish (e.g. the Moses sole, *Pardachirus mormoratus*) with its slow-changing Mottle pattern lying on the sandy sea bed, where it is well camouflaged (Figure 8.1d). Viewed against a stony reef or a seagrass patch, however, the flatfish would be vulnerable to visual detection. In contrast, picture the same scenario with the common octopus (*Octopus vulgaris*). A change in its visual environment does not render the octopus conspicuous, as it can remain cryptic against different backgrounds. The flexibility and phenotypic plasticity of dynamic camouflage enable animals that possess it to forage in a variety of habitats without increasing its risk of predation. Likewise, predators that use static camouflage behavior when hunting are restricted to environments in which they will both remain cryptic and also have a high probability of encountering prey. Thus, the dynamically camouflaging animal can find the most advantageous location for predation and adjust its body pattern according to its surroundings.

The function of dynamic coloration is not restricted to camouflage: inter- and intraspecific communication via body pattern changes is common in cephalopods (Hanlon & Messenger, 1996; Hall & Hanlon, 2002; Langridge, Broom & Osorio, 2007). Since camouflaging and communicating have opposite functions but are carried out by the same mechanism, a camouflaged individual should either signal within a certain range

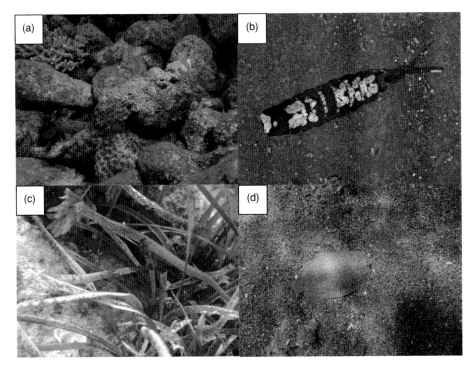

Figure 8.1 Camouflage examples in marine animals. (a) A stone fish, *Synanceia verrucosa* choosing a place to settle which matches its body pattern. (b) An isopod: displaying Disruptive coloration. (c) A Posidonia pipefish, *Syngnathus* sp. using object resemblance in hiding between seagrass leafs. (d) A Moses sole, *Pardachirus mormoratus* showing a static Mottle pattern; note partial missmatch with such a static camouflage. See plate section for color version.

of color variations or avoid the simultaneous expression of communication behavior to its conspecifics.

The main organs involved in the coleoid cephalopod's camouflaging process are the chromatophore, iridophore and leucophore cells and the complex nervous system that controls them (Boycott, 1953; Hanlon & Messenger, 1996; reviewed in Messenger, 2001; Chrachri & Williamson, 2004). Chromatophores are small, elastic saccules of pigment that reflect mainly the long-wavelength section of visible spectrum (i.e. black, brown, red, orange, etc.). During camouflaging behavior, they are expanded by the contraction of up to 24 radially arranged muscle fibers pulling the pigment sac open. The relaxation of these muscles causes the chromatophore wall to contract, thereby reducing the area visually affected by the pigment sac (Florey & Kriebel, 1969; Messenger, 2001).

Below the chromatophores lie the iridophores, which form a distinct, bright layer. Iridophore cells are themselves colorless, but they provide structural color (e.g. iridescence) via wave-length-specific reflectivity for short-wave coloration (e.g. blues and purples) in cephalopods. Iridophores are also found in the wall of the ink sac, testis and on the eye (Arnold, 1967).

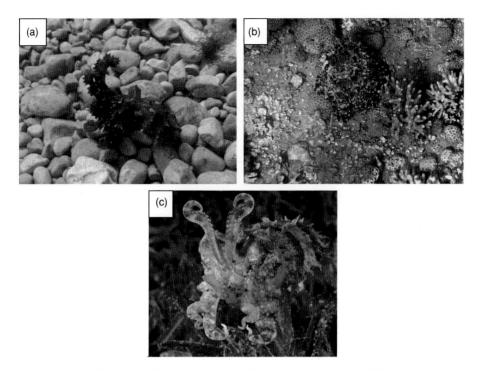

Figure 8.2 Skin spikiness in (a) *Octopus vulgaris*, (b) *Octopus cyanea* and (c) *Sepia prashadi*. Physical texture of the skin through the expression of papillae helps creating a Disruptive appearance, breaking the general outline of the animal.

The flattened leucophore cells act as diffuse reflectors and are responsible for the "white spots" seen in many cephalopods, produced by reflecting all wavelengths of scattered light (Cloney & Brocco, 1983). Leucophores, iridophores and other structures reflect the chromatic characteristics of the local light field, possibly allowing for partial color matching by passive means (Hanlon & Messenger, 1996). This may explain how cephalopods are able to match the colors around them without being able to perceive them (Mäthger, Shashar & Hanlon, 2009). Most cephalopod species so far investigated possess a single mid-wavelength visual pigment in their eyes, meaning they are effectively color-blind (Messenger, 1977; Marshall & Messenger, 1996; reviewed in Hanlon & Messenger, 1996).

In addition to the ability to alter their body patterning, many cephalopods can change the physical texture of their skin using papillae to give their skin appearances that can range from completely smooth to very spiky (Hanlon & Messenger, 1988; Allen, Mäthger, Barbosa & Hanlon, 2009). Combined with body posture, physical texture can give the animal a unique appearance (often similar to the textural attributes of its immediate surroundings), probably complicating shape-oriented searches by potential predators (Figure 8.2a–c).

8.4   Neural physiology

Controlling a complex assembly of chromatic skin cells for single-unit functionality requires a unique and precise neural control system. Electrophysiological, anatomical and behavioral studies showed that the control system is hierarchically organized (Nixon & Young, 2003). Hanlon and Messenger (1996) proposed a simplified outline of this complex system:

Eye → Optic lobe → Lateral basal lobe → Chromatophore lobe → Skin.

Anyone who has observed an octopus camouflaging or a squid signaling is probably familiar with the bilateral presentation of color on its skin (see Hanlon & Messenger, 1996 for examples). This is consistent with a bilateral organization of the system, in which each side of the body is neurally controlled by the same side of the brain (and eye). The nerve cells run, with or without limited synapses in the stellate ganglion, directly to the chromatophore muscles (Sereni & Young, 1932). Such direct neural control has several advantages:

1. Speed: entire body pattern can be altered in less than a second.
2. Continuity: as an animal moves, the environment is constantly changing around it. This system has the potential to match body pattern, color and brightness to the background at any given moment.
3. High resolution: the ability to present highly detailed expressions of patterns and texture through the precise control of fine chromatic units.
4. Polyphenism: the ability to present a wide variety of different patterns (see ethograms in Hanlon & Messenger, 1988, 1996; Hanlon, Forsythe & Joneschild, 1999).
5. Independent bilaterality: an individual may present a different pattern on each side of its body (e.g. an agonistic display on one side and a camouflage pattern on the other).
6. Stability: independent neurological control means that other motor activities do not interfere with the chromatic signals.

8.5   Body patterns

The speed, variability and complexity of cephalopod body patterning constitute an evolutionary survival strategy that is nothing less than extraordinary. The term polyphenism has been used to describe the use of multiple appearances by an individual (Mayr, 1963), and it has been proposed that this adaptation may inhibit a predator's ability to form a search image (Curio, 1976). Most coleoid cephalopods can produce around 12 body patterns (Borrelli, Fiorito & Gherardi, 2006) whose classification is at best difficult. Each body pattern comprises a combination of chromatic, textural, postural and locomotor components (Packard & Sanders, 1969; Packard & Hochberg, 1977; reviewed in Hanlon & Messenger 1996). In an effort to classify the large number of patterns, Hanlon and co-workers categorized body patterns into three main groups: Uniform, Mottled and Disruptive (Hanlon & Messenger, 1988; Hanlon et al., 2009). The simplicity of this classification has helped researchers study processes involved in camouflage and perception using new methodologies (such as image analysis) while still supporting older ethological research. However, although the findings of Hanlon and others are appealing and persuasive, a degree of uncertainty remains as many body patterns do not fall clearly into one of these categories. Furthermore, exploiting such a generalized classification system may prevent us from noticing subtle variations in body-pattern responses to a given stimulus.

8.6   Camouflage complexities

No simple task for an active cephalopod, maintaining camouflage appears to require continual visual data streaming, a color-changing mechanism, texture assessment and the ability to make predictions. For example, the immediate surroundings in which octopuses live are often heterogeneous. Vegetation, light, terrain (whether corals, gravel or sand are visible), color, texture, brightness and contrast are all subject to spatial and temporal variation. Consequently, the body patterns needed for effective concealment are equally diverse and the task of matching a specific background object is complex (Shohet, Baddeley, Anderson, Kelman & Osorio, 2006). Indeed, a camouflaging cephalopod is confronted with a set of problems and a variety of options with which to solve them:

Target species: Camouflage can be designed to hinder detection by a single species or even a specific individual. This may be especially true when a predator must prevent its detection by a specific prey. In some cases this may also involve avoiding raising the alarm in other members of the prey's group or in nearby species. The predator may need to consider the specific line of sight and field of view of the prey, the capacity of its visual system, its level of attention, and so on, to remain camouflaged. However, the situation is different for the animal exploiting camouflage to avoid detection by predators. Cephalopods are preyed upon by a wide range of animals such as fish, marine mammals and birds. Each of these predators is equipped with its own sensory (visual) system, mode of search and direction of approach. Therefore, a camouflaging cephalopod cannot limit itself to a single strategy to prevent detection (e.g. using slow motion to fool motion detectors), but instead it must avoid detection by any potential predator. Nonetheless, cuttlefish and octopuses are known to ignore previously conceived threats once it has been established that they are not under attack.

Orientation: Because a cephalopod cannot predict the position of potential predators, its camouflage pattern needs to be effective from all orientations.

Point-of-view predicament: Since there is a difference in the position of the prey/ predator and the camouflaging animal, the latter has to match itself to a background seen from a point of view it does not have (Figure 8.3). For example, if the octopus is located mostly on the seabed while the predator is located in the water column, the octopus has to match the scene as seen from above. This requires the camouflaging animal to match its surroundings as they appear from above.

General versus specific resemblance: A cephalopod may either match the general properties of its visual surroundings or it may mimic a specific object in its immediate

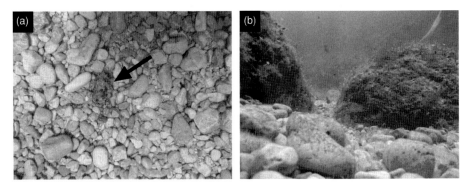

Figure 8.3 The point of view predicament: (a) Top-down view of a camouflaged *Octopus vulgaris* among bright pebbles. The octopus is marked with an arrow. (b) The same scene mentioned in (a) from the octopus's point of view.

surroundings. Neither strategy has proven superior to the other; therefore, both are widely used by cephalopods and in the greater animal kingdom.

Texture assessments: Imitating algae, coral, sand or rock, sometimes from a substantial distance from the objective, requires the cephalopod to visually assess the three-dimensional texture of its background, possibly based on previous interactions with it (Allen, Mäthger, Barbosa & Hanlon, 2009).

Color assessments: The physical lack of color perception promoted cephalopod development of the creative solution (as yet unexplained) of background matching. Color matching, which could be based as much on texture recognition as on the reflection of the animal's surroundings by its reflecting cells, remains one of the most intriguing mysteries of cephalopod camouflage.

Matching feedback: The body pattern used by a cephalopod needs to match that perceived by its visual system of its background. It would be useful (but not vital) for the animal to be able to verify that indeed it is producing a matching pattern. No such self-feedback mechanism has yet been reported (but see Hanlon & Messenger, 1988 and Allen, Mäthger, Barbosa & Hanlon, 2009, for a putative feedback path).

8.7   Camouflage limitations

The defensive behaviors of many animals fall into three categories: freezing, fleeing and fighting (Eilam, 2005). No single category alone provides an effective means of defense, and combinations of defensive behaviors that may increase the survival rate of the individual are limited (Eilam, 2005). Indeed, these categories set possible limitations on camouflage, rendering the animal, under some conditions, unable to camouflage or causing it to abandon camouflage altogether as a tactic.

Freezing is an important part in the behavior of hiding animals because most animals are very sensitive to motion in their visual fields (Land & Nilsson, 2002). For example, moving objects are often detected by the peripheral vision while a stable object goes unnoticed. Once an animal has frozen in place, it can constantly monitor the distance and activity of the target (predator or prey). If a frozen individual assumes it has been detected nonetheless, it may execute a conspicuous display (possibly as a warning or a declaration of recognition) followed by fleeing or fighting behavior (Eilam, 2005; see Hanlon, Forsythe & Joneschild, 1999 – accompanying video http://hermes.mbl.edu/mrc/hanlon/video.html for an example in octopus). Since an animal cannot freeze and flee simultaneously, these defenses are mutually exclusive and are often controlled by different motor systems (Canteras, 2002; Lamprea et al., 2002; Blanchard et al., 2003; Brandao, Troncoso, Silva & Huston, 2003; Comoli, Ribeiro-Barbosa & Canteras, 2003; Barros, Silva, Huston & Tomaz, 2004).

Movement is an obvious limitation for camouflage in animals in fleeing or chasing mode. Due to the high sensitivity of most visual systems to movement and changes in the image presented to the retina, it is likely that a fast moving animal cannot stay camouflaged. Indeed fast moving, fleeing, chasing and attacking cephalopods lose their cryptic appearance and often present a distinct pattern (Borrelli, Fiorito & Gherardi, 2006). However, cephalopods in motion are able to partially maintain crypsis while moving slowly over areas of reef or sand (Hanlon, Forsythe & Joneschild, 1999; Mather & Mather, 2004; Langridge, Broom & Osorio, 2007).

8.8 Communication and courtship

Communication requires that the signaler reveal its existence to other animals in its vicinity. In the case of visual communication this often results in camouflage being broken. Cephalopods have partially solved this limitation by two means. First, many taxa employ directional displays in the form of bilaterally asymmetrical patterns, allowing them to display a conspicuous pattern to potential mates on one side of the body while maintaining a camouflage pattern on the other (Hanlon & Messenger, 1996; Langridge, 2006). Second, by using discrete communication channels, signals are visible to conspecifics but not to most potential predators (Shashar, Rutledge & Cronin, 1996). Many cephalopod species can produce partly linearly polarized patterns on their body, which can be seen only by polarization sensitive animals, such as themselves (Cronin, Shashar & Wolff, 1995; Shashar, Rutledge & Cronin, 1996; Mäthger & Hanlon, 2006; Talbot & Marshall, 2010; Temple et al., 2012). This may allow a communicating animal to remain cryptic to polarization insensitive animals while communicating with its conspecifics. Despite the research efforts that have been invested in cephalopod behavior, however, the function of the polarization patterns is not yet fully understood (Boal et al., 2004; Mäthger, Shashar & Hanlon, 2009).

8.9 Quantifying camouflage

The challenge of measuring and quantifying camouflage is studied in a range of fields, such as image analysis, light spectrometry and animal behavior (Gretzmacher,

Table 8.2 Image parameters used to determine cuttlefish body patterns while camouflaged

Species studied	Parameters tested	Citation
Sepia officinalis	Contrast and object size	Barbosa et al. (2008)
Sepia officinalis	Edges and contrast	Chiao, Kelman and Hanlon (2005)
Sepia officinalis	Edge completion	Zylinski, Osorio, and Shohet (2009); Zylinski, Darmaillacq, and Shashar (2012)
Sepia pharaonis	Area of light objects in the substrate	Chiao and Hanlon (2001b)
Sepia officinalis	Contrast, intensity and configuration of small light elements	Chiao, Chubb, and Hanlon (2007)
Sepia pharaonis	Size, contrast and number of white squares	Chiao and Hanlon (2001a)
Sepia officinalis	Scaling	Chiao, Chubb, Buresch, Siemann, and Hanlon (2009)
Sepia officinalis	Localized visual edges	Kelman, Baddeley, Shohet and Osorio (2007)
Sepia officinalis	Granularity	Chiao et al. (2010)
Sepia officinalis	Relative size of objects in comparison to self body size	Hanlon and Messenger (1988)

Ruppert & Nyberg, 1998; Reynolds, 2011). The analysis of cryptic body patterns depends first on how we define the camouflage patterns. Trying to do so, the intricate camouflage phenomenon has been untangled into its constituent parts to figure out which environmental characteristics are reflected in the animal's body patterns (Table 8.2). For a number of cephalopod species, ethograms (Hanlon, Watson & Barbosa, 2010; Mather, Griebel & Byrne, 2010), which provide detailed catalogues of body patterns, postures and behaviors, have been devised. But lacking a numerical, measurable element, an ethogram is a dry inventory of the appearances and behaviors exhibited by a species. Another approach is to rank the strength of body pattern components used in camouflage responses as perceived by human observations (e.g. Hanlon, Forsythe & Joneschild, 1999; Barbosa et al., 2007). For example, Hanlon, Forsythe and Joneschild (1999) asked observers to rank the brightness, color, shape and skin patterning of foraging octopuses. Scores were used to quantify polyphenism and cryptic behavior and to assess camouflage. Although such methods are useful in determining how cephalopods themselves perceive their visual environment, an unbiased process that minimizes the human perspective is preferable to assess how effective body patterns are against detection by predators.

In recent years, the quest for objective examination has led to the development of automatic methods that rely on unbiased mathematical approaches (Zylinski, How, Osorio, Hanlon & Marshall, 2011; Josef, Amodio, Fiorito & Shashar, 2012). As such, they score the strength of individual components, elucidating which aspects of the pattern are influenced by different visual parameters. But this approach, too, suffers the same limitation as the subjective measures, in that it is suitable for exploring the animal's perception of its environment as opposed to evaluating the effectiveness of the pattern used. Image, spectrum and video analyses have facilitated new approaches that are superior to traditional methods in terms of speed, accuracy and objectivity. The downside of such objective methods is that they reduce the phenomenon to variables, thereby losing touch with the biological relevance of the patterns themselves. Indeed, measuring and quantifying complex cryptic behavior requires a certain amount of modesty, as the process we are trying to understand has been tested by millions of eyes of different species and evolutionarily refined to its present manifestation.

Before moving on to discuss mathematical camouflage descriptors, here we review some basic principles of image analysis. Digital images comprise thousands of pixels organized as a matrix of intensity values usually ranging from 0 to 255. Camouflage image analysis is based on examining mathematical descriptors of the pixels in areas of the animal's body and comparing them with similar descriptors of the background against which the animal is camouflaging. Three overlaying matrixes (the red, green, and blue [RGB] channels) form a color image in the RGB format. If an animal's perception of the visual world is based on a single color receptor in its eyes – as is the case with shallow water cephalopods, equipped with a single, mid-wavelength photoreceptor – the animal perceives its surroundings in grayscale due to the lack of another matrix channel with which to compare the image. Therefore, most analyses simplify the problem by using grayscale images derived from the green channel intensities. But which mathematical descriptors best describe similarity or resemblance in textures and patterns? Numerous studies in computer and machine vision have tackled similar questions (e.g. Ojala, Pietikainen & Harwood, 1996; Lowe, 2004), usually focusing on identifying differences between or within images. Although such studies provide useful tools applicable to the study of animal camouflage, these tools often tend to be too computationally complex for the task at hand. Among the image parameters that have been used to investigate cephalopod camouflage patterns (partial list, Table 8.2), each has its own advantages and limitations that cannot be neglected when analyzing the results. None of the mentioned studies claim to describe the neurological processes behind cephalopod body patterning; rather, they attempt to find the descriptors that can best quantify camouflage while remaining independent of researcher bias.

In a recent study we used previously applied image analysis pattern descriptors to investigate the camouflage patterns of *Octopus cyanea* (Josef, Amodio, Fiorito, & Shashar, 2012). Shannon's entropy, one of the most intuitive parameters to comprehend (and sometimes referred as a "measure of uncertainty"), was found to be a good proxy for pattern similarity. Other methods, including average root mean square deviation (RMSD), standard deviation (STD), fast Fourier transformation (FFT), cross-correlation, two-dimensional (2D) cross-correlation, edge detection, Hough transformation, histogram correlation, blob analysis, spectral estimation and histogram normal-fit comparisons, were all deemed inadequate for use as camouflage descriptors. In fact, we found, despite the significant loss of information they entail, that simple measuring methods were sufficient to quantify similarities between an octopus and its surroundings. Indeed, our study shows empirically that it is possible to estimate similarity between an octopus and different parts of its background even when using a relatively simple parameter such as the entropy. But, because it is insensitive to the spatial organization of pixels in the image, entropy cannot be used in all applications. Comparisons of our

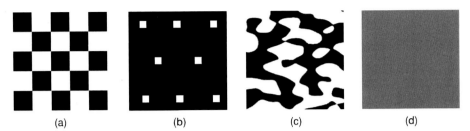

(a)   (b)   (c)   (d)

Figure 8.4 Commonly used artificial patterns. (a) Checkerboard, 50% black and white pixels eliminating color dominance effect. With relation to scale, it may evoke either Mottle or Disruptive body patterns. (b) Various size white objects over a black background, examining the effect of area and object size in eliciting patterning. (c) Holstein cow patterns composed of 50% black and white pixels, mostly evoking Disruptive body patterns. (d) Fifty-percent gray, representing neutral and uniform substrata.

results with other complex and well-established methods, however, demonstrated that entropy has both the power and the accuracy required to function as a natural scene descriptor.

The ongoing search for adequate analysis descriptors is a "hot" topic in camouflage research. Such descriptors would enable us to clearly distinguish camouflage from signaling, identify similarity zones in a given scene and quantify, possibly even grade, the quality of camouflage (Zylinski, How, Osorio, Hanlon & Marshall, 2011; Josef, Amodio, Fiorito & Shashar, 2012). Additionally, they could also lead to an automated and objective method of assessing camouflage.

8.10   How do cephalopods decide what camouflage strategy to use?

Cephalopods must rapidly and continuously assess their surroundings to determine which body pattern to use. Scientists, interested in understanding how this assessment is made and what parameters of the visual scene are taken into consideration by the animal, cannot definitively declare whether camouflage is a controlled cognitive process, during which the animal is aware of what it is matching. Conversely, it is possible that cephalopod camouflage is a reflexive response that accepts inputs from the visual, motor and memory systems to produce the desired body pattern.

The complex and diverse habitats of benthic cephalopods make field research challenging and hinder investigations of the effects of specific visual features on camouflage patterns. The use of artificial substrates in controlled settings became a popular technique among researchers, as it enabled specific visual cues used in camouflage to be examined and, in so doing, isolating the relevant image variables, which were then manipulated while the other parameters were static (Figure 8.4; Chiao & Hanlon, 2001a, 2001b; Barbosa, Florio, Chiao & Hanlon, 2004; Chiao, Kelman & Hanlon, 2005; Barbosa et al., 2007; Chiao, Chubb & Hanlon, 2007; Kelman, Baddeley, Shohet & Osorio, 2007; Barbosa, Litman & Hanlon, 2008). Among the images tested, the checkerboard pattern is an important tool that can be modified for contrast and scale and even used in experiments to assess polarization and color sensitivity (Marshall & Messenger, 1996; Grable, Shashar, Gilles, Chiao & Hanlon, 2002).

8.11   Camouflaged to resemble what?

A camouflaging cephalopod can take into account its local visual field in its entirety and execute general background matching, or it can imitate specific, selected structures or objects in its surroundings, a strategy that is known as masquerade. Alternative strategies such as Disruptive coloration may also be employed, a further testament to the animal's versatile camouflaging abilities. Indeed, the cephalopod's ability to dynamically camouflage allows it to choose the best strategy for each situation.

If using an object-oriented strategy, an animal must quickly identify an object charac- teristic of the surrounding, convincingly and accurately imitate it and remain motionless. On the other hand, the strategy of general background matching requires the animal to find the best way to describe and represent a relatively large area around it, while ensur- ing that it is properly oriented vis-à-vis its background and the seeker's field of view. A further option could involve mimicking the general characteristics of a specific object without attempting to copy it in detail, simplifying the computational requirements as all object parameters are precisely duplicated, but using camouflage to generally "belong" to the scene. Hanlon and Messenger (1988) alluded to this option in their discussion of juvenile cuttlefish mimicking pebbles.

In a recent study we attempted to determine which of these approaches is used by free ranging *O. cyanea* on a coral reef (Josef, Amodio, Fiorito & Shashar, 2012). Free-ranging octopuses were photographed from above, and the green channel of the resulting images was analyzed. First, an octopus mantle viewed from above was sampled and measured for both entropy and rotational averaged (RA)-slopes (Table 8.3). Next, the same procedure was carried out for the rest of the image on areas equal in size to the animal's mantle. By shifting the areas one pixel at a time, the entire image was examined. The differences in measurements between the octopus and its background were calculated for each position of the shifting area, and their difference values were assigned to the central pixel of the area. Comparing the octopus to the overall image creates a similarity index map, in which a low difference value signifies high similarity.

The similarity index is computed as follows (RA-slope example):

$$RAfft\ slope\ similarity\ percentage = \left[1 - \left(\frac{|Octopus_{RA-slope} - SubSample_{RA-slope}|}{Maximum\ Difference_{RA-slope}}\right)\right] \cdot 100$$

However, the RA-slope alone is not sufficient to define similarity because the slopes of two images with different intensities can be highly similar. Therefore, we used the RA-mean as an indication of intensity and only sections of the image with RA-mean similarity greater than 90% were measured for differences in RA-slopes.

Superimposing the resulting similarity maps over the original images revealed regions of animal and background similarity and others that were dissimilar (see example in Figure 8.5). We found that rather than use body patterns that represented an average of

Table 8.3 Image analysis descriptors used in the cephalopod camouflage study

Pattern descriptor	Purpose	Citation
PIV (pixel intensity variance)	Distinguishing camouflage from signaling patterns	Zylinski, How, Osorio, Hanlon and Marshall (2011)
RA-slope (rotational averaged fast Fourier transformation [FFT] slope)	Quantifying similarity between two images	Zylinski, How, Osorio, Hanlon and Marshall (2011)
Modified entropy	Comparing complexity	This paper
Contrast	Comparing either the white square to the rest of the body or to the background	Chiao and Hanlon (2001a)
Spectrum granularity	Distinguishing between Uniform/Stipple, Mottled and Disruptive body patterns	Barbosa et al. (2008)
Energy per pixel	Quantifying the influence of substrate spatial scale and the camouflager	Chiao, Chubb, Buresch, Siemann and Hanlon (2009)
Two-dimensional Fourier transform	Analyzing spatial frequency information	Chiao, Kelman and Hanlon (2005)
Spectral reflectance	Measuring the color match between animal and background	Mäthger, Chiao, Barbosa and Hanlon (2008)
Webber contrast	Comparing the animal's Disruptive body patterns and its background attributes	Hanlon et al. (2009)

their immediate environment (as in general background matching), the octopuses tended to imitate certain regions, behavior consistent with a masquerade strategy. Repeating this analysis using entropy estimation produced the same results, namely, the same regions of the images with high similarity to the octopuses were identified (Figure 8.5). The observed octopus strategy was not to precisely imitate specific objects, but, rather, to use typical traits of the relevant objects. In doing so, the octopuses reduced the likelihood of being detected by inaccurately mimicking the imitated object. Of course we do not intend to suggest that octopuses use mathematical parameters in their camouflaging decisions, merely that these descriptors assist us in understanding which habitat characteristics are being utilized in camouflage.

8.12   Concluding remarks

The dynamic camouflage of cephalopods attracts the interest of increasing numbers of researchers across multiple fields, including behavioral biology, military organizations and computer vision. The development of autonomous and increasingly sophisticated methods to assess camouflage is providing us with the power of greater insight into which elements of a visual scene are selected for matching. In turn, understanding which scene characteristics are being used by animals to determine body patterns for camouflage

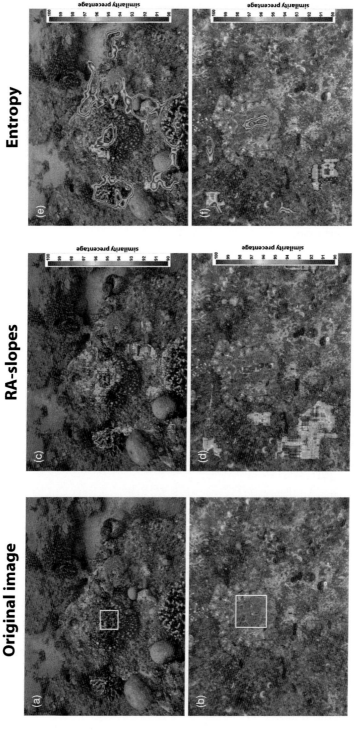

Figure 8.5 Image analysis of camouflaged octopuses. (a,b) Cryptic *Octopus cyanea* and *Octopus vulgaris* respectively in their natural habitat. The white square marks the sampled mantle for similarity comparison. (c,d) Computer-generated similarity map of the RA-slopes descriptor. For clarity reasons only 90% similarity or higher is presented. (e,f) Computer-generated similarity map of the entropy descriptor. See plate section for color version.

helps improve image analysis processes. Future research is needed to understand the neurological processes taking place, from the basics of pattern control to brain functions and neurologically mapping the body patterns.

Acknowledgments

We thank Steve MacCusker, Chris Talbot, Amit Lerner, Omer Polak and Keren Levi for their ongoing assistance, and Zvika Livnat, Ron Wolf and Ilan Ben-Tov who donated some of their high resolution images. We are grateful for the support of Israeli Science Foundation Grant No. 1081/10, the ASSEMBLE program and the Halperin and the Schechter Foundations.

References

Allen, J. J., Mäthger, L. M., Barbosa, A. and Hanlon, R. T. (2009). Cuttlefish use visual cues to control three-dimensional skin papillae for camouflage. *Journal of Comparative Physiology A*, **195**: 547–555.

Arnold, J. M. (1967). Organellogenesis of the cephalopod iridophore: cytomembranes in development. *Journal of Ultrastructure Research*, **20**: 410–420.

Bacot, A. (1907). The melanic variety of the peppered moth. *Nature*, **77**: 294–295.

Barbosa, A., Allen, J. J., Mäthger, L. M. and Hanlon, R. T. (2012). Cuttlefish use visual cues to determine arm postures for camouflage. *Proceedings of the Royal Society. B: Biological Sciences*, **279**: 84–90.

Barbosa, A., Florio, C. F., Chiao, C. C. and Hanlon, R. T. (2004). Visual background features that elicit mottled body patterns in cuttlefish *Sepia officinalis*. *The Biological Bulletin*, **207**: 154.

Barbosa, A., Litman, L. and Hanlon, R. T. (2008). Changeable cuttlefish camouflage is influenced by horizontal and vertical aspects of the visual background. *Journal of Comparative Physiology A*, **194**: 405–413.

Barbosa, A., Mäthger, L. M., Buresch, K. C., Kelly, J., Chubb, C., Chiao, C. C. and Hanlon, R. T. (2008). Cuttlefish camouflage: The effects of substrate contrast and size in evoking Uniform, Mottle or Disruptive body patterns. *Vision Research*, **48**: 1242–1253.

Barbosa, A., Mäthger, L. M., Chubb, C., Florio, C., Chiao, C. C. and Hanlon, R. T. (2007). Disruptive colouration in cuttlefish: a visual perception mechanism that regulates ontogenetic adjustment of skin patterning. *Journal of Experimental Biology*, **210**: 1139–1147.

Barros, M., Silva, M. A. D., Huston, J. P. and Tomaz, C. (2004). Multibehavioral analysis of fear and anxiety before, during, and after experimentally induced predatory stress in *Callithrix penicillata*. *Pharmacology Biochemistry and Behavior*, **78**: 357–367.

Blanchard, D. C., Li, C. I., Hubbard, D., Markham, C. M., Yang, M., Takahashi, L. K. and Blanchard, R. J. (2003). Dorsal premammillary nucleus differentially modulates defensive behaviors induced by different threat stimuli in rats. *Neuroscience Letters*, **345**: 145–148.

Boal, J. G., Shashar, N., Grable, M. M., Vaughan, K. H., Loew, E. R. and Hanlon. R. T. (2004). Behavioral evidence for intraspecific signals with monochromatic and polarized light by cuttlefish. *Behaviour*, **141**: 837–861.

Borrelli, L., Fiorito, G. and Gherardi, F. (2006). *A catalogue of body pattering in Cephalopoda*. Florence, Italy: Firenze University Press.

Boycott, B. B. (1953). The chromatophore system of cephalopods. *Proceedings of the Linnean Society of London*, **164**: 235–240.

Brandao, M. L., Troncoso, A. C., Silva, M. A. D. and Huston, J. P. (2003). The relevance of neuronal substrates of defense in the midbrain tectum to anxiety and stress: empirical and conceptual considerations. *European Journal of Pharmacology*, **463**: 225–233.

Bush, S. L., Robison, B. H. and Caldwell, R. L. (2009). Behaving in the dark: locomotor, chromatic, postural and bioluminescent behaviors of the deep-sea squid *Octopoteuthis deletron* Young 1972. *The Biological Bulletin*, **216**: 7–22.

Canteras, N. S. (2002). The medial hypothalamic defensive system: hodological organization and functional implications. *Pharmacology Biochemistry and Behavior*, **71**: 481–491.

Chiao, C. C., Chubb, C., Buresch, K. C., Barbosa, A., Allen, J. J., Mäthger, L. M. and Hanlon, R. T. (2010). Mottle camouflage patterns in cuttlefish: quantitative characterization and visual background stimuli that evoke them. *Journal of Experimental Biology*, **213**: 187–199.

Chiao, C. C., Chubb, C., Buresch, K. C., Siemann, L. and Hanlon, R. T. (2009). The scaling effects of substrate texture on camouflage patterning in cuttlefish. *Vision Research*, **49**: 1647–1656.

Chiao, C. C., Chubb, C. and Hanlon, R. T. (2007). Interactive effects of size, contrast, intensity and configuration of background objects in evoking Disruptive camouflage in cuttlefish. *Vision Research*, **47**: 2223–2235.

Chiao, C. C. and Hanlon, R. T. (2001a). Cuttlefish camouflage: visual perception of size contrast and number of white squares on artificial checkerboard substrate initiates Disruptive coloration. *Journal of Experimental Biology*, **204**: 2119–2125.

Chiao, C. C. and Hanlon, R. T. (2001b). Cuttlefish cue visually on area – not shape or aspect ratio – of light objects in the substrate to produce Disruptive body patterns for camouflage. *The Biological Bulletin*, **201**: 269–270.

Chiao, C. C., Kelman, E. J. and Hanlon, R. T. (2005). Disruptive body patterning of cuttlefish (*Sepia officinalis*) requires visual information regarding edges and contrast of objects in natural substrate backgrounds. *The Biological Bulletin*, **208**: 7–11.

Chrachri, A. and Williamson, R. (2004). Cholinergic and glutamatergic spontaneous and evoked excitatory postsynaptic currents in optic lobe neurons of cuttlefish, *Sepia officinalis*. *Brain Research*, **1020**: 178–187.

Cloney, R. A. and Brocco, S. L. (1983). Chromatophore organs, reflector cells, iridocytes and leucophores in cephalopods. *American Zoologist*, **23**: 581–592.

Comoli, E., Ribeiro-Barbosa, E. R. and Canteras, N. S. (2003). Predatory hunting and exposure to a live predator induce opposite patterns of Fos immunoreactivity in the PAG. *Behavioural Brain Research*, **138**: 17–28.

Cronin, T. W. (2005). The visual ecology of predator–prey interactions. In Barbosa, P. and Castellaris, I. (eds.) *Ecology of predator-prey interactions*. New York, NY: Oxford University Press, pp. 105–138.

Cronin, T. W., Shashar, N. and Wolff, L. (1995). Imaging technology reveals the polarized light fields that exist in nature. *Biophotonics International*, **2**: 38–41.

Curio, E. (1976). *The ethology of predation*. Berlin, Germany: Springer-Verlag.

Darwin, C. (1870). Note on the habits of the Pampas Woodpecker (*Colaptes campestris*). *Proceedings of the Zoological Society of London*, **38**: 705–706.

Eilam, D. (2005). Die hard: a blend of freezing and fleeing as a dynamic defense – implications for the control of defensive behavior. *Neuroscience and Biobehavioral Reviews*, **29**: 1181–1191.

Endler, J. A. (1981). An overview of the relationships between mimicry and crypsis. *Biology Journal of the Linnean Society*, **16**: 25–31.

Florey, E. and Kriebel, M. E. (1969). Electrical and mechanical responses of chromatophore muscle fibers of the squid, *Loligo opalescens*, to nerve stimulation and drugs. *Zeitschrift fur Vergleichende Physiologie*, **65**: 98–130.

Grable, M., Shashar, N., Gilles, N. L., Chiao, C. C. and Hanlon, R. T. (2002). Cuttlefish body patterns as a behavioral assay to determine polarization perception. *Biology Bulletin*, **203**: 232–234.

Gretzmacher, F. M., Ruppert, G. S. and Nyberg, S. (1998). Camouflage assessment considering human perception data. *Proceedings SPIE, Targets and Backgrounds: Characterization and Representation IV*, **3375**: 58–67.

Hall, K. and Hanlon, R. (2002). Principal features of the mating system of a large spawning aggregation of the giant Australian cuttlefish *Sepia apama* (Mollusca: Cephalopoda). *Marine Biology*, **140**: 533–545.

Hanlon, R. T. (1982). The functional organization of chromatophores and iridescent cells in the body patterning of *Loligo plei* (Cephalopoda: Myopsida). *Malacologia*, **23**: 89–119.

Hanlon, R. T., Chiao, C. C., Mäthger, L. M., Barbosa, A., Buresch, K. C. and Chubb, C. (2009). Cephalopod dynamic camouflage: bridging the continuum between background matching and Disruptive coloration. *Philosophical Transactions of the Royal Society of London. Series B*, **364**: 429–437.

Hanlon, R. T., Forsythe, J. W. and Joneschild, D. E. (1999). Crypsis, conspicuousness, mimicry and polyphenism as anti-predator defenses of foraging octopuses on Indo-Pacific coral reefs, with a method of quantifying crypsis from video tapes. *Biological Journal of the Linnean Society*, **66**: 1–22.

Hanlon, R. T. and Messenger, J. B. (1988). Adaptive coloration in young cuttlefish (*Sepia officinalis* L.): the morphology and development of body patterns and their relation to behaviour. *Philosophical Transactions of the Royal Society B*, **320**: 437–487.

Hanlon, R. T. and Messenger, J. B. (eds.) (1996). *Cephalopod behaviour*. Cambridge: Cambridge University Press.

Hanlon, R. T., Watson, A. C. and Barbosa, A. (2010). A "Mimic Octopus" in the Atlantic: flatfish mimicry and camouflage by *Macrotritopus defilippi. Biological Bulletin*, **218**: 15–24.

Josef, N., Amodio, P., Fiorito, G. and Shashar, N. (2012). Camouflaging in a complex environment – octopuses use specific features of their surroundings for background matching. *Public Library of Science One*, **7**: e37579.

Kelman, E. J., Baddeley, R. J., Shohet, A. J. and Osorio, D. (2007). Expression of Disruptive camouflage by the cuttlefish, *Sepia officinalis. Proceedings of the Royal Society. B: Biological Sciences*, **274**: 1369–1375.

Lamprea, M. R., Cardenas, F. P., Vianna, D. M., Castilho, V. M., Cruz-Morales, S. E. and Brandao, M. L. (2002). The distribution of fos immunoreactivity in rat brain following freezing and escape responses elicited by electrical stimulation of the inferior colliculus. *Brain Research*, **950**: 186–194.

Land, M. F. and Nilsson, D. E. (2002). *Animal eyes*. Oxford, UK: Oxford University Press.

Langridge, K. V. (2006). Symmetrical crypsis and asymmetrical signaling in the cuttlefish *Sepia officinalis. Proceedings of the Royal Society. B: Biological Sciences*, **273**: 959–967.

Langridge, K. V., Broom, M. and Osorio, D. (2007). Selective signalling by cuttlefish to predators. *Current Biology*, **17**: R1044–R1045.

Lehmann, U. (1976). *The ammonites: their life and their world*. Translation 1981. Cambridge, UK: Cambridge University Press.

Lowe, D. (2004). Distinctive image features from scale–invariant keypoints. *International Journal on Computer Vision*, **60**: 91–110.

Marshall, N. J. and Messenger, J. B. (1996). Colour-blind camouflage. *Nature*, **382**: 408–409.

Mather, J. A., Griebel, U. and Byrne, R. A. (2010). Squid dances: an ethogram of postures and actions of *Sepioteuthis sepioidea* squid with a muscular hydrostatic system. *Marine and Freshwater Behaviour and Physiology*, **43**: 45–61.

Mather, J. A. and Mather, D. L. (2004). Apparent movement in a visual display: the "passing cloud" of *Octopus cyanea* (Mollusca: Cephalopoda). *Journal of Zoology*, **263**: 89–94.

Mäthger, L. M, Chiao, C. C., Barbosa, A. and Hanlon, R. T. (2008). Color matching on natural substrates in cuttlefish, *Sepia officinalis*. *Journal of Comparative Physiology A*, **194**: 577–585.

Mäthger, L. M. and Hanlon, R. T. (2006). Anatomical basis for camouflaged polarized light communication in squid. *Biology Letters*, **2**: 494–496.

Mäthger, L. M., Shashar, N. and Hanlon, R. T. (2009). Do cephalopods communicate using polarized light reflections from their skin. *Journal of Experimental Biology*, **212**: 2133–2140.

Mayr, E. (1963). *Animal species and evolution*. Cambridge, MA: Harvard University Press.

Merilaita, S. (1998). Crypsis through Disruptive coloration in an isopod. *Proceedings of the Royal Society. B: Biological Sciences*, **265**: 1059–1064.

Messenger, J. B. (1977). Evidence that octopus is color blind. *Journal of Experimental Biology*, **70**: 49–55.

Messenger, J. B. (2001). Cephalopod chromatophores: neurobiology and natural history. *Biological Reviews*, **76**: 473–528.

Moynihan, M. (1985). *Communication and non-communication in cephalopods*. Bloomington, IL: Indiana University Press.

Nixon, M. and Young, J. Z. (2003). *The brains and lives of cephalopods*. New York, NY: Oxford University Press.

Ojala, T., Pietikainen, M. and Harwood, D. (1996). A comparative study of texture measures with classification based on feature distributions. *Pattern Recognition*, **29**: 51–59.

Packard, A. (1972). Cephalopods and fish: the limits of convergence. *Biological Reviews*, **47**: 241–307.

Packard, A. and Hochberg, F. G. (1977). Skin patterning in octopus and other genera. *Symposia of the Zoological Society of London*, **38**: 191–231.

Packard, A. and Sanders, G. D. (1969). What the octopus shows to the world. *Endeavour*, **28**: 92–99.

Parker, G. H. (1948). *Animal colour changes and their neurohumours*. Cambridge, UK: Cambridge University Press.

Reynolds, C. (2011). Interactive evolution of camouflage. *Artificial Life*, **17**: 123–136.

Sereni, E. and Young, J. Z. (1932). Nervous degeneration and regeneration in cephalopods. *Pubblicazione de la Stazione Zoologica di Napoli*, **12**: 173–208.

Shashar, N., Rutledge, P. S. and Cronin, T. W. (1996). Polarization vision in cuttlefish – a concealed communication channel. *Journal of Experimental Biology*, **199**: 2077–2084.

Shohet, A. J., Baddeley, R. J., Anderson, J. C., Kelman, E. J. and Osorio, D. (2006). Cuttlefish responses to visual orientation of substrates, water flow and a model of motion camouflage. *Journal of Experimental Biology*, **209**: 4717–4723.

Stevens, M. and Merilaita, S. (2009). Animal camouflage: current issues and new perspectives. *Philosophical Transactions of the Royal Society B*, **364**: 423–427.

Stevens, M. and Merilaita, S. (2011). *Animal camouflage*. Cambridge, UK: Cambridge University Press.

Stuart-Fox, D. and Moussalli, A. (2008). Selection for social signalling drives the evolution of chameleon colour change. *Public Library of Science One, Biology*, **6**: e25.

Talbot, C. M. and Marshall, N. J. (2010). Polarization sensitivity in two species of cuttlefish – *Sepia plangon* (Gray 1849) and *Sepia mestus* (Gray 1849) – demonstrated with polarized optomotor stimuli. *Journal of Experimental Biology*, **213**: 3364–3370.

Temple, S. E., Pignatelli, V., Cook, T., How, M. J., Chiou, T.-H., Roberts, N. W. and Marshall, N. J. (2012). High-resolution polarisation vision in a cuttlefish. *Current Biology*, **22**: R121–R122.

Zylinski, S., Darmaillacq, A.-S. and Shashar, N. (2012). Visual interpolation for contour completion by the cuttlefish *Sepia officinalis* and its use in dynamic camouflage. *Proceedings of the Royal Society. B: Biological Sciences*, **279**: 2386–2390.

Zylinski, S., How, M. J., Osorio, D., Hanlon, R. T. and Marshall, N. J. (2011). To be seen or to hide: visual characteristics of body patterns for camouflage and communication in the Australian giant cuttlefish *Sepia apama*. *The American Naturalist*, **177**: 681–690.

Zylinski, S. and Johnsen, S. (2011). Mesopelagic cephalopods switch between transparency and pigmentation to optimize camouflage in the deep. *Current Biology*, **21**: 1937–1941.

Zylinski, S., Osorio, D. and Shohet, A. J. (2009). Edge detection and texture classification by cuttlefish. *Journal of Vision*, **9**: 1–10.

9   Cuttlefish camouflage: vision and cognition

Sarah Zylinski and Daniel Osorio

Because vision is used by different animals for such a variety of purposes, it is inconceivable that all seeing animals use the same representations; each can confidently be expected to use one or more representations that are nicely tailored to the owner's purposes. (David Marr (1982))

9.1   Cephalopod camouflage and comparative cognition

Camouflage is directed at the vision of adversaries, with selection on both sides driving an evolutionary arms race. Fossils suggest that Mesozoic coleoid cephalopods moved to deep water to avoid predation and competition, with shell-loss an adaptation to overcome depth limits imposed by hydrostatic pressure on gas spaces in shells. There followed a secondary colonization of shallow waters where the soft-bodied, shell-less cephalopods acquired novel defences against fish and reptile predators (Hanlon & Messenger, 1996; Packard, 1972). A second hypothesis favours earlier colonization in the Devonian, when the predators were early fishes such as chondrosteans and placoderms (Hanlon & Messenger, 1996). Either way, fish can be described as the 'designers of cephalopod skin' (Packard, 1972), and we expect threat responses and camouflage patterns to be tuned to vertebrate vision (Hanlon & Messenger, 1988; Langridge, Broom & Osorio, 2007). These changes were probably linked to the more general evolution of large brains and complex behaviours of modern cephalopods (Budelmann, 1994; Young, Vecchione & Donovan, 1998).

Whatever its evolutionary origins we can agree that cephalopod camouflage works well for at least one species of terrestrial primate, namely humans. Camouflage relies on defeating figure-ground segregation to prevent the detection of the body as distinct from the background (Cott, 1940; Stevens, 2007). Superficially, camouflage seems unproblematic – we know a moth is camouflaged because we see that it is well matched to the tree-bark it rests on – yet substantial neural computation is required to recover information about objects from optical images. This chapter describes our current understanding of cuttlefish (*Sepia* spp.) vision, how it is used to control camouflage, and the evidence that this is a cognitive process.

This work generally falls in line with the traditions of vision science; first seeking to identify the low level (i.e. spatially local) image parameters and features that are used by

Cephalopod Cognition, eds A.-S. Darmaillacq, L. Dickel and J. Mather. Published by Cambridge University Press. © Cambridge 2014.

the animals, and then asking how this information is processed by or represented in the brain to make decisions – in this case to select a body pattern. How might this inform our understanding of cognition?

9.2   Animal visual cognition

Comparative cognition is almost universally grounded in comparisons with human intelligence (Byrne & Bates, 2006). We ask whether an animal has a mental map, consciousness, theory of mind, declarative memory and so-forth. Often for animals without language the definitions of these phenomena are unclear (Shettleworth, 2001). Instead the chief experimental question is whether the animal's behaviour can be described by a behaviourist account (Real, 1993): if not it is inferred that the behaviour requires cognition.

Unfortunately, as David Marr (1982) implied in the opening quotation, the approach to animal cognition summarized above seems flawed: the theory is flimsy, and the anthropocentric perspective is worrying. Human performance is not a gold standard for cephalopod polarization vision or motor control. Humans are good at interacting with objects, but do not have to control their body pattern. Cephalopods do things differently, and we should be open to the possibility that this applies to mental processes (Temple et al., 2012). The control of cuttlefish adaptive colouration for camouflage exemplifies this point; its remarkable versatility and sensitivity to the visual environment offers a unique approach to vision in an animal without language. We can examine how traditional approaches to visual perception (Campbell & Robson, 1968; Cavanagh, 2011; Gibson, 1979; Marr, 1982; Marr & Hildreth, 1980) apply to these remarkable animals.

The difficulty in applying existing precepts to cephalopod behaviour is exemplified by the apparent complexity of cuttlefish camouflage compared to what seems to be necessary for effective concealment! Flatfish, such as plaice (*Pleuronectes platessa*) and tropical flounders (*Bothus ocellatus*), control the level of expression of one to three basic body patterns, which they can mix to produce – for the human eye – excellent camouflage on a wide range of the sea-floor backgrounds (Kelman, Tiptus & Osorio 2006; Ramachandran et al., 1996). Similarly, it is convenient to classify cephalopod camouflage into three basic types: Uniform, Mottle and Disruptive (Hanlon, 2007; Hanlon & Messenger, 1988). However, cuttlefish almost certainly have substantially more than three types of camouflage pattern, and more than three degrees of freedom in the control of their appearance. The common cuttlefish *Sepia officinalis* controls the expression of about 40 basic behavioural components more or less independently. How their expression is coordinated, and how visual information is used to serve this behaviour is a fascinating question in cephalopod biology and comparative cognition.

The nature of cognitive processes is central to understanding neural mechanisms of behaviour. In her book *Cognition, evolution, and behavior*, Shettleworth (2010) says: 'Cognition, broadly defined, includes perception, learning, memory and decision making, in short all ways in which animals take in information about the world through the senses, process, retain and decide to act on it.' Although pragmatic, the definition is broad, and it is useful to define terms for this article. *Perception*, which is the ability to make inferences about the world from sense data (Gregory, 1997), *decision-making* and *learning* refer to behavioural capabilities, which should be distinguished from *cognition*, which refers to underlying mechanisms, and is commonly understood to entail internal representation (Tolman, 1948). It remains potentially confusing to refer to *any* type of learning or object recognition as cognitive. In a classic cognitive model, Tolman (1948) proposed that rats use a cognitive (i.e. internal) map to navigate a maze. Even though it is widely agreed that behaviourist theory faces major difficulties in accounting for animal learning (Mackintosh, 1974), the long-standing controversy about evidence for cognitive maps exemplifies the difficulties in proving the existence of an internal representation in any given experiment (Bennett, 1996; Burgess, 2006; Collett & Collett, 2002; Wang & Spelke, 2002). Similarly there is scepticism about the need for representation, especially in the field of artificial intelligence and robotics (Brooks, 1991).

Related to the distinction between cognitive and non-cognitive behaviour, vision science has long recognized a distinction between low-level processes informed purely by bottom-up, scene-based information such as edge detection, and high-level processes that take account of global organization and involve long-range top-down, viewer-informed, decision-based analyses that combine low-level retinal input with prior knowledge to generate representation and are (probably) cognitive (Cavanagh, 2011). Cognitive mechanisms are thought to be computationally demanding and, hence, costly for neural processing, but they offer flexible processing and interpretation of sensory information.

Marr's (1982) emphasis on internal representations and computation has been especially influential and controversial. Marr proposed that vision is a multi-stage process based on successive neural representations of the retinal image. In the first stage, local (i.e. low-level) mechanisms, such as linear spatial filters, and edge and detectors, produce a primal sketch, which is elaborated by more global and contextual information to produce a 2½-dimensional representation of a scene. Marr also made a well-known distinction between the algorithmic, computational and hardware (i.e. physiological) levels of understanding of the brain, which is especially relevant to comparisons between remotely related species.

Marr contrasted his cognitive account with Gibson's (1979) theory of direct perception. Gibson largely rejected the need for representation, and instead emphasized how the interaction of an actively moving agent with the visual world can constrain and simplify visual computation. Subsequent work on animal and robotic vision has often favoured a Gibsonian perspective; it emphasizes the interaction between the actively moving animal and its visual world, and argues that Marr overstated the amount of computation necessary and significance of representations for vision (Brooks, 1991; Krapp & Hengstenberg, 1997; Srinivasan & Venkatesh, 1997).

As they cannot verbally report their experience, animal experiments often rely on binary-choice tests of behaviour. Such tests are poorly suited to investigating cognition, because a simpler account is normally possible. The study of cuttlefish camouflage

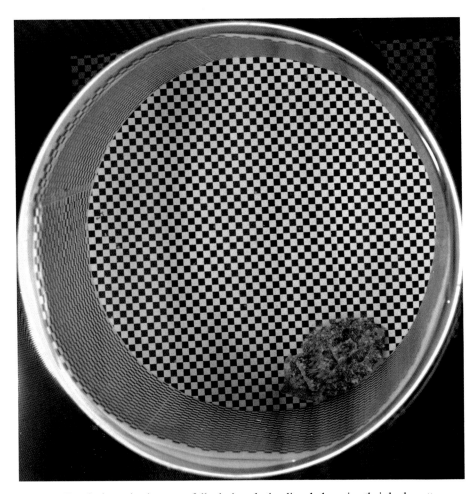

Figure 9.1 By placing animals on carefully designed stimuli and observing their body-pattern responses we can gain unique insight into their perception of the visual world. Here, an individual *Sepia officinalis* is settled in a test arena with a small chequerboard stimulus. The animal uses a Mottle-type body pattern containing light and dark elements that are spatially similar to those in the stimulus.

echoes broader debates on animal cognition, but the richness of the behaviour offers new insights into how animals perceive complex images (Crook, Baddeley & Osorio, 2002). Recent work has moved from identifying low-level mechanisms towards more cognitive accounts. Experiments set out to relate the choice of body pattern directly to local image parameters and features, such as spatial frequency and edges (Figure 9.1); yet, as we will see, it is often easier to conceive that the animals use an object-based representation to select the right body pattern for the environment. Marr's (1982) primal sketch theory is important here because of its bottom-up approach to visual processing: it shows how scene representation can be achieved in the absence of knowledge or experience of the contents.

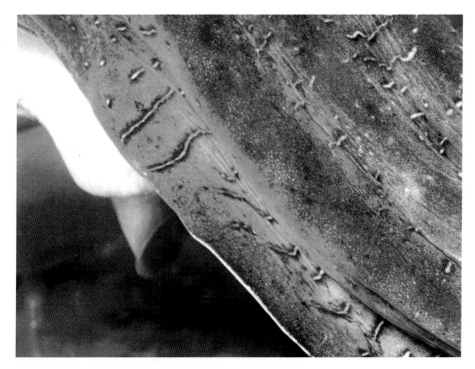

Figure 9.2 The bright blues and greens in the mating displays of the Australian giant cuttlefish *Sepia apama* are primarily due to wavelength specific reflectors. The animals themselves are most likely colour-blind. See plate section for colour version.

9.3   Expression of body patterns

The wealth of patterns used by cuttlefish is compelling evidence for the visual sophistication of their potential predators and prey. This section outlines the basic biology of cephalopod adaptive camouflage and goes on to outline how we can study this behaviour.

9.3.1   Skin pigmentation

Cephalopod skin is a remarkable organ, which compensates for the animals' lack of physical defences with control of both colour and physical texture (Hanlon, Forsythe & Joneschild, 1999; Hanlon & Messenger, 1988, 1996). The skin is multi-layered: chromatophores, which contain ommochrome pigments that produce blacks, browns, reds and yellows, overlie white leucophores, while iridophores contain wavelength-specific reflectors that result in vibrant blues and greens (Mäthger & Hanlon, 2007; Messenger, 2001) (Figure 9.2). Chromatophore density varies considerably between taxa, but on *Octopus vulgaris* mantle chromatophore density reaches 230 per mm^2 (Messenger 2001). The chromatophores pigment sacs are opened by supporting muscles, which are innervated directly from the brain, allowing rapid colour changes and precise control of the visible area of pigment. In theory the animal could control these individual chromatophores like pixels on a computer monitor. Patterns could then be expressed in response to the visual environment via a mechanism akin to an output of a retinotopic map, with photoreceptor-to-chromatophore mapping of the background.

In fact the expression of chromatophores is coordinated, sometimes as a localized group, and sometimes as more global patterns. These form the basic behavioural elements known as 'chromatic components' (Hanlon & Messenger, 1988; Packard & Hochberg, 1977; Packard & Sanders, 1971). Chromatic components in turn tend to be expressed, along with textural and postural components, in common suites to form complete body patterns (Hanlon & Messenger, 1996). The suite of 50 or so behavioural components identified in *Sepia* has obvious equivalents in other coleoid cephalopods, but is unmatched in any other animal group (Kelman, Tiptus & Osorio, 2006; Stuart-Fox & Moussalli, 2009; Stuart-Fox, Whiting & Moussalli, 2006). Measurement of their expression is central to characterizing cephalopod visual behaviour. The potential for independent expression of the behavioural components offers the cuttlefish an enormous repertoire of body patterns, especially as the animal can precisely regulate the intensity of each component. The extent to which the animals can realize this potential is poorly known.

To facilitate understanding of the patterns that are typically expressed in response to a set of basic visual stimuli, we will refer to the three main *classes* of body pattern in Hanlon's UMD (Uniform, Mottle, Disruptive; Figure 9.3) scheme (Hanlon, 2007). However, the reader should bear in mind that the animal has enormous – and largely unexplored – flexibility: each class contains many different body patterns distinguished by the relative expression of individual components and overall luminance. Equally, different body pattern classes are often mixed (see Figure 9.3, below). How *Sepia* determines what body pattern components to express in order to achieve effective camouflage, given local visual cues, forms the crux of our research and the core of this chapter.

9.3.2   Principal component analysis and other descriptors of body patterns

It is readily apparent that to study cuttlefish adaptive camouflage requires a rigorous, efficient and meaningful method to describe body patterns. Most methods deal with the appearance in single images (e.g. Barbosa et al., 2008; Chiao, Chubb, Buresch & Siemann, 2009; Shohet, Baddeley, Anderson & Osorio, 2007), but the patterns of change over time are also of considerable interest (Langridge, Broom & Osorio, 2007; Zylinski, Osorio & Shohet, 2009a). At present two main methods are used to describe body patterns. One is to measure the spatial properties of the body pattern, much as one can characterize a visual texture, in terms of the responses of a set of tuned spatial filters (Allen et al., 2010; e.g. Barbosa et al., 2008; Chiao et al., 2010). Such measures can be run on photographs of the animals in a semi-automated manner, and they can be compared directly to measures of the background allowing a direct evaluation of the quality of camouflage. A disadvantage is that they are normally one-dimensional; the pattern is defined by a single parameter, and so does not represent the full range of patterns that can be produced. An alternative and more labour-intensive method is to score the level of expression of a large number (or all) of the body pattern components

(Kelman, Baddeley, Shohet & Osorio, 2007; Kelman, Osorio & Baddeley, 2008). This method potentially allows the investigation of how camouflage patterns are fine-tuned in response to visual stimuli. However, large multivariate data sets are unwieldy to analyse and difficult to interpret, and as a result biological relevance and patterns within the data can become lost. Principal component analysis (PCA) allows for such multivariate data sets to be reduced with a minimum loss of information, effectively transforming data of high dimensionality to one of fewer dimensions (Manly, 1994). PCA creates a set of new independent orthogonal variables based on the degree of covariance between sets of original variables. The first principal component (PC) is derived from an eigen-vector that accounts for as much of the variance within the original data as possible, with each following PC accounting for successively smaller proportions of the observed variance. Ideally for further analysis, the significant variation of the data is adequately described in the first few PCs (Jolliffe, 1986).

   In our work on cuttlefish colouration a data set for PCA is produced by assessing the strength of expression of up to 42 chromatic, textural and postural components, which were identified by Hanlon and Messenger (1988). Each component is scored on a four-point scale from not expressed (0) to strongly expressed (3) (e.g. Kelman, Baddeley, Shohet & Osorio, 2007; Zylinski, Darmaillacq & Shashar, 2012). The number of components ultimately included in the analysis varies as uninformative components can be excluded. The data set of component scores is subsequently reduced by PCA. A decision must next be made regarding the number of PCs retained for further analysis, commonly determined from a scree plot and/or the Kaiser criterion (Jolliffe, 1986). Eigen-vectors can be rotated to maximize the distance between PCs, but in practice unrotated PCs tend to provide variables that are biologically relevant and easily interpretable – with relevance to cuttlefish camouflage responses: in our experiments PCs 1 and 2 typically and broadly equate to Disruptive and Mottle body patterns (Figure 9.3; and see Figure 9.4 later in the chapter). Consideration of the original body pattern components that contribute to the retained PCs allows us to visualize which body pattern components tend to be correlated in their expression (e.g. Kelman, Baddeley, Shohet & Osorio, 2007; Kelman, Osorio & Baddeley, 2008; Zylinski, Osorio & Shohet, 2009b). The response to test stimuli can then be assessed using the new PC scores through common statistical tests.

9.4   Cuttlefish vision

Cephalopods have large, single chambered camera-type eyes (with the notable exception of the nautiloids, which have a unique pin-hole eye) whose optics and overall structure resembles that of fish, providing a striking example of convergence driven by a shared ecology (Land & Nilsson, 2002; Packard, 1972). Similarities include eye size range, lenses with a varying refractive index to minimize spherical aberration, variable pupils and migrating screening pigments. There are also differences: cephalopods photoreceptors face towards the light (i.e. unlike ours they are the 'right way around', meaning there is no blind spot); they have rhabdomeric rather than ciliary photoreceptors, and

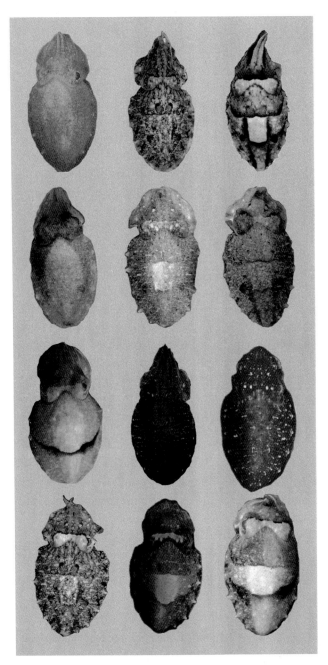

Figure 9.3 Demonstration of just some of the body pattern variation *Sepia officinalis* uses in camouflage body-pattern responses to the visual environment. The top row shows the primary characteristics of the main three *classes* of body pattern referred to in the text: Uniform (left), Mottle (centre) and Disruptive (right). The remaining images show how individual chromatic components patterns can be varied in their expression, along with the overall contrast of the body pattern, to give a wide range of body patterns that cannot always be readily identified as Uniform, Mottle or Disruptive. See plate section for colour version.

most species have only a single photopigment type (Marshall & Messenger, 1996). Differences are also apparent in the location of early neuronal processing; while vertebrates process a lot of visual information in the retina via the selective receptive fields of ganglion cells, the cephalopod retina lacks such cells and therefore does little processing. It is believed that the types of processing done in the vertebrate retina occurs instead in the large optic lobe (Williamson & Chrachri, 2004).

Studies of neural receptive fields from vertebrate retinal ganglion cells and primary visual cortex, along with human psychophysical studies, show that the vertebrate visual system first encodes the retinal image via local processes, operating on small regions of the retinal image. The local operations in the low-level stage of vision have been modelled as linear spatio-temporal filters, and as non-linear operations such as edge and motion detectors and, perhaps, to local texture analyzers (Bruce, Green & Georgeson, 1996). These non-linear processes are sometimes identified as feature detectors. Apart from local processing all stages of the visual pathway (but especially beyond the retina) have long-range interactions and receive feedback from higher centres. Such processes are probably crucial for figure-ground segregation: for example object borders can be identified by intensity differences, colour, texture, motion and depth (Zipser, Lamme & Schiller, 1996). Typically these processes which are sensitive to global context and are thought to occur at (or involve via feedback) later stages of processing; for example, pre-striate cortical areas, and they are classified as 'high-level'. In addition to the integration of multiple low-level cues this involves long-range interactions, contextual information, memory and attention. High-level vision is conceived as involving representations of the visual world and, hence, is cognitive (Cavanagh, 2011; Marr, 1982).

Findings on cephalopod spatial-vision fit into the foregoing scheme where low-level local processing involving linear-spatial filtering and local-feature detection is followed by higher-level (putatively cognitive) processes that integrate information from multiple sources. The animals are sensitive to a similar set of low-level spatial-image parameters to humans (Snowden, Thompson & Troscianko, 2006); namely mean reflectance, contrast, spatial frequency, orientation, spatial phase and depth, but not colour. The way in which the animals integrate this low level information to select camouflage then gives evidence for the existence of some type of higher level internal representation about the organization of the world into objects.

The next sections of this chapter outline experiments that support such conclusions, and indicate how findings are important for higher order visual tasks such as object detection and texture discrimination. We then go on to explore experiments that add to these basic findings to tackle potentially more cognitive processes.

9.4.1   Camouflage and low-level vision

Unfortunately there are few electrophysiological studies of cephalopod vision (Saidel, Shashar, Schmolesky & Hanlon, 2005), but we can study vision via body patterns. The approach is exemplified by Marshall and Messenger's (1996) demonstration that cuttlefish are colour blind. They placed the animals on substrates of either uniformly coloured gravel, gravel with stones varying in achromatic brightness (i.e. black and white) or gravel with stones whose reflectance spectra differed (they looked blue and yellow to the human eye) but were predicted to be of equal brightness to the cuttlefish photoreceptor. The animals behaved as if the latter background was uniform, consistent with their being colour-blind, a finding that has since been confirmed by a more detailed study (Mäthger, Barbosa, Miner & Hanlon, 2006).

About five years after Marshall and Messenger's (1996) work on colour vision, Chiao, Hanlon and their co-workers began a systematic study of responses to artificial backgrounds by *Sepia officinalis* and the tropical species *Sepia pharaonis* (Chiao & Hanlon, 2001a, 2001b). A key innovation was the use of a simple chequerboard stimulus (see below and Figure 9.1). The choice seems natural to those who are familiar with the use of stimuli such as gratings in human psychophysics, but there is a concern that a 2D chequerboard is such an impoverished stimulus compared to the visual environment of the shallow sea-floor habitat that the animals would not display meaningful responses. However, chequerboards have the advantages that they can be viewed from multiple orientations (see Shohet, Baddeley, Anderson, Kelman & Osorio (2006) for responses to gratings) and they contain completed 'objects' in the form of individual checks. In fact as this and subsequent studies have shown the animals respond meaningfully to chequerboards and other simple patterns with well-defined spatial characteristics (Zylinski & Osorio, 2011).

Chiao and Hanlon (2001a) found that for pharaoh cuttlefish (*S. pharaonis*), whose patterns closely resemble those of *S. officinalis;* both check size and achromatic contrast affected the body patterns. They characterized the body pattern by scoring the expression of a limited number of coarse-scale components that contribute to the 'Disruptive' body pattern (Hanlon & Messenger 1988, 1996), of which the most obvious is the so-called 'White Square' component, henceforth referred to as WS (see Figure 9.3). In keeping with what we might expect for camouflage, animals increased the expression of coarse, higher-contrast components as the checks increased in size and contrast.

In human psychophysics grating thresholds can be related to the modulation transfer function (MTF), which is a convenient measure of the optical quality of the eye and of spatial resolution (Campbell & Robson, 1968). What do Chiao and Hanlon's (2001a, 2001b) results imply about the acuity and contrast discrimination thresholds of *S. pharaonis*? A complication is that patterns used for smaller checks and lower contrast stimuli are not discoverable by scoring the Disruptive components. Chequerboards of intermediate sizes (relative to the WS) and contrasts result in the expression of components typical of the so-called 'Mottle' body pattern (see Figure 9.1), as explored by Barbosa and co-workers and by us (Barbosa et al., 2008; Zylinski, Osorio & Shohet, 2009b). As with human grating detection (Campbell & Robson, 1968) both contrast and spatial scale affect visibility, thus very small checks at high contrast are treated as a Uniform pattern, and elicit the Uniform body pattern, with the contrast thresholds falling as dimensions increase, up to a maximum and low contrasts (Zylinski, Osorio & Shohet, 2009b).

So can we say that these fine spatial and low contrast patterns, which elicit a Uniform body pattern, are below the visual acuity and contrast discrimination thresholds of the cuttlefish? Well possibly, but not conclusively, because this might be reflecting the animals decision about the best choice of pattern rather than a psychophysical threshold imposed by the eye or low-level neural mechanisms. In other words, the cuttlefish might be able to see that a fine chequerboard stimulus is made up of individual small checks, and the most effective match to this within its body pattern repertoire is the Uniform pattern. We return to these experiments in the account of edge detection below.

9.4.2 Edge detection and spatial phase

Whereas detection thresholds for spatial patterns – whether gratings, chequerboards or opticians test-charts – can generally be modelled by treating the visual pathway as a linear spatial system (e.g. as a set of spatial filters), the detection of local features such as motion and edges requires a non-linear mechanism (Bruce, Green & Georgeson, 1996). Edges and objects turn out to be of considerable significance to cuttlefish camouflage.

The experiments described above involved chequerboards with sharply defined edges separating adjacent checks. However, Barbosa et al. (2008) found that varying check contrast affects the choice of body pattern even for stimuli that cuttlefish can easily detect. They found that reducing contrast did not cause the animals to resort to the Uniform body pattern, as for a uniform background, but rather they display a Mottle pattern. As contrast differences between objects decrease, edges become less distinct (the step-difference becomes less) so these results suggest that object *edginess* might be important in the animal's choice between Disruptive and Mottle body patterns. Chiao, Kelman and Hanlon (2005) explored a related question using manipulated photographs of a gravel substrate that elicited the expression of Disruptive components. They found that, while an un-manipulated photograph of the gravel resulted in the same levels of expression in the measured components as the real gravel, when they removed the edge information in the image using a low-pass (Gaussian) filter the expression of these components was significantly reduced, even though information pertaining to object area and contrast was retained. Mäthger et al. (2007) demonstrated the same phenomenon using real substrates: by filling in the spaces around pebbles that elicited a Disruptive body pattern with sand, thereby reducing the strength of the edge information (as demonstrated using a computer-based edge detector), they showed that the animals reduced the expression of Disruptive components.

Any spatial pattern can be completely represented by a Fourier transform, which includes both spatial frequency and spatial phase information. Kelman, Baddeley, Shohet & Osorio (2007) tested phase sensitivity by comparing responses to conventional chequerboard patterns with those to patterns with identical spatial power-spectra but randomized phase. These phase-randomized chequerboards look like normal chequerboards without clearly defined edges. This treatment, like reduction of contrast, essentially caused the animals to switch from the Disruptive components they had used on the original chequerboards to a Mottle. It seems that cuttlefish, like humans, are sensitive to phase. All of these findings point to the existence of specialized edge detectors in cuttlefish vision, with the presence of edges favouring the expression of Disruptive components. Edges are of course a characteristic of object boundaries. By comparison patterns lacking edges but with an otherwise comparable spatial frequency power-spectrum favour Mottle body pattern components.

Can the relationship between the animal's background and the pattern that is displayed be summarized by the simple set of relations:

$$\text{Objects} \rightarrow \text{Disruptive, Texture} \rightarrow \text{Mottle, Uniform} \rightarrow \text{Uniform,}$$

and can it be more rigorously defined? We have proposed (Zylinski, Osorio & Shohet, 2009b) that, while Disruptive patterns are used in response to edgy, low-contrast stimuli, Mottle patterns are used where objects are small or edges are poorly defined (either through the visual attributes of the objects or the physiological limitations of the animal's visual system). We suggested a model based on the ability or inability of the cuttlefish to distinguish higher Fourier components within a given stimulus. Edges occur where sinusoidal components of different frequencies are in phase at their zero-crossings (Morrone & Burr, 1988). In a two-dimensional (2D) Fourier transform a square wave can be approximated by a low-frequency fundamental sinusoid with the addition of the third and fifth harmonics – these are in phase with the fundamental wave –and the more sinusoidal terms added the more representative of the original signal it becomes. According to this *MTF + minimal edges* model, if a stimulus is of high enough spatial frequency that only the fundamental component is resolvable, *or* if the edge information is not well defined so that higher harmonics are not in phase with the fundamental then the cuttlefish will respond with a Mottle-type pattern. If, however, the stimulus contains spatial frequency information low enough for higher harmonics to be resolved *and* there is phase congruency between the fundamental and (at least) the third harmonic, characterizing edges, then the animal will respond with Disruptive-type body patterns. We demonstrated that, by independently modulating the spatial characteristics and the contrast of checks in a chequerboard background and analyzing the resulting body-pattern responses of cuttlefish, thresholds between body patterns could be distinguished that were consistent with this model.

9.4.3   Objects and object completion

Human vision has powerful mechanisms for separating objects from their background that combine both local and more global cues (Bruce, Green & Georgeson, 1996; Zipser, Lamme & Schiller, 1996). The underlying mechanisms, especially where they implicate long-range interactions, have attracted considerable attention in work on visual processing in the cortex (Lamme & Roelfsema, 2000; Zipser, Lamme & Schiller, 1996); for example, the studies of illusory contours in visual area 2 of primates by Peterhans and co-workers (e.g. Peterhans & von der Heydt, 1989, 1991). It is, therefore, interesting to ask how cuttlefish use local visual cues in figure-ground segregation.

Chiao and Hanlon (2001a, 2001b) suggested that the overall area of objects in the visual environment is important in determining the cuttlefish's body pattern. How might the animals measure object area? As previously mentioned, human vision can identify step edges that indicate object boundaries by local edge detectors (Marr & Hildreth, 1980; Morrone & Burr, 1988). In a series of experiments designed specifically to investigate the importance of edges in determining camouflage body patterns (Zylinski, Osorio & Shohet, 2009c), we first asked: if the animals express a given body pattern in response to a whole object (in this case a 2D white circle on a grey background), will just the edges of these same objects provide sufficient information for the animals to respond in the same way? The approach was to produce images where regions where defined by edges but with no mean intensity difference between the figure and the ground; this is done simply by high-pass filtering an image (Figure 9.4). It turns out that the responses of the animals to the whole objects and to the high-pass outlines of the circles were not statistically separable. By comparison if the contrast of a figure (such as light circle on a dark background) is reduced, the animals suppress Disruptive components and use a Uniform body pattern.

What does the finding that outlines appear to substitute for whole objects say about the importance of object area as a cue for determining the animals' choice of camouflage pattern? An obvious interpretation is that, in the real world, objects without area do not occur: edges are indicative of the presence of objects, which is exactly why they are important. Bearing this in mind, we wondered if the presence of isolated edge segments, or fragments, might be sufficient for the animal to infer the presence of an associated object (also known as contour completion). Our rationale was that, in the real world, objects that the cuttlefish wants to use in its decision about camouflage patterns might be partially occluded by other objects in the three-dimensional (3D) environment, or perhaps partially buried in finer substrate (e.g. white pebbles partly hidden from the animal's view by seaweed, or partly buried in darker sand), and correctly interpreting these visual ambiguities may be the difference between being well camouflaged, and, hence, protected from visual predation, and being conspicuous.

We tested half-circle, quarter-circle and eighth-circle high-pass filtered edge fragments and found that indeed cuttlefish interpreted the presence of edges as evidence for the presence of corresponding objects, as determined by the animal's use of Disruptive components being indistinguishable from those used in response to whole circles (Figure 9.5a,b). Strikingly this was the case even for quarter-circle edge fragments, in which the white area of each fragment was less than one would predict was needed to elicit such as response (Figure 9.5c). Clearly the animal is choosing camouflage by inferring the size of the objects in the background rather than direct measurement. The extrapolation of object presence ceased when edge fragments were further reduced: the animals responses were in keeping with those expected for individual small objects, using Mottle-type body patterns, when edge fragments were eighth-circles.

We see from the experiments outlined above that, as in vertebrate and machine vision, edges are very important to cuttlefish. Not only are they using edges to gain information about objects in their environment, but also, additionally, they are translating this information back into their body patterns in order to achieve effective camouflage.

9.4.4   Contour completion

The finding that *Sepia* can use isolated edge segments to infer the presence of whole objects (Zylinski, Osorio & Shohet, 2009c) suggests a way to test a distinct set of visual

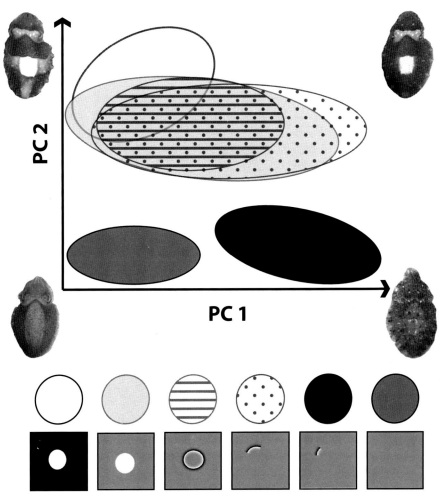

Figure 9.4 Example of how scores from two principal components (PC 1 and PC 2) can be used to visualize how different stimuli influence body patterning beyond simple classifications. The example here is based on the experiment described in section 9.3.3, using high-pass filtered 'objects' and edge fragments to explore edge detection mechanisms in *S. officinalis* (see Zylinski, Osorio & Shohet, 2009c for futher detail). Different patterned and shaded areas show the range of PC scores for 20 cuttlefish responses to the stimuli shown below (presented as multiple printed objects across the floor and walls of the test arena) and are presented as such to allow the reader to easily see the separation and overlap in the responses to the various stimuli. Cuttlefish images on the axes give examples of typical responses at extremes. For example, high-contrast white objects on a black background (open circle) result in responses characterized by low PC 1 scores and high PC 2 scores, equating to a Disruptive-type body-pattern response. By contrast, quarter-edge segments (black-tinted circle) result in high PC 1 scores and low PC 2 scores, equating to more Mottle-type responses. Low PC 1 and PC 2 scores equate to a Uniform body pattern, as seen in response to a homogenous grey stimulus (dark-grey circle).

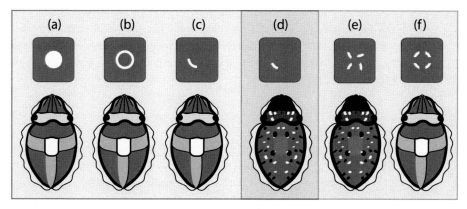

Figure 9.5 (a) Cuttlefish respond with body patterns containing blocky, high contrast Disruptive components in response to white 'objects' (two-dimensional printed filled-in circles on a mid-grey background) of an area 40–120% of the white square (WS) component. (b) The same response is given to the outline of the circle alone. (c) Animals also give the same response when edge fragments down to ~¼ of the circle are presented. (d) When edges are reduced further the animals change from the blocky Disruptive response and instead use a Mottle-type response. (e) When edge fragments are clustered but anomalously configured the same Mottle-type response is used. (f) When the same fragments are shown in the correct configuration then the cuttlefish once again use Disruptive components. Adapted from Zylinski, Darmaillacq and Shashar (2012).

phenomena associated with the reconstruction of fragmented information of which best known are modal and amodal completion. Modal completion refers to that which occurs when a foreground object is viewed against a background with predominantly similar intensity properties, such as the classic Kanisza Triangle (Pessoa, Thompson & Noë, 1998). In this case boundaries of the object are completed by the percept of illusory contours accompanied by a concurrent brightness enhancement. Amodal completion refers to the situation when a foreground figure appears to partially occlude a target figure, but the visual system is nevertheless able to perceive the object in its entirety by linking the visually fragmented parts of the target, completing it without a sensation of the occurrence of the borders (Halko, Mingolla & Somers, 2008; Pessoa, Thompson & Noë, 1998; Peterhans & von der Heydt, 1989).

Based on the knowledge gained from the edge detection experiment described above (Zylinski, Osorio & Shohet, 2009c), Zylinski, Darmaillacq and Shashar (2012) took the outline (edges) of an 'object' (a white circle) to which *S. officinalis* responded with Disruptive components (Figure 9.5b) and disassembled it into edge fragments smaller than those from which the animals infer the presence of larger objects (Figure 9.5d). In other words, these fragments resulted in the use of a Mottle- or Uniform-type body pattern when randomly scattered across a mid-grey background (printed 2D stimuli; Figure 9.5d). However, when these same fragments were presented in a configuration that was in keeping with the outline of the original circle, the animals responded with Disruptive components (Figure 9.5f). In other words, the animals were able to recon-struct the fragmented visual information and respond as if the complete object was present when these fragment edges were configured thus. To ensure this response was not a response to the clustering of high contrast objects (see section 9.3.5) the same fragments were tested in the same global positions but in an anomalous configuration: the fragments were rotated on their axes. The cuttlefish responded to this stimulus with non-Disruptive body patterns similar to the responses to the scattered fragments (Figure 9.5e). This strengthens the interpretation of these results as a demonstration of boundary completion.

9.4.5   Texture

We can consider visual texture a property of 'stuff' in a scene, in contradistinction with 'things' such as lines and objects (Adelson & Bergen, 1991; Landy & Graham, 2004). This might be analogous to the linguistic differences between the mass noun 'water' and the count noun 'cuttlefish'. Another analogy is the separation of sketchable and non-sketchable image regions, where non-sketchable is equivalent to texture.

Often boundaries between image regions are not formed by distinct intensity changes, represented by step edges, but are instead separated by textural differences that have no associated intensity differences. What makes one texture easily distinguishable from another is not straightforward and is incompletely understood, even in human vision. Texture discrimination has been the subject of much research for human and machine vision (Julesz, 1981; Julesz & Schumer, 1981; Portilla & Simoncelli, 2000). In cuttlefish visual perception and camouflage it seems that the Mottle body pattern is used largely in response to image texture, just as the use of Disruptive components seems to be strongly correlated with the presence of objects (within a given size range) with distinct edges. Indeed, the pattern components themselves are much more 'textural' than the blocky, distinct Disruptive components.

Chiao, Chubb, Buresch and Siemann (2009) used a set of well-defined artificial substrates to take a closer look at the interaction between textural background features and body-pattern responses. They used a random noise matrix, filtered at various spatial scales, to keep the overall characteristics the same but changed the scale of the background attributes. They showed that, as with the closed objects created by chequerboards, these random shapes (which still contained strong edge information) evoked a transition from Uniform- to Mottle- to Disruptive-type patterns with increased scale (or relative area of black and white in the background). Interestingly, they noted that some of the backgrounds that were expected to elicit a Mottle response also contained Disruptive components. They suggested that spatial scale is more important than defined objects in determining which body pattern will be used, but given that in real visual scenes substrates containing such defined edges and high contrast components will usually be associated with distinct objects, it is not clear to what extent scale and object can be decoupled. We suspect, based on the findings outlined above, that cuttlefish interpolate and extrapolate information; the final outcome of the body pattern is likely based on the integration of multiple cues of which scale is just one. For example, these random noise patterns retain the equal ratios of black and white seen in chequerboards; although it becomes harder to define, design and interpret more complex patterns, these seem to be necessary to unravel the complete story of visual cues in cuttlefish camouflage.

We carried out experiments to attempt to explicitly test the responses of juvenile *S. officinalis* to objects defined by local texture rather than by overall luminance (Zylinski,

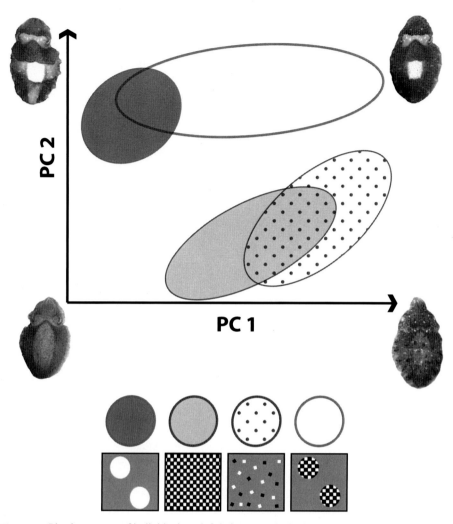

Figure 9.6 Plotting scores of individual cuttlefish for two principal components (PC 1 and PC 2) enables us to visualize how the animals use textural information. Patterned and tinted areas show the range of responses for individual cuttlefish to the stimuli tested, as given below. Cuttlefish images show the general body pattern characteristics associated with the high/low scores on each axis. We see from this that the body-pattern response to objects formed as textural 'clumps' of chequerboard (white circle) is distinct from that of continuous chequerboard (light grey circle) and untextured objects (dark grey circle). Unclumped individual textural components (dotted circle) result in a similar, but not identical, response as the continuous chequerboard.

Osorio & Shohet, 2009c). To do this we designed a mid-grey printed background scattered randomly with 'objects' made up of circular patches of small black and white checks (Figure 9.6). This meant the overall luminance of the objects was identical to that of the background, but that the objects, unlike the background, had a distinct texture. The size of the patch circles was predetermined to elicit a Disruptive-type response when displayed as white objects on a mid-grey background. We also assayed the body-pattern responses of cuttlefish to these small checks configured as a continuous chequerboard, and as individual checks scattered across the grey background rather than clustered into objects (Figure 9.6). Interestingly, we found that these latter two stimuli resulted in a similar (but not identical) Mottle-type response, with the scattered individual squares resulting in a much stronger Mottle than the continuous chequerboard.

Contrary to expectations based on the responses to the latter two stimuli described above, the main test stimulus (patches of objects) resulted in responses consistently containing high-contrast Disruptive components (PC 2 in this study), such as the White Square and White Head Bar. In other words, the animals used a significantly different response to the same small black and white squares depending on whether they were scattered across the background or clustered into objects, suggesting perceptual grouping. However, the animals appeared to integrate aspects of the textural nature of the patches, and expressed Mottle-type components (PC 1 in this study) in addition to the Disruptive components. Such results can be compared to the responses to both white circles and a mixture of black and white circles, which scored high on PC 2 but low on PC 1 (i.e. similar strength of Disruptive components but fewer Mottle components). These findings show that: (a) the cuttlefish cue in on global attributes of the visual environment, not just absolute local features; and (b) texture, distinct from objects, lines and features, drive Mottle-type body patterns and associated components.

The responses of animals to some stimuli tested by Chiao, Chubb and Hanlon (2007) point to similar findings, but not explicitly so. For example, one experiment tested something akin to the opposite to our test: they tested cuttlefish body-pattern responses to square white 'objects' on a background composed of smaller textural components. Although in their paper they interpret this in terms of size predominating over contrast, an alternative interpretation would be that reducing the integrity of the edge information (in terms of contrast difference) between the large white figure and the small chequerboard background resulted in the suppression of Disruptive components. This is in keeping with our findings that the loss of edge information results in the animal responding with Mottle or Uniform patterns, even in the presence of objects typically associated with Disruptive type patterns.

9.5   Making decisions about body patterns

Do cuttlefish make active choices about camouflage? Do they show preference for backgrounds or substrates over others, and is this preference based on the visual attributes? When faced with a background containing multiple options for camouflage, how do the animals solve the dilemma of what they should camouflage to? Laboratory and field studies have tackled these questions in several species.

Zylinski, How, Osorio, Hanlon and Marshall (2011) analysed the characteristics of body patterns and backgrounds of images of the Australian giant cuttlefish, *Sepia apama*, in the near-shore benthic habitats that form their breeding grounds. Here, males embark in conspicuous agonistic kinetic displays (i.e. moving stripes) with other males and direct similar displays to females (Figure 9.7a). When not involved in mating behaviours, both

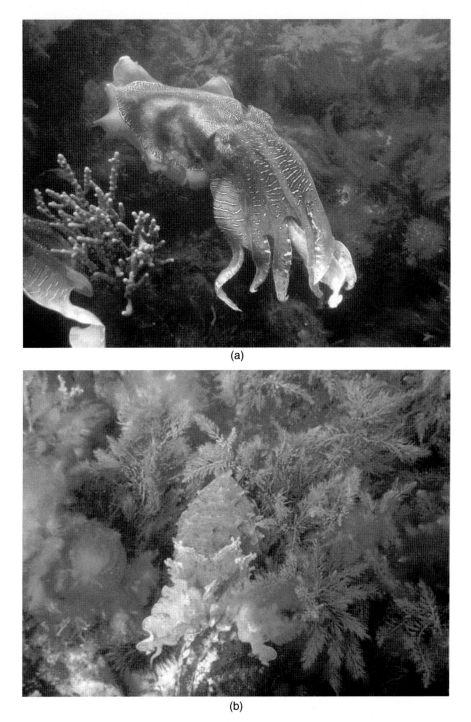

(a)

(b)

Figure 9.7 The giant Australian cuttlefish, *Sepia apama*, chooses simple backgrounds to display against, which probably acts to increase signal efficacy, and more complex backgrounds to camouflage against making visual search more difficult for potential predators. (a) A male engaged in an agonistic display to another male. (b) A camouflaging individual uses chromatic and textural components. (c) Plot of intensity variances (a measure of visual complexity) from image analysis of the mantle patterns of signalling and camouflaging animals compared background areas against which they were photographed, along with those for a random set of habitats (control). Adapted from Zylinski, How, Osorio, Hanlon and Marshall (2011). See plate section for colour version of (a) and (b).

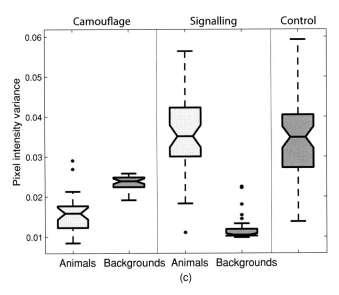

Figure 9.7 (*cont.*)

sexes use camouflaged body patterns (Figure 9.7b). The study clearly showed that there were differences not just between the spatial characteristics of the body patterns an animal used during these different behaviours, but also in the visual characteristics of the backgrounds used when camouflaging compared to when signalling. Backgrounds used for camouflage typically have a significantly higher variance in intensity, suggesting that they were more visually complex, while backgrounds used for signalling against were more homogenous (Figure 9.7c). This suggests that the cuttlefish actively choose a simple background reducing noise to improve signal efficacy and, conversely, a more visually complex area for camouflage in order to improve its effectiveness.

Allen et al. (2010) investigated background choice and camouflage pattern use in *S. officinalis* in a series of laboratory-based experiments. These experiments focused on camouflage pattern choice in the presence of multiple visual background types. They found that, within the small range of artificial and natural backgrounds used and the relatively small area within which they were tested, when given a choice of substrates designed to elicit different classes of body patterns the animals did not show a preference to settle on a specific substrate (suggesting they have no preference for using a particular class of body pattern). The only significant finding with regards to choice was that, in the case of loose natural substrates, the cuttlefish showed a preference for substrates into which they could bury over those substrates they could not. Buresch et al. (2011) found that *S. officinalis* made choices as to which aspect of the visual environment to match in order to obtain camouflage. They tested the body-pattern responses of cuttlefish to 3D objects on a 2D substrate at varying levels of contrast. They found that 3D objects were salient for camouflage when they were of a higher contrast than the substrate.

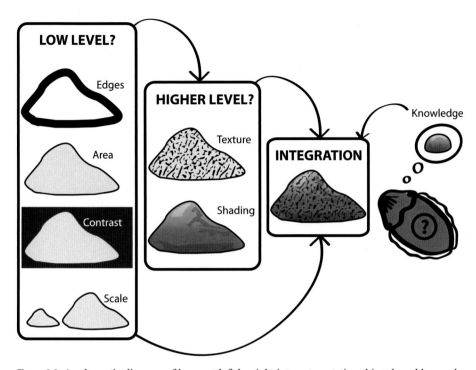

Figure 9.8 A schematic diagram of how cuttlefish might integrate putative object-based low and higher level (bottom-up) and viewer-based scene knowledge (top-down) information about the local visual environment in order to make decisions about what body pattern to use.

9.6   Concluding remarks

Here we have discussed just those aspects of cuttlefish vision and camouflage for which we have a reasonable level of understanding. Little is yet known about the mechanisms used by cuttlefish in other aspects of vision that are crucial in vertebrate vision, such as the processing of motion (Zylinski, Osorio & Shohet, 2009a) and the perception of depth (Allen, Mäthger, Barbosa & Hanlon, 2009; Barbosa, Allen, Mäthger & Hanlon, 2012; Buresch et al., 2011). Much evidence points to the conclusion that the body patterns used by cuttlefish for camouflage are not hard-wired responses to specific cues (Figure 9.8). By following the input to eye, to optic lobe, to brain, to the chromatophore output, we encounter cognitive processes.

Cephalopods have large brains that have evolved independently of vertebrates and it is, therefore, interesting to ask to what extent they share similar principles of operation. At one level this can concern relatively low-level phenomena, such as the evidence that cuttlefish have local edge detectors that resemble those thought to be used by humans (Kelman, Baddeley, Shohet & Osorio, 2007; Kelman, Osorio & Baddeley, 2008; Morrone & Burr, 1988; Zylinski, Osorio & Shohet, 2009b). On the other hand, cephalopods mostly lack colour vision (Marshall & Messenger, 1996; Mäthger, Barbosa, Miner & Hanlon, 2006), but make much greater use of polarization (Temple et al., 2012), giving them a different phenomenal world from ours; we have hardly begun to understand their cognitive worlds.

Acknowledgements

We would like to acknowledge support from Office of Naval Research MURI grant no. N00014–09–1–1053 to S. Z.

References

Adelson, E. and Bergen, J. (1991). The plenoptic function and elements of early vision. In *Computational models of visual processing* M. Landy and J. A. Movshon (Eds.). Cambridge, MA: MIT Press.

Allen, J. J., Mäthger, L. M., Barbosa, A., Buresch, K. C., Sogin, E., Schwartz, J., Chubb, C. and Hanlon, R. T. (2010). Cuttlefish dynamic camouflage: responses to substrate choice and integration of multiple visual cues. *Proceedings of the Royal Society. B: Biological Sciences*, **277**(1684): 1031–1039.

Allen, J. J., Mäthger, L. M., Barbosa, A. and Hanlon, R. T. (2009). Cuttlefish use visual cues to control three-dimensional skin papillae for camouflage. *Journal of Comparative Physiology A*, **195**(6): 547–555.

Barbosa, A., Allen, J. J., Mäthger, L. M. and Hanlon, R. T. (2012). Cuttlefish use visual cues to determine arm postures for camouflage. *Proceedings of the Royal Society. B: Biological Sciences*, **279**: 84–90.

Barbosa, A., Mäthger, L. M., Buresch, K. C., Kelly, J., Chubb, C., Chiao, C.-C. and Hanlon, R. T. (2008). Cuttlefish camouflage: the effects of substrate contrast and size in evoking Uniform, Mottle or Disruptive body patterns. *Vision Research*, **48**(10): 1242–1253.

Bennett, A. T. (1996). Do animals have cognitive maps? *Journal of Experimental Biology*, **199**(1): 219–224.

Brooks, R. (1991). Intelligence without representation. *Artificial Intelligence*, **47**: 139–159.

Bruce, V., Green, P. R. and Georgeson, M. A. (1996). *Visual perception: physiology, psychology and ecology* (3rd edn). Hove, UK: Psychology Press.

Budelmann, B. U. (1994). Cephalopod sense organs, nerves and the brain: adaptations for high performance and life style. *Marine and Freshwater Behaviour and Physiology*, **25**(1–3): 13–33.

Buresch, K., Mäthger, L., Allen, J., Bennice, C., Smith, N., Schram, J., Chiao, C.-C., Chubb, C. and Hanlon, R. (2011). The use of background matching vs. masquerade for camouflage in cuttlefish *Sepia officinalis*. *Vision Research*, **51**(23–24): 2362–2368.

Burgess, N. (2006). Spatial memory: how egocentric and allocentric combine. *Trends in Cognitive Sciences*, **10**(12): 551–557.

Byrne, R. W. and Bates, L. A. (2006). Why are animals cognitive? *Current Biology*, **16**(12): R445–448.

Campbell, F. W. and Robson, J. G. (1968). Application of Fourier analysis to the visibility of gratings. *Journal of Physiology*, **197**: 551–566.

Cavanagh, P. (2011). Visual cognition. *Vision Research*, **51**: 408–416.

Chiao, C.-C., Chubb, C., Buresch, K. C., Barbosa, A., Allen, J. J., Mäthger, L. M. and Hanlon, R. T. (2010). Mottle camouflage patterns in cuttlefish: quantitative characterization and visual background stimuli that evoke them. *Journal of Experimental Biology*, **213**(2): 187–199.

Chiao, C.-C., Chubb, C., Buresch, K. C. and Siemann, L. (2009). The scaling effects of substrate texture on camouflage patterning in cuttlefish. *Vision Research*, **49**: 1647–1656.

Chiao, C.-C., Chubb, C. and Hanlon, R. T. (2007). Interactive effects of size, contrast, intensity and configuration of background objects in evoking Disruptive camouflage in cuttlefish. *Vision Research*, **47**: 2223–2235.

Chiao, C.-C. and Hanlon, R. T. (2001a). Cuttlefish camouflage: visual perception of size, contrast and number of white squares on artificial chequerboard substrata initiates Disruptive coloration. *Journal of Experimental Biology*, **204**(12): 2119–2125.

Chiao, C.-C. and Hanlon, R. T. (2001b). Cuttlefish cue visually on area- not shape or aspect ratio -of light objects in the substrate to produce Disruptive body patterns for camouflage. *The Biological Bulletin*, **201**(2): 269–270.

Chiao, C.-C., Kelman, E. J. and Hanlon, R. T. (2005). Disruptive body patterning of cuttlefish (*Sepia officinalis*) requires visual information regarding edges and contrast of objects in natural substrate backgrounds. *The Biological Bulletin*, **208**(1): 7–11.

Collett, T. S. and Collett, M. (2002). Memory use in insect visual navigation. *Nature reviews. Neuroscience*, **3**(7): 542–552.

Cott, H. B. (1940). *Adaptive colouration in animals*. London, UK: Methuen Publishing.

Crook, A. C., Baddeley, R. and Osorio, D. (2002). Identifying the structure in cuttlefish visual signals. *Philosophical Transactions of the Royal Society B*, **357**(1427): 1617–1624.

Gibson, J. J. (1979). *The ecological approach to visual perception*. Boston, MA: Houghton Mifflin.

Gregory, R. L. (1997). Knowledge in perception and illusion. *Philosophical Transactions of the Royal Society B*, **352**(1358): 1121–1127.

Halko, M. A., Mingolla, E. and Somers, D. C. (2008). Multiple mechanisms of illusory contour perception. *Journal of Vision*, **8**(11): 1–17.

Hanlon, R. T. (2007). Cephalopod dynamic camouflage. *Current Biology*, **17**(11): R400–R404.

Hanlon, R. T., Forsythe, J. W. and Joneschild, D. E. (1999). Crypsis, conspicuousness, mimicry and polyphenism as antipredator defences of foraging octopuses on Indo-Pacific coral reefs, with a method of quantifying crypsis from video tapes. *Biological Journal of the Linnean Society*, **66**: 1–22.

Hanlon, R. T. and Messenger, J. B. (1988). Adaptive coloration in young cuttlefish (*Sepia officinalis* L) – the morphology and development of body patterns and their relation to behavior. *Philosophical Transactions of the Royal Society B*, **320**(1200): 437–487.

Hanlon, R. T. and Messenger, J. B. (1996). *Cephalopod behaviour*. New York, NY: Cambridge University Press.

Jolliffe, I. T. (1986). *Principal component analysis*. New York, NY: Springer-Verlag.

Julesz, B. (1981). Textons, the elements of texture perception, and their interactions. *Nature*, **290**(5802): 91–97.

Julesz, B. and Schumer, R. A. (1981). Early visual perception. *Annual Review of Psychology*, **32**: 575–627.

Kelman, E. J., Baddeley, R. J., Shohet, A. J. and Osorio, D. (2007). Perception of visual texture and the expression of Disruptive camouflage by the cuttlefish *Sepia officinalis*. *Proceedings of the Royal Society. B: Biological Sciences*, **274**: 1369–1375.

Kelman, E. J., Osorio, D. and Baddeley, R. J. (2008). A review of cuttlefish camouflage and object recognition and evidence for depth perception. *Journal of Experimental Biology*, **211**(11): 1757–1763.

Kelman, E. J., Tiptus, P. and Osorio, D. (2006). Juvenile plaice (*Pleuronectes platessa*) produce camouflage by flexibly combining two separate patterns. *Journal of Experimental Biology*, **209**: 3288–3292.

Krapp, H. G. and Hengstenberg, R. (1997). Estimation of self-motion by optic flow processing in single visual interneurons. *Nature*, **384**: 463–466.

Lamme, V. A. F. and Roelfsema, P. R. (2000). The distinct modes of vision offered by feedforward and recurrent processing. *Trends in Neurosciences*, **23**: 571–579.

Land, M. F. and Nilsson, D.-E. (2002). *Animal eyes*. Oxford, UK: Oxford University Press.

Landy, M. S. and Graham, N. (2004). Visual perception of texture. In *The visual neurosciences* L. M. Chalupa & J. S. Werner (Eds.). Cambridge, MA: MIT Press.

Langridge, K. V., Broom, M. and Osorio, D. (2007). Selective signalling by cuttlefish to predators. *Current Biology*, **17**(24): R1044–R1045.

Mackintosh, N. J. (1974). *Psychology of animal learning*. Oxford, UK: Academic Press.

Manly, B. F. J. (1994). *Multivariate statistical methods – a primer* (2nd edn). London, UK: Chapman and Hall.

Marr, D. (1982). *Vision: a computational investigation into the human representation and processing of visual information*. New York, NY: Henry Holt and Co.

Marr, D. and Hildreth, E. (1980). Theory of edge detection. *Proceedings of the Royal Society. B: Biological Sciences*, **207**(1167): 187–217.

Marshall, N. J. and Messenger, J. B. (1996). Colour-blind camouflage. *Nature*, **382**: 408–409.

Mäthger, L. M., Barbosa, A., Miner, S. and Hanlon, R. T. (2006). Color blindness and contrast perception in cuttlefish (*Sepia officinalis*) determined by a visual sensorimotor assay. *Vision Research*, **46**(11): 1746–1753.

Mäthger, L. M., Chiao, C. C., Barbosa, A., Buresch, K. C., Kaye, S. and Hanlon, R. T. (2007). Disruptive coloration elicited on controlled natural substrates in cuttlefish, *Sepia officinalis*. *Journal of Experimental Biology*, **210**(15): 2657–2666.

Mäthger, L. M. and Hanlon, R. T. (2007). Malleable skin coloration in cephalopods: selective reflectance, transmission and absorbance of light by chromatophores and iridophores. *Cell and Tissue Research*, **329**(1): 179–186.

Messenger, J. B. (2001). Cephalopod chromatophores: neurobiology and natural history. *Biological Reviews*, **76**: 473–528.

Morrone, M. C. and Burr, D. C. (1988). Feature detection in human vision: a phase-dependent energy model. *Proceedings of the Royal Society. B: Biological Sciences*, **235**: 221–245.

Packard, A. (1972). Cephalopods and fish: the limits of convergence. *Biological Reviews*, **47**(2): 241–307.

Packard, A. and Hochberg, F. G. (1977). Skin patterning in *Octopus* and other genera. *Symposium of the Zoological Society of London*, **38**: 191–231.

Packard, A. and Sanders, G. D. (1971). Body patterns of *Octopus vulgaris* and maturation of the response to disturbance. *Animal Behaviour*, **19**(4): 780–790.

Pessoa, L., Thompson, E. and Noë, A. (1998). Finding out about filling-in: a guide to perceptual completion for visual science and the philosophy of perception. *Behavioral and Brain Sciences*, **21**(6): 723–802.

Peterhans, E. and von der Heydt, R. (1989). Mechanisms of contour perception in monkey visual cortex. II. Contours bridging gaps. *Journal of Neuroscience*, **9**(5): 1749–1763.

Peterhans, E. and von der Heydt, R. (1991). Subjective contours-bridging the gap between psychophysics and physiology. *Trends in Neurosciences*, **14**(3): 112–119.

Portilla, J. and Simoncelli, E. P. (2000). A parametric texture model based on joint statistics of complex wavelet coefficients. *International Journal of Computer Vision*, **40**(1): 49–71.

Ramachandran, V. S., Tyler, C. W., Gregory, R. L., Rogers-Ramachandran, D., Duensing, S., Pillsbury, C. and Ramachandran, C. (1996). Rapid adaptive camouflage in tropical flounders. *Nature*, **379**: 815–818.

Real, L. A. (1993). Toward a cognitive ecology. *Trends in Ecology and Evolution*, **8**(11): 413–417.

Saidel, W. M., Shashar, N., Schmolesky, M. T. and Hanlon, R. T. (2005). Discriminative responses of squid (*Loligo pealeii*) photoreceptors to polarized light. *Comparative Biochemistry and Physiology A*, **142**: 340–346.

Shettleworth, S. (2001). Animal cognition and animal behaviour. *Animal Behaviour*, **61**(2): 277–286.

Shettleworth, S. (2010). *Cognition, evolution, and behavior* (2nd edn). Oxford, UK: Oxford University Press.

Shohet, A. J., Baddeley, R. J., Anderson, J. C., Kelman, E. J. and Osorio, D. (2006). Cuttlefish responses to visual orientation, water flow and a model of motion camouflage. *Journal of Experimental Biology*, **209**: 4717–4723.

Shohet, A., Baddeley, R. J., Anderson, J. C. and Osorio, D. (2007). Cuttlefish camouflage: a quantitative study of patterning. *Biological Journal of the Linnean Society*, **92**(2): 335–345.

Snowden, R. J., Thompson, P. and Troscianko, T. (2006). *Basic vision: an introduction to visual perception*. Oxford, UK: Oxford University Press.

Srinivasan, M. V. and Venkatesh, S. (1997). *Living eyes to seeing machines*. Oxford, UK: Oxford University Press.

Stevens, M. (2007). Predator perception and the interrelation between different forms of protective coloration. *Proceedings of the Royal Society. B: Biological Sciences*, **274**: 1457–1464.

Stuart-Fox, D. and Moussalli, A. (2009). Camouflage, communication and thermoregulation: lessons from colour changing organisms. *Philosophical Transactions of the Royal Society B*, **364**(1516): 463–470.

Stuart-Fox, D., Whiting, M. J. and Moussalli, A. (2006). Camouflage and colour change: antipredator responses to bird and snake predators across multiple populations in a dwarf chameleon. *Biological Journal of the Linnean Society*, **88**: 437–446.

Temple, S. E., Pignatelli, V., Cook, T., How, M. J., Chiou, T. H., Roberts, N. W. and Marshall, N. J. (2012). High-resolution polarisation vision in a cuttlefish. *Current Biology*, **22**(4): R121–R122.

Tolman, E. C. (1948). Cognitive maps in rats and men. *Psychological Review*, **55**: 189–208.

Wang, R. F. and Spelke, E. S. (2002). Human spatial representation: insights from animals. *Trends in Cognitive Sciences*, **6**(9): 376–382.

Williamson, R. and Chrachri, A. (2004). Cephalopod neural networks. *Neurosignals*, **13**(1–2): 87–98.

Young, R. E., Vecchione, M. and Donovan, D. T. (1998). The evolution of coleoid cephalopods and their present biodiversity and ecology. *South African Journal of Marine Science*, **20**(1): 393–420.

Zipser, K., Lamme, V. A. F. and Schiller, P. H. (1996). Contextual modulation in primary visual cortex. *Journal of Neuroscience*, **16**(22): 7376–7389.

Zylinski, S., Darmaillacq, A.-S. and Shashar, N. (2012). Visual interpolation for contour completion by the European cuttlefish (*Sepia officinalis*) and its use in dynamic camouflage. *Proceedings of the Royal Society. B: Biological Sciences*, **279**(1737): 2386–2390.

Zylinski, S., How, M. J., Osorio, D., Hanlon, R. T. and Marshall, N. J. (2011). To be seen or to hide: visual characteristics of body patterns for camouflage and communication in the Australian giant cuttlefish *Sepia apama*. *The American Naturalist*, **177**(5): 681–690.

Zylinski, S. and Osorio, D. (2011). What can camouflage tell us about non-human visual perception? A case study of multiple cue use in the cuttlefish *Sepia officinalis*. In *Animal camouflage: mechanisms and function* M. Stevens & S. Merilaita (Eds.). Cambridge, UK: Cambridge University Press.

Zylinski, S., Osorio, D. and Shohet, A. J. (2009a). Cuttlefish camouflage: context-dependent body pattern use during motion. *Proceedings of the Royal Society. B: Biological Sciences*, **276**(1675): 3963–3969.

Zylinski, S., Osorio, D. and Shohet, A. J. (2009b). Edge detection and texture classification by cuttlefish. *Journal of Vision*, **9**(13): 1–10.

Zylinski, S., Osorio, D. and Shohet, A. J. (2009c). Perception of edges and visual texture in the camouflage of the common cuttlefish, *Sepia officinalis*. *Philosophical Transactions of the Royal Society B*, **364**(1516): 439–448.

10 Visual cognition in deep-sea cephalopods: what we don't know and why we don't know it

Sarah Zylinski and Sönke Johnsen

10.1 The other cephalopods

A quick glance at the recent cephalopod literature, or even at the chapters of this book, tells us that when we talk about cephalopod cognition we are really considering cognition in a handful of genera. There can be no argument that studies of these animals have led to remarkable results that have challenged the traditional view of invertebrate intelligence. Yet when we consider that less than 10 species of cephalopod are commonly seen as the focus of behavioural studies, let alone in studies specifically about cognition, it becomes apparent that claims regarding the cognitive capabilities of cephalopods are generalizations drawn from work on a handful of genera. The majority of the 800 or so described species of cephalopod do not share the neritic and near-shore benthic habitats of the taxa with which we are most familiar; virtually unknown in terms of their behaviour and ecology, these species inhabit a different world in the deep, dark waters of the open ocean (Figure 10.1).

In this chapter, we introduce and discuss the neglected cephalopods of the deep sea, many of which are not so distantly related to the species with which we are familiar, but whose existence in the deep sea has little in common with the complex reefs and near-shore habitats associated with taxa such as *Octopus* and *Sepia*. What effect might these differences in ecology have on the cognitive abilities of deep-sea cephalopods compared with their shallow water relatives? Chapter 9 of this volume (by Zylinski & Osorio) explored what we can deduce about cuttlefish visual cognition from the body patterns they use for camouflage. In this chapter we revisit the theme of making inferences about visual perceptive and cognitive abilities via body patterning in the handful of epipelagic and mesopelagic species that have been studied to date. Prior to that, we consider how the cognitive needs of these animals might differ from those of near-shore or shallow benthic environments. We explore what is known about the potential for visual cognition in deep-sea cephalopods and discuss why we know so little. Readers might find this chapter heavier on natural history and observation than the others in this book, but we hope that it will serve as a reminder that most cephalopods are essentially unknown beyond their descriptions.

Cephalopod Cognition, eds A.-S. Darmaillacq, L. Dickel and J. Mather. Published by Cambridge University Press. © Cambridge 2014.

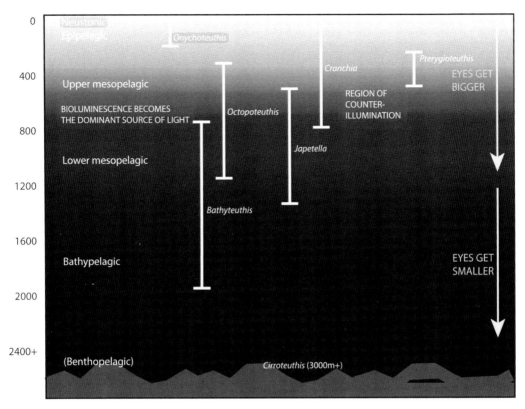

Figure 10.1 Approximate depths in metres of habitat zones for clear oceanic waters. Benthopelagic realm is close to the ocean floor at any depth of the pelagic realm. Vertical lines show approximate depth ranges for some of the species referred to in this chapter, taken from daytime trawl data for adults (Arkhipin, 1996; Arkhipkin & Nigmatullin, 1997; Roper & Young, 1975).

10.2   Why do we know so little about the other 95%?

Although notoriously 'moody' (Talbot & Marshall, 2010) the coastal cephalopod taxa with which we are familiar (e.g. *Sepia* and *Octopus*) can be hatched and/or kept in the laboratory with some level of expertise and patience (e.g. Domingues, Dimarco, Andrade & Lee, 2005; Forsythe, Lee & Walsh, 2002). This has led to the volume of well-controlled visual behavioural research we have for these animals (e.g. Barbosa, Allen, Mäthger & Hanlon, 2012; Chiao, Chubb, Buresch, Siemann & Hanlon, 2009; Mäthger, Chiao, Barbosa & Hanlon, 2008; Shashar, Rutledge & Cronin, 1996; Shohet, Baddeley, Anderson, Kelman & Osorio, 2006; Zylinski, Osorio & Shohet, 2009), supplemented by field observations and experiments where data can be obtained with relative ease with scuba (e.g. Hall & Hanlon, 2002; Zylinski, How, Osorio, Hanlon & Marshall, 2011) or even by snorkelling (e.g. Hanlon, Forsythe & Joneschild, 1999). Behavioural observations, let alone controlled behavioural experiments, are few and far between for mesopelagic animals. Collecting animals from mesopelagic depths requires either the use of specialized trawl nets or undersea vehicles (e.g. a remotely operated vehicle (ROV) or manned submersible). ROVs and submersibles enable *in situ* observations of animals, which have greatly improved our knowledge of interactions, behaviour and physiology of deep-sea animals, as well as enabling the gentle capture of specimens (Hunt & Seibel, 2000; Robison, 2004; Vecchione & Roper, 1991). However, experimental behavioural biology requires a rigorous framework beyond these natural history observations, and there are some concerns about the influence of motor vibrations and viewing lights on *in situ* behavioural observations (for example, animals living in perpetual near-darkness are probably literally and permanently blinded by these lights). The collection of animals using trawl nets has been aided by the use of thermally-insulated and light-tight closing cod ends (Childress, Barnes, Quetin & Robison, 1978), which enables the recovery of specimens in collection-depth temperatures and light conditions, and prevents excessive mechanical damage. However, in both cases, there is no guarantee that the animals required for a planned experiment will be caught. Weeks at sea can be spent in frustration as each trawl returns to the surface without the target taxa for a specific study. Luck and patience are both critical for the deep-sea biologist!

Trends in data from vertebrates and hymenopteran insects suggest that certain lifestyles and the need to deal with specific tasks predispose the evolution of complex behaviour. Ecological complexity is generally associated with cognition, be it the need to forage for cache-specific foods (e.g. Clayton, Dally & Emery, 2007; Hills, 2006), navigate using cues and landmarks (e.g. Collett & Collett, 2002) or interact with conspecifics (e.g. Bergman, Beehner, Cheney & Seyfarth, 2003; Grosenick, Clement & Fernald, 2007). The ecology of shallow-water, benthic species of cephalopods such as members of *Sepia* and *Octopus* is such that we see clear evidence for complexity in their life histories: octopuses move through complex rocky reef or coral habitats to forage for food (Forsythe & Hanlon, 1997; Hanlon, Forsythe & Joneschild, 1999) and navigate to and from their lairs (Mather, 1991); cuttlefish signal to conspecifics when hunting and during courtship (Hall & Hanlon, 2002; Langridge, Broom & Osorio, 2007; Zylinski, How, Osorio, Hanlon & Marshall, 2011). Species from both genera are well known for the complex body patterns they employ for both signalling and camouflage (Hanlon & Messenger, 1988; Packard & Sanders, 1971).

The mesopelagic habitat offers a different set of ecological requirements: animals can pass their entire lives without coming in contact with any abiotic structure, with hundreds (if not thousands) of metres of water above and below them. Underwater light decreases exponentially with depth, and by 150 m in clear, oceanic water more than 99% of surface light has been scattered or absorbed (Jerlov, 1976) (this said, it should be noted that this can result in surprisingly bright conditions in which the human eye can still function perfectly well). Many species live at greater depths where the amount of downwelling light is so small that it is no longer useful for vision, and here biological light (bioluminescence) is used in many capacities such as signalling, hunting and camouflage (e.g. silhouette reduction via counterillumination) (Haddock, Moline & Case, 2010). Temperatures here tend to be cold (typically between 0 and 6°C) and constant due to the lack of mixing with surface waters (Robison, 2004). The

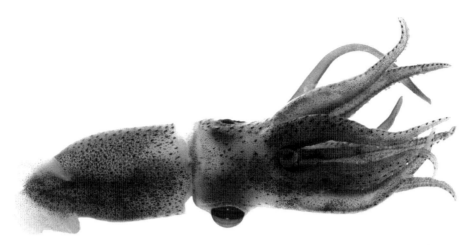

Figure 10.2 The lower-mesopelagic squid *Histeoteuthis* has asymmetrical eyes and optic lobes, with a large left eye for looking up for passing silhouettes of potential prey against the weak downwelling light, and a small right eye orientated downwards, probably specialized for detecting point-source bioluminescence. See plate section for colour version.

mesopelagic habitat is virtually globally continuous, with the same species found in similar conditions around the world, with absolute depths changing with corresponding differences in temperature, oxygen minimum zone depths and light levels.

In the vast three-dimensional habitat that is the deep-sea pelagic realm, the diversity and quantity of animals decrease in parallel with depth. It is renowned for being a hard place to find a mate, and many non-broadcast spawning deep-sea taxa have evolved unusual reproductive methods, such as male parasitism of females in deep-sea angler-fish (Marshall, 1958). Cephalopods also appear to use some quirky tactics to maximize the chances of reproduction when solitary individuals meet. For example, males of the mesopelagic squid *Octopoteuthis* apparently mate (implant sperm packages) indiscriminately when they encounter both males and females of the same species, presumably because sex differences are hard to determine in low-light conditions and the cost of failing to mate given the opportunity is high (Hoving, Bush & Robison, 2012).

There is also a trend for relative eye size of many taxa to increase as light gets dimmer from the surface waters to the lower-mesopelagic realm, where the downwelling surface light can still be useful if the eye is sensitive enough (Figure 10.1). In the bathypelagic zone (below ~1000 m) the trend reverses, and eye size tends to decrease as ambient light becomes not detectable. In general, eyes in the mesopelagic realm are either designed to maximize the possible light capture and make use of the small amounts of light available at the cost of reducing spatial acuity, or they are optimized to detect point sources (to enable them to see flashes of bioluminescence) at the cost of reduced sensitivity to the ambient light (Warrant & Locket, 2004). Aside from such general trends, evolution has found varied and novel ways to obtain visual information in dim light, and the cephalopods offer some of the most interesting of these. Take, for example, the deep mesopelagic squid *Histioteuthis* (Figure 10.2), which has highly asymmetrical eyes and correspondingly asymmetrical optic lobes (Maddock & Young, 1987; Wentworth & Muntz, 1989). This animal has a large left eye, probably specialized for gaining information from the dim downwelling light as the animal swims on its side with this large eye facing upwards. Meanwhile, the smaller, downward-facing right eye is probably specialized for detecting point-source bioluminescence in the darker waters below.

10.3   Do mesopelagic cephalopods need to be visually cognitive? Is there evidence to suggest that they are?

Much emphasis has been placed on the large brains and well-developed sense organs in cephalopods as adaptations for their 'high performance' lifestyles (Budelmann, 1994, 1995). They are typically viewed as fast animals moving in complex environments, actively predating and evading predation, and often loosely social. However, as with many deep-sea taxa, the metabolic rate of deep-sea cephalopods is greatly reduced compared to their shallow water counterparts, likely a response to relaxed pressure from visual predation (Childress, 1995; Seibel & Carlini, 2001; Seibel, Thuesen, Childress & Gorodezky, 1997). Large brains are metabolically costly to maintain, and there is evidence in mammals that brain size will be reduced where lifestyle allows for it (Safi, Seid & Dechmann, 2005).

Godfrey-Smith (2002) described aspects of environmental complexity as an attempt to give a general functional explanation of cognition. He used the term cognition to describe 'a collection of capabilities which, in combination, allow organisms to achieve certain kinds of coordination between their actions and the world' that 'has the function of making possible patterns of behaviour which enable organisms to effectively deal with complex patterns and conditions in their environments'. In their consideration of body pattern richness and habitat complexity (see below), Hanlon and Messenger (1996) describe the pelagic realm as a uniform habitat, and it seems reasonable to accept that the open ocean contains less structural complexity than a near-shore reef habitat. However, if we use habitat to include the wider physical and biological characteristics of a species' interactions, then we must consider what habitat complexity means on an individual species basis. Given the characteristics of the mesopelagic realm, is there sufficient selective pressure for the evolution or maintenance of higher-level visual processes?

Complex behaviours and corresponding large brains tend to evolve in response to the selective pressure of complex ecologies, including trophic and social interactions (Lefebvre & Sol, 2008). Brain areas that receive direct input from sensory systems or are responsible for complex cognitive function are under strong selective pressure, with neural development often reflecting these behavioural adaptations and sensory special-izations. For example, in primates both an increasing reliance on frugivory (indicating complex foraging behaviour) and social group size (indicating social complexity) are independently positively correlated with the size of the neocortex brain region. Research from multiple vertebrate groups, for example primates (Barton & Harvey, 2000), cichlid fish (Pollen et al., 2007) and bats (Safi & Dechmann, 2005), suggest that the cognitive centres in the brain are under specific pressure according to mosaic theory, whereby localized changes in functionally distinct regions are mediated by selection on a specific set of behaviours according to a given species' ecology (Barton & Harvey, 2000). In a comparative analysis controlling for phylogeny, bat species foraging in complex habitats, which must distinguish prey from background noise whilst avoiding obstacles, were shown to have larger brain regions associated with hearing and memory than species that hunting in open spaces (Safi & Dechmann, 2005).

Neuroecology is the study of the adaptive variation in cognition and the brain, often by employing behavioural and anatomical techniques to examine the neural correlates of cognition (Sherry, 2006). There are few studies directly investigating the correlation between pelagic versus benthic ecologies and brain structure independent of phylogeny. Yopak (2012) reviewed the neuroecology of cartilaginous fishes and found, irrespective of phylogenetic history, larger brains with well-developed telencephala and highly foliated cerebella occurred in reef-associated species, suggesting brain structures may have developed in conjunction with enhanced cognitive capabilities. In contrast, deep-sea species had relatively smaller brains, which the author suggested might be indicative of specialization of non-visual senses.

Maddock and Young (1987) measured 30 optic and chromatophore lobes of the brains of 63 species of cephalopod from all types of habitats, providing the most comprehensive data on the neuroecology of cephalopods currently available. However, this study did not control for phylogeny, meaning phylogenetic effects may confound the observed differences and similarities between taxa. We can nonetheless identify some general trends in the correlation between habitat and brain regions associated with vision and body patterning (Figure 10.3). These data suggest that the mosaic theory proposed for mammalian brains (Barton & Harvey, 2000), may be relevant for cephalopods; specific brain regions apparently associated with particular ecologies have a greater volume than would be accounted for by allometric scaling. In Figure 10.3, we show these data for 42 of these species for which complete records for mantle length, absolute brain volume, optic-lobe volume and chromatophore-lobe volume were given.

10.4   Body pattern repertoire in the open ocean and deep sea

For shallow-water cephalopods there is a clear link between vision and body patterning via the expression of chromatic components; there is no doubt that the visual system of species such as *Sepia officinalis* plays a vital role in making decisions about what body pattern to use in order to achieve effective camouflage in a given environment (see chapter 9, this volume, by Zylinski & Osorio). Hanlon and Messenger (1996) put forward a hypothesis of 'ecological correlates of body patterning' (ECBP) that suggested a strong correlation between habitat complexity and patterning richness (number of chromatic components). They proposed that diurnal cephalopod species occurring in complex habitats such as coral reefs or kelp environments have a richer array of body patterns at their disposal than near-reef or 'murky habitat' species, with a positive correlation between the two. With this correlation they extrapolated and predicted that species

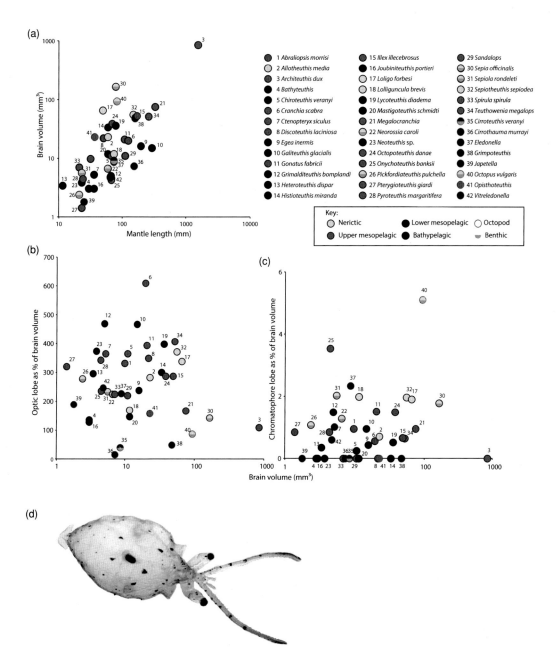

Figure 10.3 Brain size and brain regions in a range of cephalopods from different habitats (data taken from Maddock & Young, 1987). The 34 species of decapods plotted on each graph are listed on the right in alphabetical order. A further eight species of octopods are then listed in alphabetical order and are distinguished by a red marker ring. Numbers relate to the placement on the plot. The colour of marker represents a common habitat type (or usual collection depth range) for adults during daylight hours (the depth occurrence of many species changes with size and life-stage, and many of the species listed undergo vertical migration so will be found in shallower waters at night), as given in the key. (a) Absolute brain volume plotted against mantle

in the less-complex 'open ocean' habitat would have the lowest number of chromatic components, but conceded: 'we can only make educated guesses about species living on the deeper continental shelf, the deep fore-reef, on bland substrates like mud or in oceanic and deep-water habitats'.

Accepting that Hanlon and Messenger's (1996) ECBP was presented as a first attempt to develop the correlation between habitat and body pattern richness, it should be noted that it overweighs the significance of this correlation, because it assumes phylogenetic independence between the data points. In other words, the correlation between patterning richness and habitat complexity may be an artifact of the fact that most of the species for which data exists are closely related. For example, of the 12 coral reef, rocky reef or kelp environment species included, four are from the genus *Octopus*, while all of the 'social squids near reefs' are loliginids. It might, therefore, be that the common ancestor of *Octopus* had a richer range of body patterns compared with the common shared ancestor of *Loligo* and, therefore, the apparent trend between body pattern number and habitat could be largely explained by relatedness rather than by habitat complexity. A more thorough investigation using independent contrasts would correct for this (Felsenstein, 1985; Purvis & Rambaut, 1995; Seibel & Carlini, 2001). However, before this can prove useful we need to greatly increase and improve our knowledge and expand our data set with quality behavioural and physiological data, particularly for mesopelagic and bathypelagic taxa. Furthermore, while headway is being made in resolving phylogenetic relationships within the cephalopods, these are (not surprisingly) biased towards neritic taxa at the species level.

An important consideration for future work assessing the correlation between habitat and body pattern richness is defining sensible and applicable metrics for habitat complexity and chromatic components/body pattern richness. As Packard and Sanders (1971) pointed out: 'if we ask "How many patterns are there in an octopus?" the best, though hardly satisfactory, answer is, "There are as many patterns as can be recognized by the classifier"'. The large research effort on the body patterning of *Sepia* compared to any other group is unsurprising given the extraordinary camouflage capabilities of these animals (Hanlon, 2007; Zylinski & Osorio, 2011), but it has the potential to overweigh

---

Figure 10.3 (*cont.*) length, showing a positive correlation between brain volume and body length, although there is a tendency for shallow-water benthic taxa (namely *Loligo*, *Sepia* and *Octopus*) to fall above the trend, and bathypelagic/bathybenthic species to fall below the trend, be they octopod or decapod (note log scales). (b) Plotting optic lobe volume (given as a percentage of brain volume, measured separately because of location and large size (d)) against absolute brain volume shows that optic lobe volume varies greatly and is not correlated with overall brain volume. Interestingly, many pelagic and mesopelagic species have comparatively larger optic lobes than neritic/benthic species that are considered highly visual. (c) Plotting the chromatophore lobe volume against brain volume shows chromatophore lobe volume varies greatly between species. There is a trend for shallow-water species to have relatively larger chromatophore lobes, with notable exceptions (e.g. the deep-water pelagic octopod *Eledonella*). Many deep-sea species had no chromatophore lobes or lobes too small to be measured. (d) An oegopsid squid paralarva showing eye stalks with the large optic lobe located behind the eye on the stalk and separate from the brain. See plate section for colour version.

the number of chromatic components used by *Sepia*. Additionally, much work on *Sepia* has been carried out under controlled laboratory conditions (this said, we still have an incomplete description of their body patterning; see chapter 9, this volume, by Zylinski & Osorio). Conversely, observations in mesopelagic taxa (see below) are typically made from video footage under ROV lights, resulting in problems discriminating true physiological changes under artificial lighting, rapid changes in body position and unnatural behaviours. Issues such as these make sensible comparisons of body pattern richness between species difficult. At a more basic level, the ECBP as it stands considers only the structural aspects of the tangible environment; as discussed above, a more typical definition of a species' habitat includes all aspects of physical and biological conditions. While habitat *structural* complexity might drive a diverse range of body patterns for camouflage, social interactions might drive a wider range of body patterns for communication.

10.5   Evidence for complex visual behaviours and body patterning in mesopelagic cephalopods

10.5.1   *Octopoteuthis deletron*

Bush, Robison and Caldwell (2009) used ROV footage from Monterey Bay Aquarium Research Institute's (MBARI's) video archive (which records the occurrence of taxa filmed during the Institute's ROV deployments) to analyze the behaviour of the large pelagic squid, *Octopoteuthis deletron*. They analyzed observations of 76 (presumed) individuals recorded at depths between 344 and 1841 m and produced an ethogram of behavioural components that were displayed by more than one individual. These included 17 light and dark chromatophore-based components (see chapter 9, this volume, by Zylinski & Osorio and Hanlon & Messenger, 1996), some of which are surprisingly complex given the low-light environment, such as fine arm bands and ventral mantle bands. In addition to these chromatic components, the authors described a further 42 postural and bioluminescent components, giving a total of 59 components. This number is comparable to those for several neritic and reef squid for which ethograms exist, for example 59 in the broadfin squid *Sepioteuthis affinis* (Mauris, 1989), 39 in *Loligo opalescens* (Hunt, Zeidberg, Hamner & Robison, 2000) and 56 in *Loligo pealeii* (Hanlon, Maxwell, Shashar, Loew & Boyle, 1999). Bush, Robison and Caldwell (2009) suggest these behavioural components might serve to impede search image formation, disrupt hydrodynamic signatures and camouflage via Disruptive colouration and illumination, as well as being used in conspecific communication and offensive behaviour.

10.5.2   *Dosidicus gigas*

Following the study of *Octopoteuthis* by Bush, Robison and Caldwell (2009; see above), L. Trueblood, B. H. Robison and B. A. Seibel (unpublished data) used footage from the MBARI's ROV video library to produce an ethogram of behaviour and body patterning of the Humboldt squid *Dosidicus gigas* at depths greater than 150 m. They described

29 putative chromatic components as well as 15 postural components and 6 locomotory components. The authors suggest that of the 29 chromatic components described, 15 contained body countershading elements, making camouflage an important role in body pattern usage. Individual squid were observed to use chromatic component changes more when aggregated than when solitary, suggesting that body patterning is used for intraspecific communication in this species.

10.5.3   *Taningia danae*

Kubodera, Koyama and Mori (2007) used a mid-water high definition baited camera rig to record footage of the large eight-armed squid *Taningia danae* 'hunting' for suspended bait between 240 m (night) and 940 m (day). They did not report any body pattern colouration changes, but did observe arm-tip bioluminescence emissions associated with bait attacks. The authors suggest these might function to both blind prey and provide illumination to accurately determine target distance.

10.5.4   *Japetella heathi*

The pelagic octopus *Japetella* is caught in deep day trawls, with smaller individuals occurring in shallow waters (600–800 m) and mature adults in deeper waters (800 m+) (Roper & Young, 1975). This sluggish creature looks like a gelatinous ball with small arms – very different from the fast-moving, protean octopuses we are familiar with. However, we recently found that not all aspects of this small octopus are as slow as they first appear. These animals are rather transparent when left undisturbed (with reflective guts and eyes that are often associated with transparency), but are capable of expanding a layer of red–orange chromatophores over the mantle (Zylinski & Johnsen, 2011; Figure 10.4). We found that, while shadows and passing objects did not elicit the expansion of chromatophores in *Japetella*, a sudden onset of blue light caused these red-orange chromatophores to be expanded. This is consistent with the hypothesis that these and other cephalopods (e.g. *Onychoteuthis banksii*) can maintain camouflage under both ambient light conditions and bioluminescent searchlights. Interestingly, we found that they tracked passing objects, an observation made possible by their prominent, swivelling eyes. Sweeney, Haddock and Johnsen (2007) suggesting that *Japetella* may have poor visual acuity compared with other measured pelagic cephalopods. However, at four cycles per degree, this is comparable to the acuity of a rainbow trout, which seems rather good for an animal assumed to have very little visual stimulation within its habitat, and which appears to have limited abilities to evade or respond to visual threat compared with the rapid responses typical of many cephalopods.

10.6   Bioluminescence: using and detecting

In their discussion of ecological correlates of body patterning Hanlon and Messenger (1988) stated: 'We might . . . predict that cephalopods with light organs inhabiting the

(a)

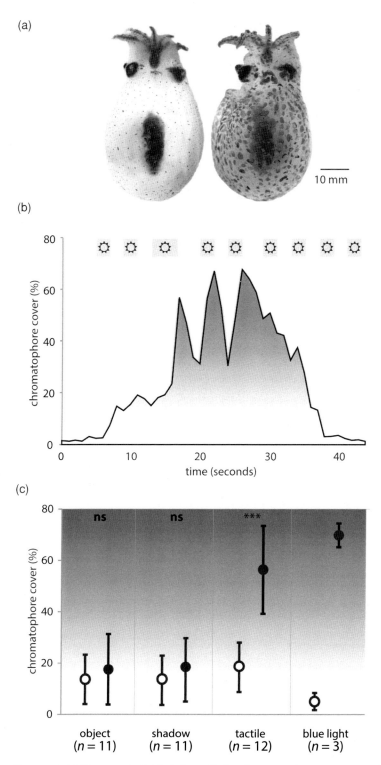

10 mm

(b)

(c)

Figure 10.4 (a) The same individual *Japetella heathi* octopus in transparent mode (left) and pigmented mode (right). (b) Responses of a single *J. heathi* to directed blue light. Yellow boxes

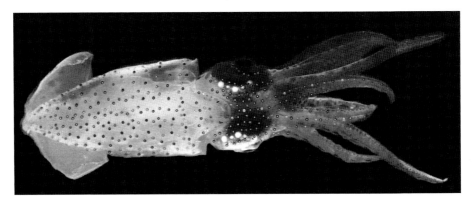

Figure 10.5 Ventral and ocular photophores on the ventral surface of an *Abraliopsis* squid. See plate section for colour version.

oceanic mid-waters could signal with bioluminescent body patterns'. As the intensity of the ambient downwelling light decreases, the occurrence and importance of biolumi- nescence increases. At depths greater than around 800 m (the exact depth being defined by local conditions) bioluminescence becomes the dominant source of light (Young, 1983), present in every major taxonomic group represented. Haddock, Moline and Case (2010) discuss the functions, diversity and physiology of bioluminescence in an excel- lent review, and we direct the interested reader to this. Here, we draw attention to the fact that almost half of cephalopod genera (66 of 139) possess bioluminescent organs (Hastings & Morin, 1991), and a vast majority of the taxa possessing such organs are mesopelagic (Figure 10.5). A well-known exception to this is the near-shore sepiolid squid *Euprymna scolopes*, which produces bioluminescence via the luminescent bacte- rial symbiont *Vibrio fischeri* (Ruby, 1996). The apparent functions of bioluminescence in cephalopods are varied, including sexual signalling, biological searchlights, counter- illumination and hunting behaviour (Clarke, 1963; Haddock, Moline and Case, 2010; Johnsen, Widder & Mobley, 2004; Johnsen, 2005; Young, 1978, 1983). Biolumines- cence seems to have evolved multiple times in cephalopods, with some species utilizing

---

Figure 10.4 (*cont.*) and icon indicate onset and cessation of individual lighting 'bouts', consisting of a flashing blue light at one flash per second. Most bouts lasted for 3 seconds and, therefore, subjected the animal to three flashes. Chromatophores can be seen to expand seconds after initial exposure. After continued exposure the animal ceased reacting to the light with chromatophore responses, and instead displayed evasive behaviour such as swimming away from the light-source and retraction of the head into the mantle. (c) Responses of *J. heathi* to four different stimuli. Objects passed in front of the animals, and shadows passed overhead, failed to evoke a significant increase in chromatophore expression. A tactile stimulus (touching the arms with a blunt needle) resulted in the rapid expansion of chromatophores. By comparison, directed blue light resulted in a rapid and strong expression of chromatophores. White circles = pre-stimulus, black circles = post-stimulus. Error bars show standard deviation from mean. From Zylinski & Johnsen 2011. See plate section for colour version.

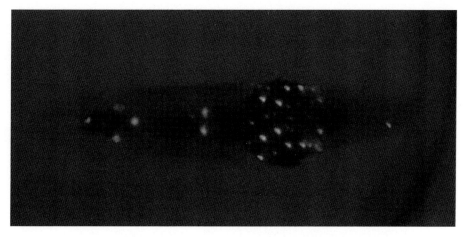

Figure 10.6 Counterilluminating photophores in the squid *Pterygioteuthis*. Here, during shipboard experiments, the very low downwelling blue light was been turned off and the animal photographed from below under dim red light.

symbiotic luminescent bacteria (e.g. *Euprymna*), while most deep-sea taxa have intrinsic bioluminescence.

Counterillumination is an important function of bioluminescence in pelagic cephalopods (Johnsen, Widder & Mobley, 2004; McFall-Ngai, 1990; Widder, 2010). Many predators visually hunting in the mesopelagic have upward-pointing eyes positioned to take advantage of the conspicuousness of the silhouettes against the downwelling ambient light. Many animals get around this by being transparent, which provides the advantage of being effective from all viewing angles. Yet this is not a complete solution to camouflage in the pelagic (see section 10.5.4. on *Japetella heathi* above). Another solution is to use counterilluminating photophores that obliterate a silhouette by emitting light at the wavelength and intensity of the downwelling light from ventral photophores (Figure 10.6). Many cephalopods have extra-ocular photosensitive vesicles, which are presumed to play a role in determining the output of ventral photophores. Young (1978) conducted shipboard experiments where they used opaque 'shutters' to block information about the intensity of downwelling light to a species of *Abraliopsis* squid over the dorsal photosensitive vesicles, the eyes, or both. They demonstrated that the intensity of the ventral photophores was independently affected by covering both eyes and photosensitive vesicles, but that the latter had a greater effect. It would be interesting indeed to know how information regarding downwelling light and the intensity of the photophore output is processed.

The deep sea is often considered to be a lightless environment, but biological light provides a method for communication that has the potential to be information rich as well as spatially and temporally complex. Matching the spectral and intensity characteristics of the ambient downwelling light for counterillumination is non-trivial. These are two potential ways in which bioluminescence could support complex visual processing in the pelagic realm.

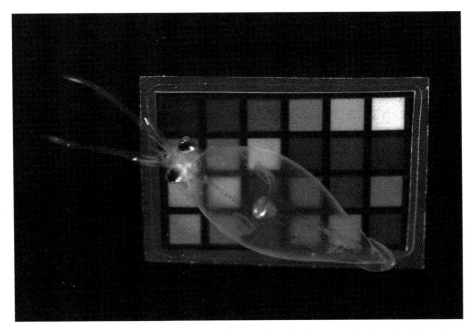

Figure 10.7 Transparency is a common form of camouflage in the mesopelagic realm. Here the transparency of a chranchiid squid is demonstrated as it rests over a colour standard. See plate section for colour version.

10.7   Concluding remarks

Gaping holes exist in our knowledge of the basic behaviour of most cephalopods, many of which inhabit the vast, three-dimensional wilderness that is the deep sea. Gaining insight to potential complex behaviours in mesopelagic taxa is difficult for numerous reasons.

The need for a wide body pattern repertoire for camouflage via chromatic components is reduced in the mesopelagic realm. Body patterning is probably less useful at depth for two main reasons: (1) light is more monochromatic; and (2) the visual resolution of most animals is far worse due to spatial summation. Although camouflage is still important, it is more commonly achieved in deep-sea cephalopods by passive means, such as reflectors, transparency (Figure 10.7) or overall red/black colouration. Counterillumination via bioluminescence to obliterate silhouettes must match the ambient downwelling light in order to be effective, and the means by which this is achieved is not well understood. However, it seems unlikely it will require cognitive processes in the traditional sense. Cognition is needed when adaptive responses depend on changing conditions. When an environment is highly constant – such as the deep sea – there is no selective pressure for cognitive responses, as fixed responses are sufficient. In addition the environment is colder, darker and food-limited, meaning that visual cognition and the brainpower needed to mediate it are unlikely to evolve.

At present, attempts to correlate body pattern richness with habitat (or environmental) complexity seem fraught with difficulties of assessing either in a comparable or repeatable way. Pelagic habitats from well-lit surface waters to deep, cold waters, although indeed equally low in habitat (structural) complexity, perhaps offer more variable and complex environmental conditions than is often appreciated. A metric of complexity that accounts for interactions with conspecifics and predators, the level of usable ambient light, the degree of bioluminescence available for visual tasks and factors regarding metabolic constraints should be developed to enable comparisons between pelagic species. Similarly, phylogenetic relatedness may be a confounding factor in apparent correlations between body pattern richness and habitat complexity, and between body patterning and visual cognition.

Chapter 9 of this volume (by Zylinski & Osorio) introduced concepts about what makes vision cognitive, and emphasized that internal representation is likely an important determinant here. The lack of a body pattern output that directly relates to aspects of the visual environment in mesopelagic taxa invalidates the use of this assay for evidence of internal representation. Many aspects of the ecology and physiology of a majority of mesopelagic cephalopod taxa lead us to doubt the need or presence of cognitive vision. However, ROV footage of some species suggests complex behaviours and a surprisingly large body pattern repertoire. Furthermore, brain measurements show a large investment in optic lobes (coupled with large eyes) and learning centres (e.g. the vertical lobe system) in some taxa, which tantalize us with the potential for complex visual processing. Finally, the complex species-specific photophore patterns found in many mesopelagic squids provide another avenue for visual communication that is so far poorly understood.

Chapter 9 of this volume (by Zylinski & Osorio) highlights similarities between visual processing in the neritic cuttlefish *S. officinalis* and vertebrates (including humans). The visual environment in the well-lit shallow-water benthic environment is not dissimilar to our own visual world in many respects, and the body patterns used by *S. officinalis* for camouflage are designed primarily to defeat shallow-water vertebrate (including mammalian) predators. It is, therefore, perhaps unsurprising that evolution has provided similar solutions to shared problems. In contrast, it is harder to imagine the visual tasks facing cephalopods and their predators in a low-light world where biological light might be the most important source of illumination. We hope time and research effort will shed light on this. As new technologies allow us better access than ever to the world's largest and least understood habitat we will surely be treated to many more fascinating cephalopod stories. Whether visual cognition is ultimately an interesting avenue of research to pursue for the majority of these taxa, any behavioural data obtained can only be an asset given the current level of knowledge.

Acknowledgements

We would like to acknowledge support from Office of Naval Research MURI grant no. N00014–09–1–1053.

References

Arkhipkin, A. (1996). Age and growth of planktonic squids *Cranchia scabra* and *Liocranchia reinhardti* (Cephalopoda, Cranchiidae) in epipelagic waters of the central-east Atlantic. *Journal of Plankton Research*, **18**: 1675–1683.

Arkhipkin, A. I. and Nigmatullin, C. M. (1997). Ecology of the oceanic squid *Onychoteuthis banksi* and the relationship between the genera Onychoteuthis and Chaunoteuthis (Cephalopoda: Onychoteuthidae). *Journal of the Marine Biological Association of the United Kingdom*, **77**: 839–869.

Barbosa, A., Allen, J. J., Mäthger, L. M. and Hanlon, R. T. (2012). Cuttlefish use visual cues to determine arm postures for camouflage. *Proceedings of the Royal Society. B: Biological Sciences*, **279**: 84–90.

Barton, R. A. and Harvey, P. H. (2000). Mosaic evolution of brain structure in mammals. *Nature*, **405**: 1055–1058.

Bergman, T. J., Beehner, J. C., Cheney, D. L. and Seyfarth, R. M. (2003). Hierarchical classification by rank and kinship in baboons. *Science*, **302**: 1234–1236.

Budelmann, B. U. (1994). Cephalopod sense organs, nerves and the brain: adaptations for high performance and life style. *Marine and Freshwater Behaviour and Physiology*, **25**: 13–33.

Budelmann, B. U. (1995). The cephalopod nervous system: what evolution has made of the molluscan design. In *The Nervous Systems of Invertebrates: An Evolutionary and Comparative Approach* O. Breidbach and W. Kutsch (Eds.). Basel, Switzerland: Birkhäuser Verlag.

Bush, S. L., Robison, B. H. and Caldwell, R. L. (2009). Behaving in the dark: locomotor, chromatic, postural, and bioluminescent behaviors of the deep-sea squid *Octopoteuthis deletron* Young 1972. *The Biological Bulletin*, **216**: 7–22.

Chiao, C.-C., Chubb, C., Buresch, K., Siemann, L. and Hanlon, R. T. (2009). The scaling effects of substrate texture on camouflage patterning in cuttlefish. *Vision Research*, **49**: 1647–1656.

Childress, J. J. (1995). Are there physiological and biochemical adaptations of metabolism in deep-sea animals? *Trends in Ecology and Evolution*, **10**: 30–36.

Childress, J. J., Barnes, A. T., Quetin, L. B. and Robison, B. H. (1978). Thermally protecting cod ends for the recovery of living deep-sea animals. *Deep Sea Research*, **25**: 419–422.

Clarke, W. (1963). Function of bioluminescence in mesopelagic organisms. *Nature*, **198**: 1244–1246.

Clayton, N. S., Dally, J. M. and Emery, N. J. (2007). Social cognition by food-caching corvids. The Western Scrub-Jay as a natural psychologist. *Philosophical Transactions of the Royal Society of London. Series B*, **362**: 507–522.

Collett, T. S. and Collett, M. (2002). Memory use in insect visual navigation. *Nature Reviews Neuroscience*, **3**: 542–552.

Domingues, P. M., Dimarco, F. P., Andrade, J. P. and Lee, P. G. (2005). Effect of artificial diets on growth, survival and condition of adult cuttlefish, *Sepia officinalis* Linnaeus, 1758. *Aquaculture International*, **13**: 423–440.

Felsenstein, J. (1985). Phylogenies and the comparative method. *The American Naturalist*, **125**: 1–15.

Forsythe, J. W. and Hanlon, R. T. (1997). Foraging and associated behavior by *Octopus cyanea* Gray, 1849 on a coral atoll, French Polynesia. *Journal of Experimental Marine Biology and Ecology*, **209**: 15–31.

Forsythe, J. W., Lee, P. and Walsh, L. (2002). The effects of crowding on growth of the European cuttlefish, *Sepia officinalis* Linnaeus, 1758 reared at two temperatures. *Journal of Experimental Marine Biology and Ecology*, **269**: 173–185.

Godfrey-Smith, P. (2002). Environmental complexity and the evolution of cognition. In *The Evolution of Intelligence* R. J. Sternberg and J. C. Kaufman (Eds.). New York, NY: Psychology Press.

Grosenick, L., Clement, T. S. and Fernald, R. D. (2007). Fish can infer social rank by observation alone. *Nature*, **445**: 429–432.

Haddock, S. H. D., Moline, M. A. and Case, J. F. (2010). Bioluminescence in the sea. *Annual Review of Marine Science*, **2**: 443–493.

Hall, K. C. and Hanlon, R. T. (2002). Principal features of the mating system of a large spawning aggregation of the giant Australian cuttlefish *Sepia apama* (Mollusca: Cephalopoda). *Marine Biology*, **140**: 533–545.

Hanlon, R. T. (2007). Cephalopod dynamic camouflage. *Current Biology*, **17**: R400–R404.

Hanlon, R. T., Forsythe, J. W. and Joneschild, D. E. (1999). Crypsis, conspicuousness, mimicry and polyphenism as antipredator defences of foraging octopuses on Indo-Pacific coral reefs, with a method of quantifying crypsis from video tapes. *Biological Journal of the Linnean Society*, **66**: 1–22.

Hanlon, R. T., Maxwell, M. R., Shashar, N., Loew, E. R. and Boyle, K. L. (1999). An ethogram of body patterning behavior in the biomedically and commercially valuable squid *Loligo pealei* off Cape Cod, Massachusetts. *The Biological Bulletin*, **197**: 49–62.

Hanlon, R. T. and Messenger, J. B. (1988). Adaptive coloration in young cuttlefish (*Sepia officinalis* L) – the morphology and development of body patterns and their relation to behavior. *Philosophical Transactions of the Royal Society of London. Series B*, **320**: 437–487.

Hanlon, R. T. and Messenger, J. B. (1996). *Cephalopod Behaviour*. New York, NY: Cambridge University Press.

Hastings, J. W. and Morin, J. G. (1991). Bioluminescence. In *Neural and Integrative Animal Physiology*, 4th edn, C. L. Prosser (Ed.). New York, NY: Wiley-Liss.

Hills, T. T. (2006). Animal foraging and the evolution of goal-directed cognition. *Cognitive Science*, **30**: 3–41.

Hoving, H. J. T., Bush, S. L. and Robison, B. H. (2012). A shot in the dark: same-sex sexual behaviour in a deep-sea squid. *Biology Letters*, **8**: 287–290.

Hunt, J. C. and Seibel, B. A. (2000). Life history of *Gonatus onyx* (Cephalopoda: Teuthoidea): ontogenetic changes in habitat, behavior and physiology. *Marine Biology*, **136**: 543–552.

Hunt, J. C., Zeidberg, L. D., Hamner, W. M. and Robison, B. H. (2000). The behaviour of *Loligo opalescens* (Mollusca: Cephalopoda) as observed by a remotely operated vehicle (ROV). *Journal of the Marine Biological Association of the United Kingdom*, **80**: 873–883.

Jerlov, N. G. (1976). *Marine Optics*. Amsterdam, the Netherlands: Elsevier.

Johnsen, S. (2005). The red and the black: bioluminescence and the color of animals in the deep sea. *Integrative and Comparative Biology*, **45**: 234–246.

Johnsen, S., Widder, E. A. and Mobley, C. D. (2004). Propagation and perception of bioluminescence: factors affecting counterillumination as a cryptic strategy. *The Biological Bulletin*, **207**: 1–16.

Kubodera, T., Koyama, Y. and Mori, K. (2007). Observations of wild hunting behaviour and bioluminescence of a large deep-sea, eight-armed squid, *Taningia danae*. *Proceedings of the Royal Society. B: Biological Sciences*, **274**: 1029–1034.

Langridge, K. V., Broom, M. and Osorio, D. (2007). Selective signalling by cuttlefish to predators. *Current Biology*, **17**: R1044–R1045.

Lefebvre, L. and Sol, D. (2008). Brains, lifestyles and cognition: are there general trends? *Brain, Behavior and Evolution*, **72**: 135–144.

Maddock, L. and Young, J. Z. (1987). Quantitative differences among the brains of cephalopods. *Journal of Zoology*, **212**: 739–767.

Marshall, N. B. (1958). *Aspects of Deep Sea Biology*, 2nd edn. London, UK: Huchinson.

Mather, J. A. (1991). Navigation by spatial memory and use of visual landmarks in octopuses. *Journal of Comparative Physiology A*, **168**: 491–497.

Mäthger, L. M., Chiao, C.-C., Barbosa, A. and Hanlon, R. T. (2008). Color matching on natural substrates in cuttlefish, *Sepia officinalis*. *Journal of Comparative Physiology, A*, **194**: 577–585.

Mauris, E. (1989). Colour patterns and body postures related to prey capture in *Sepiola affinis* (Mollusca: Cephalopoda). *Marine Behaviour and Physiology*, **14**: 189–200.

McFall-Ngai, M. J. (1990). Crypsis in the pelagic environment. *American Zoologist*, **30**: 175–188.

Packard, A. and Sanders, G. D. (1971). Body patterns of *Octopus vulgaris* and maturation of the response to disturbance. *Animal Behaviour*, **19**: 780–790.

Pollen, A. A., Dobberfuhl, A. P., Scace, J., Igulu, M. M., Renn, S. C. P., Shumway, C. A. and Hofmann, H. A. (2007). Environmental complexity and social organization sculpt the brain in Lake Tanganyikan cichlid fish. *Brain, Behavior and Evolution*, **70**: 21–39.

Purvis, A. and Rambaut, A. (1995). Comparative analysis by independent contrasts (CAIC): an Apple Macintosh application for analysing comparative data. *Computer Applications in the Biosciences*, **11**: 247–251.

Robison, B. H. (2004). Deep pelagic biology. *Journal of Experimental Marine Biology and Ecology*, **300**: 253–272.

Roper, C. F. E. and Young, R. E. (1975). *Vertical Distribution of Pelagic Cephalopods*. Washington, DC, USA: Smithsonian Institution Press.

Ruby, E. G. (1996). Lessons from a cooperative, bacterial-animal association: the *Vibrio fischeri-Euprymna scolopes* light organ symbiosis. *Annual Review of Microbiology*, **50**: 591–624.

Safi, K. and Dechmann, D. K. N. (2005). Adaptation of brain regions to habitat complexity: a comparative analysis in bats (Chiroptera). *Proceedings of the Royal Society. B: Biological Sciences*, **272**: 179–186.

Safi, K., Seid, M. A. and Dechmann, D. K. N. (2005). Bigger is not always better: when brains get smaller. *Biology Letters*, **1**: 283–286.

Seibel, B. A. and Carlini, D. B. (2001). Metabolism of pelagic cephalopods as a function of habitat depth: a reanalysis using phylogenetically independent contrasts. *The Biological Bulletin*, **201**: 1–5.

Seibel, B. A., Thuesen, E. V., Childress, J. J. and Gorodezky, L. A. (1997). Decline in pelagic cephalopod metabolism with habitat depth reflects differences in locomotory efficiency. *The Biological Bulletin*, **192**: 262–278.

Shashar, N., Rutledge, P. S. and Cronin, T. W. (1996). Polarization vision in cuttlefish – a concealed communication channel? *Journal of Experimental Biology*, **199**: 2077–2084.

Sherry, D. F. (2006). Neuroecology. *Annual Review of Psychology*, **57**: 167–197.

Shohet, A. J., Baddeley, R. J., Anderson, J. C., Kelman, E. J. and Osorio, D. (2006). Cuttlefish responses to visual orientation, water flow and a model of motion camouflage. *Journal of Experimental Biology*, **209**: 4717–4723.

Sweeney, A. M., Haddock, S. H. D. and Johnsen, S. (2007). Comparative visual acuity of coleoid cephalopods. *Integrative and Comparative Biology*, **47**: 808–814.

Talbot, C. M. and Marshall, N. J. (2010). Polarization sensitivity in two species of cuttlefish, *Sepia plangon* (Gray 1849) and *Sepia mestus* (Gray 1849), demonstrated with polarized optomotor stimuli. *Journal of Experimental Biology*, **213**: 3364–3370.

Vecchione, M. and Roper, C. F. E. (1991). Cephalopods observed from submersibles in the western north Atlantic. *Bulletin of Marine Science*, **49**: 433–445.

Warrant, E. J. and Locket, N. A. (2004). Vision in the deep sea. *Biological Reviews*, **79**: 671–712.

Wentworth, S. L. and Muntz, W. R. A. (1989). Asymmetries in the sense organs and central nervous system of the squid *Histioteuthis*. *Journal of the Zoological Society, London*, **219**: 607–619.

Widder, E. A. (2010). Bioluminescence in the ocean: origins of biological, chemical, and ecological diversity. *Science*, **328**: 704–708.

Yopak, K. E. (2012). Neuroecology of cartilaginous fishes: the functional implications of brain scaling. *Journal of Fish Biology*, **80**: 1968–2023.

Young, R. (1978). Vertical distribution and photosensitive vesicles of pelagic cephalopods from Hawaiian waters. *Fishery Bulletin*, **76**: 583–616.

Young, R. (1983). Oceanic bioluminescence: an overview of general functions. *Bulletin of Marine Science*, **33**: 829–845.

Zylinski, S., How, M. J., Osorio, D., Hanlon, R. T. and Marshall, N. J. (2011). To be seen or to hide: visual characteristics of body patterns for camouflage and communication in the Australian giant cuttlefish *Sepia apama*. *The American Naturalist*, **177**: 681–690.

Zylinski, S. and Johnsen, S. (2011). Mesopelagic cephalopods switch between transparency and pigmentation to optimize camouflage in the deep. *Current Biology*, **21**: 1937–1941.

Zylinski, S. and Osorio, D. (2011). What can camouflage tell us about non-human visual perception? A case study of multiple cue use in the cuttlefish *Sepia officinalis*. In *Animal Camouflage: Mechanisms and Function* M. Stevens and S. Merilaita (Eds.). Cambridge, UK: Cambridge University Press.

Zylinski, S., Osorio, D. and Shohet, A. J. (2009). Perception of edges and visual texture in the camouflage of the common cuttlefish, *Sepia officinalis*. *Philosophical Transactions of the Royal Society of London. Series B*, **364**: 439–448.

Index of species

Index

Printed in the United States
By Bookmasters